Palliative Nursing

Palliative Nursing
Across the Spectrum of Care

Edited by

Elaine Stevens
Susan Jackson
Stuart Milligan

WILEY-BLACKWELL

A John Wiley & Sons, Ltd., Publication

This edition first published 2009
© 2009 by Blackwell Publishing Ltd

Blackwell Publishing was acquired by John Wiley & Sons in February 2007. Blackwell's publishing programme has been merged with Wiley's global Scientific, Technical, and Medical business to form Wiley-Blackwell.

Registered office
John Wiley & Sons Ltd, The Atrium, Southern Gate, Chichester, West Sussex, PO19 8SQ, United Kingdom

Editorial offices
9600 Garsington Road, Oxford, OX4 2DQ, United Kingdom
2121 State Avenue, Ames, Iowa 50014-8300, USA

For details of our global editorial offices, for customer services and for information about how to apply for permission to reuse the copyright material in this book please see our website at www.wiley.com/wiley-blackwell.

The right of the author to be identified as the author of this work has been asserted in accordance with the Copyright, Designs and Patents Act 1988.

Wiley also publishes its books in a variety of electronic formats. Some content that appears in print may not be available in electronic books.

Designations used by companies to distinguish their products are often claimed as trademarks. All brand names and product names used in this book are trade names, service marks, trademarks or registered trademarks of their respective owners. The publisher is not associated with any product or vendor mentioned in this book. This publication is designed to provide accurate and authoritative information in regard to the subject matter covered. It is sold on the understanding that the publisher is not engaged in rendering professional services. If professional advice or other expert assistance is required, the services of a competent professional should be sought.

Library of Congress Cataloging-in-Publication Data

Palliative nursing : across the spectrum of care / edited by Elaine Stevens, Susan Jackson, Stuart Milligan.
     p. ; cm.
   Includes bibliographical references and index.
   ISBN 978-1-4051-6997-4 (pbk. : alk. paper)   1. Palliative treatment.   2. Terminal care.
3. Nursing.   I. Stevens, Elaine M., 1960-   II. Jackson, Susan.   III. Milligan, Stuart.
   [DNLM: 1. Nursing Care–methods.   2. Palliative Care–methods.   3. Nursing Care–trends.
   WY 152 P1674 2009]
   RT87.T45P41   2009
   616'.029–dc22   2008039844

A catalogue record for this book is available from the British Library.

Set in 10/12.5pt Palatino by Aptara® Inc., New Delhi, India
Printed and bound in Malaysia by KHL Printing Co Sdn Bhd

1   2009

Contents

Contributors

John Atkinson is a community nurse by background. Originally from London he has lived and worked in Scotland since 1984, achieving all of his higher education during that time. His work has mainly been with marginalised people: the homeless, people with HIV, prisoners and those with drugs problems. Before coming into academic life he was Health Care Manager at HM Prison Barlinnie. Since 1999. he has worked at the University of Paisley (now the University of the West of Scotland) as a Senior Lecturer and now Professor and Associate Dean for Research and Commercialisation. He has published widely including a collaborative venture with other academics *Interdisciplinary Research: Diverse Approaches in Science, Technology, Health and Society* published by Wiley in 2006.

Jane Belmore has worked in paediatric oncology for the past 20 years in the Royal Hospital for Sick Children, Glasgow. She was appointed as the first paediatric Macmillan nurse in Scotland in 1995 and now works as a paediatric oncology outreach nurse specialist. Jane was the recipient of a Florence Nightingale scholarship in 1998 and visited North America and Canada looking at their paediatric oncology services. Jane is a member of RCN paediatric oncology outreach nurses' group, a member of the steering committee for the MCN for children and young people's services in Scotland and a member of the recently formed Scottish children and young people's palliative care network.

Helen de Renzie-Brett qualified as a registered nurse in 1985 and spent much of her early nursing career working with older people both within the hospital and community environments. Since 1993, she has been involved in education and staff development, with experience of planning and delivering programmes within a range of settings including the NHS, Higher Education and the independent sector. Helen is currently the Head of Education at Dorothy House Hospice Care. Her particular areas of interest include older people and end of life care, practice development and staff development. Helen is a member of the RCN and education, research and older people forums.

Carole Ferguson trained as a general nurse in the mid 1970s and then as a midwife. She specialised in genetics then health visiting. Working in genetics again in the early 1990s Carole learned about Motor Neurone Disease (MND), in 1994 changed career path to work with MND patients their families and carers. Carole has now worked with MND patients and their families for 14 years, closely associated with the Scottish Motor Neurone Disease that has funded the post since its inception in 1983. During this period Carole has gained a wealth of knowledge not only of MND but also of the importance of good palliative care. Carole is a member of the Royal College of Nursing.

Elizabeth-Anne Gold, (Libby) is from Children's Hospice Association Scotland (CHAS); she is Director of Care at Robin House Children's Hospice. She has been working at CHAS since Rachel House opened in 1996. Robin House is Scotland's second children's hospice and opened in 2005. Libby qualified as a children's nurse in 1986 and a general nurse in 1987. She worked in adult medical nursing for a number of years and during this time gained a Post Graduate Diploma in Palliative Nursing Care. In 2005 she completed a Masters Degree in Nursing. Libby is a member of the Royal College of Nursing.

Dorothy Hardyway qualified as a registered nurse in the Belfast City Hospital in 1979 and her career has involved experience in hospital, community and also working in the voluntary sector, in posts throughout the UK and New Zealand. She was appointed to her present post of Parkinson's Disease Nurse Specialist with the remit of palliative care in 2007. This is a new role and she has been employed by Northern Ireland Hospice to identify the palliative care needs of people with Parkinson's disease, and to establish a service which will recognise and support the palliative care needs of these people and their carers throughout the disease trajectory.

Felicity Hasson is Senior Lecturer in the Institute of Nursing Research at the University of Ulster. She has undertaken a number of research projects exploring the palliative care needs of people with non-malignant conditions and exploring the role and preparation of unqualified assistants (commonly referred to as health care assistants) in clinical and community settings. She is currently involved in doctoral research into the role and impact of the health care assistant upon nursing students' clinical learning experience. She is also member of a number of ethical committees and is a reviewer for a number of journals including *Journal of Advanced Nursing, Quality and Safety in Health Care* and *Nurse Education Today*.

Denise Heals is a registered nurse with an interest and considerable experience in specialist palliative care and more latterly education. She is an Education Facilitator at Dorothy House Hospice Care, a role which includes working with a variety of agencies including Primary Care Trusts, Acute Hospital Trusts, Social Care Organisations and the independent sector to deliver palliative care education. Denise's professional interests include the development of practice in the area of palliative care in care homes, people with learning disabilities and those with dementia. Denise is a member of the RCN and education, ethics and palliative care forums

Susan Jackson works in a combined role of lecturer in cancer and palliative care within the School of Health, Nursing and Midwifery of the University of West of Scotland and education facilitator with ACCORD Hospice in Paisley. Within the School, she is programme leader for the Post Graduate Certificate in Cancer and Palliative Care and also takes a leading role in the delivery of the undergraduate cancer education provision. Within the hospice she is the Chair of the Clinical Governance Education and Training Group and has the responsibility for provision of in-house education and training. She has many years' experience as a Macmillan Oncology Nurse Specialist and has maintained her interest in the area of haematology–oncology and lung cancer.

Vikki Knowles has been Respiratory Nurse Specialist for 18 years, and is currently working for Surrey PCT and Asthma, UK. Within Surrey PCT she is developing a community multidisciplinary respiratory care team to support patients across primary and secondary care. The team cares for patients with chronic respiratory disease aiming to avoid unplanned emergency admissions and supporting early discharge from the acute sector. The team provides chronic disease management within nurse-led clinics, pulmonary rehabilitation, palliative care and home/telephone support. As Clinical Lead for Asthma UK Vikki is responsible for providing clinical leadership for the organisation and supporting Asthma Nurse Specialists running the advice line service. Vikki's main interests include management of COPD with particular emphasis on palliative care. She was a member of the group looking at management of end-stage respiratory disease as part of the work on the NSF for COPD. Vikki is also a Committee Member, Association of Respiratory Nurse Specialists

Margaret Kendall has been Macmillan Consultant Nurse in Palliative Care for North Cheshire since in 2001, although her clinical career in palliative care began in 1989 as a Macmillan CNS in the Merseyside area. Since 2003, Margaret has been Independent Nurse Prescriber and holds outpatient clinics twice weekly. She has contributed to consultations on the nursing perspective of Palliative Care for the Renal NSF and to the workings of National Prescribing Centre on the safe disposal of Controlled Drugs in the Community following the Shipman Inquiry. Margaret has a place on several National Committees including the RCN Palliative Nursing Forum and NICE. Margaret has given evidence to the Committee of Safety of Medicines regarding the further expansion of the formulary for Independent Nurse Prescribers. She also sits on the Editorial board for the *End of Life Care* journal.

George Kernohan is active in health research with interests in palliative care, health technology assessment, evaluation of innovation in health, health informatics and computing. He chairs the research group at Northern Ireland Hospice Care. He works on user involvement with the Northern Health and Social Services Council. He teaches evidence-based practice and advanced health research at the postgraduate level. He holds a combined science degree and a doctorate in orthopaedic research. He has previously worked with the (NHS) Research and Development Office for Northern Ireland. He is currently Professor of Health Research with University of Ulster.

Carol Komaromy is Head of Department and Director of the Health and Social Care programme at the Open University. Prior to joining the Open University, she worked for many years in the NHS as a nurse and midwife. Carol has published in the area of the sociology of death and dying and, more recently, extended her research into birth and death, focussing on the way that parents and professionals cope with stillbirth and neonatal death at the time of and shortly after death. Carol is the course chair of the Open University's popular course, 'Death and Dying'.

May McCreaddie is Research Associate in Nursing Studies at the University of Edinburgh and a part-time doctoral student at the University of Strathclyde. She is the Acute and Supportive Care RCN Scottish Board member and an ex-executive member of NHIVNA. May has worked in a variety of settings including clinical (medical, surgical, infectious diseases), research (e.g. needlestick injuries, sexuality needs in HIV, and HCV palliative care needs) and education (e.g. Education and Training Manager for the Greater Glasgow Bloodborne Viruses programme). She has undertaken development work in Romania and established an HIV nursing course in Chennai, India, for which she won the RCN/Nursing Standard Robert Tiffany International Award.

Stuart Milligan originally followed a career in biological research and achieved his PhD degree in 1986. However, the bulk of his working life has been spent as a nurse, firstly, in general surgery but since 1993 in hospice and palliative care. He is currently jointly employed by the University of the West of Scotland (as Lecturer in Palliative Care) and Ardgowan Hospice, Greenock (as Education Facilitator). Stuart's main professional interest is in the therapeutic relationships which exist between health care professionals and those they care for. He conducted his Masters research on 'The Attitudes of Hospice Nurses to Spirituality' and has also written articles on ritual and symbolism at the end of life and spiritual care giving.

Helen Noble has experience with renal patients dating back to 1990. In 1995 she completed her degree in nursing and a diploma in management. Following an appointment as Modern Matron of Renal Inpatient Services she took on the role of Senior Clinical Nurse Specialist, Renal Supportive Care, and has been responsible for establishing The Renal Supportive Care Service at Barts and The London NHS Trust, London, for those renal patients who have opted not to have dialysis. She is presently undertaking her PhD, researching the experiences of these patients and the resulting impact on, and needs of their carers alongside their trajectory to death. Helen was previously the English Co-Editor and later the Editor of the *European Dialysis and Transplant Nurses Association* journal until 2006. She is a member of the Editorial Board of a new journal launched last year titled *End of Life Care* specifically aimed at non-specialist nurses caring for dying patients in hospital, community and nursing home settings.

Shirley Potts is Senior Lecturer at Liverpool Hope University where she heads Disability Studies and also contributes to Early Childhood Studies. Following an early career in social care, Shirley trained as a counsellor, and prior to lecturing at Liverpool Hope, was Family Support Coordinator in a children's hospice, creating and sustaining a bereavement support service for all generations of a family, as well as working with dying children. Whilst there, she undertook her Masters degree incorporating research with bereaved parents. She maintains an interest in palliative care and bereavement through her trusteeship of Hospice23.

Sarah Russell has worked in cancer and palliative care for over 15 years. Her interest in the area began in her pre-nursing history and sociology degree and developed through her training. Sarah is Director of Education at the Hospice of St Francis, Berkhamsted, and a part-time doctoral research student at the University of Hertfordshire. She also leads the end-stage respiratory care module at Education for Health's MSc in Respiratory Care and teaches at the University of Hertfordshire and University of Bedfordshire Degrees and Masters in Palliative Care. Sarah's research interests include palliative care education, respiratory palliative care and communication at the end of life.

Philip Saltmarsh qualified as Registered Nurse at Warrington Hospital in 1993. He has since worked in a variety of settings from ICU to community before settling into a varied career in palliative care, beginning at the Marie Curie Hospice Liverpool, then as Community Macmillan Nurse and Hospital Macmillan Nurse in Palliative Care. As a member of the Marie Curie Palliative Care Institute, Liverpool, Philip has been involved in the dissemination of the Liverpool Care Pathway for the Dying Patient. In 2003 Philip completed his MA in The Ethics of Cancer and Palliative Care. His special areas of interest are ethics, spiritual care and integration of specialist palliative care services.

Stephen DM Smith trained as a general and mental health nurse and for the last 15 years has worked in palliative care. This has involved clinical, research and managerial experience within the voluntary hospice sector as well as working in the NHS as Clinical Nurse Specialist. Stephen has been Chair of NHS Lothian's Palliative Care Managed Clinical Network and worked with Quality Improvement Scotland in the development of national palliative care standards. Stephen led and coordinated the West Lothian Dementia Palliative Care Project, a three-year action research project and is currently Lead Nurse for Napier University and NHS Lothian's Leadership in Compassionate Care Project.

Elaine Stevens holds a joint appointment between The Ayrshire Hospice and The University of The West of Scotland. She manages the education service at the Hospice and is the programme leader for the palliative care named award at degree level within the University. Before this Elaine held a number of nursing posts in hospices, including managing palliative day services. She remains lead for education and research for The Association of Palliative Day Care Leaders. Elaine is also the current Chair of The Palliative Nursing Forum of The Royal College of Nursing. This forum has over 8000 members and the steering group acts as a voice for palliative nurses within the UK. The steering group is regularly involved in commenting on palliative care guidance at international, national and local levels to ensure nurses influence new policies, protocols and standards.

Anne Thomson started her nursing career in Glasgow in the early 1980s. She then moved on to paediatrics, before training to be District Nurse. It was whilst working in the community that Anne first became interested in palliative care. She was fortunate to join the team at the Ayrshire Hospice in 1993 as a Community Specialist Palliative Care Nurse. She worked in this team for 12 years. Anne's role within the Scottish Huntington's Association to promote a palliative care approach to the management of families affected by this illness proved to be the most challenging and thought provoking of my career. Anne is a member of the RCN.

Richard Warner works as Nurse Consultant for Gloucestershire Hospitals NHS Foundation Trust. His field of practice is multiple sclerosis and he has a research interest in fatigue. Following completion of pre-registration training in Birmingham he worked within general medicine and stroke rehabilitation within a hospital environment before entering MS care.

Wendy Wesson is Assistant Head of Subject in the Nursing and Health Care Practice Department of the University of Derby. She has worked in community nursing since 1987 as a community staff nurse, district nurse, practice teacher and practice educator. She currently leads the BSc/MSc Community Specialist Practice programme at the University of Derby, alongside her clinical role in palliative care as a hospice at home nurse for a local hospice. Wendy is a member of the Association of District Nurse Educators, and is currently carrying out research into the assessment of higher levels of practice as part of a Doctorate in Education programme.

Foreword

'In ordinary moments of care – extraordinary things do happen'

I often use this phrase when I am talking to students about the value of compassion in care. I never need to explain to them what it means. When we say it was 'a privilege' to have been with a particular patient at a particular moment, then we are affirming this truth. I certainly do not need to expand on it to patients. They have experienced the moment and it has nourished their spirits. It is hugely enriching to think that we have entered the lives of our patients in such a manner and although we may not remember them all, they will never forget. Although this is the case for all encounters with patients, I think that in palliative care in particular, our patients show us such examples of love, compassion, courage and humanity that it cannot fail to lift our spirits and validate for us that humanity is indeed made for great things. The ordinary man or woman can be an extraordinary teacher.

I have been a nurse, academic and fellow cancer traveller for most of my life. Although I would not have wished for such 'in vivo' learning, there is no doubt that my personal experience of cancer has given me valuable insights to share with younger practitioners. I hope they enjoyed this narrative and not felt it too self-satisfying. Being a cancer sufferer and a teacher has also given me a chance to articulate the needs of patients and I have always felt it my duty to advocate on their behalf.

Elaine, Susan, Stuart and I have worked together for 8 years to provide the palliative component of courses delivered by the University of the West of Scotland at its Paisley campus and elsewhere. It seems fitting, therefore, to use the analogy of the 'Paisley pattern' to reflect on the developments which brought about that collaboration and culminated in the production of this book.

The Paisley Pattern

The town of Paisley was renowned for its weavers and the mills that produced the thread for their cloth. When I first approached our local hospices to invite them to consider joint appointments with the university to increase our capacity and ability to deliver high quality palliative care education, they immediately warmed to the idea, and with very little prompting the plan was approved and the process completed. Thus, the Palliative Care Development Group was established as a powerful partnership between three hospices (ACCORD Hospice, Paisley, Ardgowan Hospice, Greenock and Ayrshire Hospice, Ayr) and the School of Health, Nursing and Midwifery at Paisley. What developed was, and still is, a model of good practice, joining together the various elements of palliative education into a weave that is more effective than the various threads that make it up. I know that other hospices and universities admire the mutual trust and respect that cements this relationship.

The Paisley Pallium

It is interesting to reflect that the word 'Pallium' not only refers to a cloak to give protection from the elements – hence the term 'palliative' care – it was also the name given to a garment that academics wore in the middle ages. This connection confirmed for me the absolute validity of what we were doing within the Palliative Care Development Group, protecting our patients with compassionate care, but also underpinning this practice with clinical expertise and a sound research base. To be able to call upon expert clinicians, from Consultants to Chaplains, and to deliver university courses in the Hospice Education Centres, only served to reinforce the link between education and practice. There was to be no dissonance in our group between the classroom and the clinical area – our expert colleagues made sure of that.

The Paisley Philosophy

As we planned our group, it became clear that we would need a 'mission statement' – a philosophy that would unite us and sustain us and become a focus for renewal when difficulties arose. We found in the work of Abraham Maslow a philosophy that seemed to echo our own. His 'Hierarchy of Needs' is a testament to his own belief in the value of the human person. He was the son of Russian Jewish immigrants to the US. When the full horror of the Holocaust was revealed after the Second World War, we might have expected him to have developed a hatred for his fellow man – but he actually did the opposite. He stated that what happened under the Nazis was an aberration and that man was meant for good: he was striving for 'self-actualisation' – to be all he could be. As people move through their life journey, they have a variety of needs, from basic needs like shelter and food to higher order needs like knowledge. But they also have 'aesthetic needs' – the need to find meaning and value in their lives. Surely the purpose of palliative care is not just to relieve suffering, but also to be a witness to the underlying value of the human spirit in sickness and health. Our patient's thirst for this recognition – our objective must be to help satisfy that need so that even in extremes, they can still strive to be more than they ever thought possible.

The Paisley Partnership

Elaine, Susan and Stuart, together with many other clinical colleagues, have been fundamental to the success of the Palliative Care Development Group, and this book enables their efforts to benefit nurses and other readers much further afield. However, it is the patients who are our greatest teachers. By their experiences we learn so much about what we need to know – their honesty, fortitude and good humour are central to sustaining us all in the partnership. They are so grateful for what we do for them. I would like to thank them for all they give to us.

Finally, I was much moved when I first read the poem 'Not waving, but Drowning' by the late English poetess Stevie Smith. Reading her words – 'I was much further out than I thought and not waving but drowning' – I got transported back to my student nurse days at Stobhill Hospital in the north of Glasgow in the mid 1970s. In those days, patients were nursed in the long Nightingale wards and I always remember going off shift and turning back to wave a cheery 'bye-bye' to the patients. I can see them now in my mind's eye – all of them waving back at me. How many were waving? How many were drowning? I am ashamed to say that then I could not have told you. I hope that palliative care education in general, and this book in particular, will encourage a new generation of professionals to see who is waving and who is drowning, and to provide the lifeline of appropriate and effective care which is so desperately needed.

Simon Carr
Academic Director
Department of Health, Nursing and Midwifery
Professional and Community Education
University of the West of Scotland

Introduction

'You matter because you are you. You matter to the last moment of your life and we will do all we can, not only to help you die peacefully, but also to live until you die.'

Dame Cicely Saunders

This is the essence of palliative nursing: seeing people as human beings and recognising that each individual will live and die differently depending on many different factors. Palliative nursing is both an art and a science, which when practised together allow the nurse to provide truly holistic, empathetic palliative care.

With this in mind this book has been developed for nurses working in areas of practice where general palliative care is provided. This may be in hospitals, nursing homes, dementia units, the community and any other clinical areas which are not classified as specialist palliative care.

The book is divided into three parts. The first part is concerned with adult palliative care, while the second part focusses on palliative care for children and young people. Finally, the third part investigates palliative care education and research.

Chapter 1 provides an overview of the history of the hospice movement as well as the development of contemporary palliative care services. The second chapter then discusses current palliative care terminology used within the health care arena before examining the aims of palliative care, as defined by the World Health Organization. The final chapter of Part I reviews issues of providing palliative care to marginalised and disenfranchised groups. It challenges our preconceptions of who these people are and where they can be found as well as showing how palliative care can be provided to these groups.

The second section of Part I focusses on the challenges of providing palliative care across the different care settings where most people die, namely hospital, home and care home. Each chapter identifies the barriers to providing palliative care within the setting as well as the benefits that good palliative nursing care can offer patients who are dying in these settings. The final chapter in this section discusses nursing care for dying people and their families within the hospice setting. This has been included to show the reader what hospices can provide as there is evidence that many health care workers do not have a clear idea of what hospices do and as a result do not refer their dying patients to such services.

With the recognition that the palliative care approach can be applied not just to cancer patients but also to anyone diagnosed with a life-limiting illness, Section 3 of Part I considers a number of specific illnesses. In each of these chapters evidence is presented to show how palliative nursing care can improve the care of the dying person to allow them to live as actively as possible within their illness and also to enable a peaceful death. These chapters will allow the reader to look in more depth at the palliative phase of these illnesses and at how they can provide effective palliative care to those diagnosed with a range of conditions.

Part II of the book then focusses on palliative care for children and young people. The first chapter reviews the history and ethos of palliative care in these groups. The second chapter addresses the challenge of providing paediatric palliative care in the hospital setting. The third chapter then focusses on the role of children's hospices and how palliative care can be provided to dying children in the community.

The final part of the book considers issues relating to palliative care education and research. The first chapter, on palliative nursing education, looks at the education needs of nurses working in different roles within palliative care and describes how the nurse can utilise the knowledge and skills framework to ensure he or she has the correct level of skill and knowledge to ensure optimal palliative care provision in their current post. The chapter also looks at how to improve knowledge and skills with a view to working towards further career opportunities in palliative care. Some more senior nursing posts are described to highlight the career opportunities that exist in clinical palliative care. The second chapter in this part focusses on palliative care research. It begins by reviewing the current need for research in this field before examining the barriers and challenges faced by those conducting research around the end of life.

Within each chapter the reader will find a number of practice points. These are intended to encourage the reader to reflect on the information provided and link this to their own clinical situation. By undertaking these practice points, the nurse can incorporate the new information gained into their practice. In this way it is intended that practitioners will develop the confidence and ability to provide the palliative care approach to their patients and families whenever it is required.

PART ONE

ADULT PALLIATIVE CARE

Section One

History and Ethos of Palliative Care

Chapter 1

The history of palliative care

Stuart Milligan and Shirley Potts

Introduction

The history of palliative care is a fascinating story of how ideas and practices around the care of people with life-threatening illnesses have evolved against a background of social trends, changing public opinion and policy developments. Central to that story is the history of modern hospice care, from a promise of a window to a worldwide movement. This chapter will focus primarily on the UK, but will also locate that story within an international context.

Learning outcomes

Once you have read this chapter and completed the associated practice points you will be able to:

- Discuss the origins of palliative care
- Describe the influence of the modern hospice movement in the development of palliative care
- Identify ways in which palliative care is responding to contemporary challenges

The origins of palliative care

Whilst only recognised as an area of medical specialty in 1987, palliative care has a much longer history than that date would imply. The evolution into the services seen today can be traced to a few inspirational figures whose determination and dynamism spurred radical change in the care of the dying. Chief among these was Dame Cicely Saunders who is largely credited with inspiring the modern hospice movement. However, the origins of palliative care can be traced back considerably further.

The word palliative derives from the Latin *pallium*, meaning cloak or covering – reflected in the Middle Eastern blessing, 'may you be wrapped in tenderness, you my brother, as in a cloak'. The original meaning of the word 'hospice' was not derived, as many assume, from 'hospital', but was a term familiar to those on pilgrimages, meaning 'a resting place for weary travellers'.

The first use of the term hospice as a home for dying people is attributed to Madame Jeanne Garnier who, in 1842, created L'Association des Dames du Calvaire in Lyon, France (Clark et al. 2005). From her own experience as a widow and bereaved mother, she identified a need and strived to meet it.

In the nineteenth century, societal and medical developments were resulting in a gradual transition in both causes and places of death. Where death had once occurred, almost inevitably, at home, it became more commonplace in hospital or other institutions. Causes of death were changing too, as infection control, public hygiene services and medical innovations dramatically reduced the rate of fatal infections that had previously been the common precursor to a rapid death. Skills of prognosis advanced and awareness developed, in some quarters, of a need for explicit 'care of the dying'. Unsurprisingly, this resource did not initiate from within mainstream medical care – whose pronouncement was to remain for some years 'there is no more we can do for you'. Rather, it was religious orders that founded the first of these 'homes for the dying'. Our Lady's Hospice in Harold's Cross, Dublin, was opened by the Irish Sisters of Charity in 1879, and the same order sent five of its number to the East End of London in 1900 to care for the terminally ill there. As a consequence, St Joseph's Hospice, Hackney, London, was opened in 1905 – an establishment that would come to inspire the work of Cicely Saunders.

In the 1950s an upsurge of concern began to materialise, as an understanding of the medical profession's abandonment of dying people was acknowledged. This was not necessarily a wilful neglect but an understandable response from doctors who were consumed with such enthusiasm for evolving curative approaches that those patients seen as incurable would be either discharged or overlooked. The emerging profession of social work, coupled with social science research, identified the value of specific care for those with terminal illnesses. A greater understanding of the mind/body relationship, together with hitherto neglected philosophies such as patient autonomy and dignity, heralded a new perspective on the needs of dying people. One significant catalyst was a survey conducted by the Marie Curie Memorial Foundation in the mid 1950s (Doyle et al. 2005). Having interviewed thousands of cancer patients living at home, the survey report recommended more residential and convalescent homes, as well as improved equipment and clearer information for cancer patients. The Marie Curie Memorial Foundation responded by opening its own homes for terminally ill cancer patients. Within a short time, further research by Bailey (1959), Glynn Hughes (1960) and Hinton (1964), amongst others, confirmed that the issue of improved care for dying people was in the public arena, offering a challenge to the NHS as well as charitable and religious organisations. Much of the research had been conducted from a specific perspective, be that medical, social or epidemiological. One of the features of the remarkable influence of Cicely Saunders was her ability to unite these perspectives through rigorous research, linked with studious observations and innovative clinical practice.

The modern hospice movement

The explosion of hospices across the UK over the past 40 years is largely attributable to the work and influence of Cicely Saunders. She originally trained as a nurse in the 1940s but back problems prevented her continuing, so she retrained as a medical social worker (then called almoners) and returned to work at St Thomas's Hospital, London. It was here that she encountered David Tasma, a terminally ill, 40-year-old Polish. The relationship, which began as professional, rapidly became close friendship as Cicely Saunders accompanied this lonesome man on his journey towards death. This journey sowed the seeds of Saunders' lifelong determination to improve and develop suitable services for dying people. In conversation with David Tasma, when offering to read to him, he responded to her, 'I only want what is in your mind and in your heart'. Cicely Saunders discussed with David Tasma what might have helped him on his journey and she tellingly comments:

> 'Not necessarily so much better on symptoms, because he didn't have a terribly difficult dying, but somewhere that could have helped him with what I was trying to do, which was to assure him that he was a worthwhile person, dying at the end of what he thought of as a rather empty life.'
>
> (Clark et al. 2005, p. 16)

This poignant comment offers a prelude to a statement now endorsed by many hospices which was first published in the *Nursing Times* in 1976 –

> 'You matter because you are you and we will do all we can, not only to help you die peacefully, but to live until you die.'
>
> (Thompson 2002, p. 27)

Through further conversations with patients, and meticulous record keeping, Saunders also developed the concept of 'total pain' (triggered by a female patient who told her, 'all of me is wrong'). This encapsulates the understanding that physical, spiritual and psychological pain can be interwoven, therefore suggesting the futility and counter-productivity of only responding to one area of need in a patient's life (Lloyd-Williams 2003).

Cicely Saunders appreciated the spiritual, emotional and psychological needs of the dying, as well as their physical care, and vowed to open the country's first purpose-built hospice. Beginning with £500 left to her by David Tasma ('I'll be a window in your hospice'), Saunders fund-raised doggedly, trained as a medical doctor in order to develop expertise in pain control, and opened St Christopher's Hospice, London, in 1967, where there is, indeed, a window dedicated to David Tasma (Potts 2005). Saunders herself was to comment years later, 'It took me 19 years to build a home around the window, but the core principles of our approach were borne out of my conversations with him as he was dying' (Booth 2002). Today, St Christopher's is recognised as the model for the modern hospice movement and has a flourishing Education Centre that extends the evidence-based practice and research-informed theory emanating from twenty-first century palliative care.

Other early developments

Although the towering influence of Cicely Saunders in the modern develop-ment of palliative care cannot be denied, hers was one of the many important contributions. For instance, in 1911, Douglas Macmillan witnessed the pain and suffering experienced by his father and other people dying of cancer and es-tablished the Society for the Prevention and Relief of Cancer (later to become Macmillan Cancer Support). His vision, to bring expert symptom relief and sup-port to those in most need, was realised with the creation of the first Macmillan Nurse post in 1975 (Macmillan Cancer Support 2006). Thirty years later, the charity has funded over 3000 Macmillan Nurse posts and 500 other health care professionals (Macmillan Cancer Support 2007).

Saunders also worked alongside and influenced a generation of clinicians in the field of pain and symptom relief. Robert Twycross, for instance, carried out important early studies on the most appropriate use of strong opioids (Saunders 2000). Colin Murray Parkes explored the psychosocial needs of family carers and their experiences of loss and grief. And Saunders' concerns for the psycho-spiritual needs of dying people were shared by Michael Kearney, later Medical Director at Our Lady's Hospice, Dublin. His conclusions were published in *Mortally Wounded: Stories of Soul Pain, Death and Healing* (Kearney 1996).

Much attention invariably focuses on Britain and Ireland when discussing the origins of palliative care. However, similar developments, albeit heavily influ-enced by events in the UK, took place in the US around the same time. Between 1967 and 1969, Elizabeth Kubler-Ross, a Swiss-born psychiatrist, interviewed dying patients at the University of Chicago's Billings Hospital (Newman 2004). Her findings, written up in the unlikely bestseller *On Death and Dying*, shocked many who regarded death as taboo, but also raised awareness of the com-plex communication needs associated with the end of life (Kubler-Ross 1970). Kubler-Ross, together with Florence Wald, former Dean of Yale School of Nurs-ing, was influential in establishing the US hospice movement in the early 1970s (Hoffmann 2005).

Many other countries around the world have embraced the hospice ethos. Often, the catalyst for the process has been the vision and determination of a few individuals. For instance, the early growth of hospice care in Russia was in no small part due to the efforts of Victor Zorza, an English journalist, and Andrei Gneszdilov, a St Petersburg psychiatrist (Wright 2007). The support of palliative care experts from countries such as the UK where palliative care is well established is also beneficial, and will no doubt be aided by the recently formed Worldwide Palliative Care Alliance (Prail and Pahl 2007).

Practice Point 1.1

Hospices usually form only part of the palliative care provision available in any one lo-cality. Find out which agencies provide palliative care services in your health authority, and what those services are.

Commentary:

What you will probably have discovered that palliative care is provided by different agencies in your area. Some of these may be part of the independent hospice movement while others may be part of the NHS. The intention of Saunders and the other early hospice pioneers was to move the care of the dying out of the NHS 'so that attitudes and knowledge could move back in' (Saunders 1993). In practice, that process began almost immediately. The first home care service, in which care was shared between the hospice and primary care teams, was launched by St Christopher's in 1969 (Help the Hospices 2005). Thereafter, the first hospital palliative care service in the UK was established at St Thomas' Hospital, London, in 1977. Prior to that, in Ontario, Canada, a little-known urology surgeon, Balfour Mount, established a ward for dying people in 1973. The Royal Victoria Hospital Palliative Care Service he subsequently founded became an important centre of palliative care development in North America (Clark 2007). Balfour Mount's place in this history is particularly important because he is credited with the first use of the term 'palliative care' (Hospice History Project 2001).

Gaining recognition and setting standards for palliative care

In the early years of the UK hospice movement, professional attitudes to hospice philosophy and hospice care were mixed. Some pioneering hospices encoun-tered reluctance from the health care establishment to refer patients or even to seek advice. However, several developments ushered in a more enlightened view of hospice and palliative care. Firstly, Cicely Saunders' vision of an ev-idence base for palliative care began to come to fruition, and the publication of the landmark textbook *The Management of Terminal Disease* in 1978 marked an important milestone in that process (Saunders 1978). Secondly, NHS-funded palliative care services continued to be established, leading to greater integration between palliative and established services. Thirdly, and perhaps most signifi-cantly, the public wanted hospices. By 1981 there were already 58 inpatient units and 32 home care teams in the UK, and by the mid 1980s, the rate of hospice building had risen to 10 new hospices per month (Clark et al. 2005). All of these developments also no doubt contributed to the momentum which ultimately led, in 1987, to the recognition by the Royal College of Physicians of the new sub-specialty of Palliative Medicine.

The increase in palliative care services in the UK and Ireland has continued to the present day, although the rate of that increase has slowed considerably, and there is more evidence of infilling of gaps, particularly in hospital-based services. By 2008, the Hospice and Palliative Care Directory was listing 223 inpatient units, 304 hospital support teams, 283 day care services and 316 home care (community) services (Hospice Information Service 2008).

Those years of local expansion of hospice and palliative care services were swiftly followed by attempts to organise and regulate services, and to follow a more strategic course. The Help the Hospices charity was established in 1984 'to help hospices ensure that the best possible care is provided to all those affected by terminal illness' (Help the Hospices 2008). A move to Europe-wide coordination followed in 1988 with the establishment of the European Association for Palliative Care. Then, in 1991, the National Council for Hospice and Specialist Palliative Care Services (NCHSPCS) (now the National Council for Palliative Care, NCPC) in England, Wales and Northern Ireland, and the Scottish Partnership Agency for Palliative and Cancer Care (now the Scottish Partnership for Palliative Care, SPPC) were set up as national umbrella bodies.

In 1990, the World Health Organization (WHO) set its first standards for palliative care. These were particularly significant in that they both cemented the ethos of palliative care and established internationally recognised benchmarks for palliative care services. What is particularly interesting is the very obvious influence of Cicely Saunders, particularly in the statements relating to active living and multi-disciplinary teamwork. The WHO guidelines were revised in 2002 (Sepulveda et al. 2002), but remain, quite unusually, a striking statement of the underlying philosophy for an approach to care.

National standards were also agreed in the UK. *The Principles and Provision of Palliative Care* was produced by the Standing Medical Advisory Committee and the Standing Nursing and Midwifery Advisory Committee in 1993, closely followed in 1994 by the *Palliative Cancer Care Guidelines* produced by the Scottish Partnership Agency and the Clinical Resource and Audit Group. Of major significance, around that time, was the recommendation by the National Council (and later endorsed by the NHS Executive) to distinguish three levels of palliative care: the palliative care approach, palliative interventions and specialist palliative care (NCHSPCS 1995; NHS Executive 1996). This development meant that two sets of benchmarks were now recognised: one applying to specialist services and one applying to other care providers. In Scotland, specialist standards were devised by the Clinical Standards Board (now Quality Improvement Scotland) and used to carry out the first national performance evaluation for specialist services in 2003 (NHS Quality Improvement Scotland 2004).

In the 40 years since the opening of St Christopher's Hospice, palliative care has come to be recognised as an important element of service provision, not only within the voluntary sector but also across the spectrum of UK health and social services (Matthew et al. 2003). In addition, over that period, palliative care has edged its way into national government's health and social policy. Recommendations over the period from 1986 to 2000, for instance, have included increasing the provision of palliative care services for people with non-malignant diseases, introducing palliative care at earlier stages in the disease process and promoting greater partnership working across agencies and sectors (Mathew et al. 2003).

Contemporary issues and future challenges

Those policy changes mentioned above have contributed to the numerous developments in UK palliative care practice witnessed over the last decade. Some of the most far reaching of these have been the introduction of the Liverpool Care Pathway, the Gold Standards Framework and the 'Preferred priorities of care' document, and their inclusion in the Department of Health's End of Life Care Strategy (Department of Health 2007).

Practice Point 1.2

Find out what progress your local health authority has made towards implementing palliative care pathways and service models.

Commentary:

The driving force behind the development of new care pathways and service models for palliative care has been the need to improve standards for all patients. The perception of hospices as being 'a little bit of heaven for the few' (Clark et al. 2005) has been borne out by studies which suggest differences in the quality of end of life care received by patients in these and other settings (Seale and Kelly 1997). Addressing this discrepancy is one of the principal priorities of palliative care today.

The Liverpool Care Pathway was developed specifically to transfer best practices from hospices into acute hospital settings (Ellershaw and Wilkinson 2003). The resulting document (together with its associated education programme) has been modified in the intervening years and is now available in hospital, community, care home and hospice versions (Marie Curie Palliative Care Institute Liverpool 2008).

The Gold Standards Framework was devised to improve cancer and palliative care in the community by tackling shortcomings in communication and planning. Early results suggest that dying at home can be improved if services and agencies are properly coordinated, and if family carers are kept informed and involved (Gold Standards Framework Scotland Project Team 2007).

One of the most contentious issues around the care of the dying has been choice of place to die (Gomes and Higginson 2004). Studies consistently report a wide discrepancy between patients' stated chosen place of death and their ultimate destination (House of Commons Select Committee on Health 2004). This situation has greatly exercised practitioners and policy makers alike, and resulted, in 2004, in the launch of the 'Preferred place of care' document (now modified to 'Preferred priorities of care') (Lancashire and South Cumbria Cancer Services Network Project Team 2004). This patient-held, advanced care plan offers a ready means of recording peoples' preferences and priorities for their end of life care (National Preferred Priorities of Care Team 2007).

In 2006, the Department of Health proposed an End of Life Care Strategy with the ambitious aim of meeting 'the health and social care needs and preferences of all adult patients in where they live and die' (National Council for Palliative Care 2006). The strategy included a commitment to roll out the three tools already discussed here. Early progress towards the realisation of the strategy has been positive (Department of Health 2007). In Scotland, palliative care services are currently coordinated by a framework of managed clinical networks (Scottish Partnership Agency for Palliative and Cancer Care 2000). However, in 2008, the Scottish Government accepted the recommendation of the Scottish Partnership for Palliative Care to implement a comprehensive palliative and end of life care strategy (SPPC 2007, 2008).

The case for improving the care of dying people across every care setting has already been successfully made – although the challenge of delivery has only just begun (Cooley 2007). An equally strong case has been made to make palliative care available to people across the spectrum of life limiting diseases. As will have become apparent, much of the early provision of palliative care in the UK was restricted to people with cancer. However that position has become increasingly indefensible, and current policy is strongly directed towards care on the basis of need, not diagnosis (NCHSPCS 1998, 2003; SPPC 2006).

There are other inequities of access related to ethnic background, old age, learning disability and so on which equally require to be tackled if the provision of palliative care is to be fair and equitable (Roscoe and Schonwetter 2006). Internationally too, we are far from meeting even the limited demand of Ahmedzai et al. (2004) that there should be guaranteed access to palliative care for every person with cancer. Unfortunately there are still areas of the world where affordable palliative care is completely unknown (Costello 2005; Milicevic 2002).

Palliative care at 40

If the birth of modern palliative care is agreed to have coincided with the opening of St Christopher's Hospice in 1967, then palliative care has now reached its early forties. But what does the future hold for a speciality which describes itself as 'an approach' and claims to be applicable across the spectrum of care settings and diagnoses, but (in the UK at least) is substantially provided by the voluntary sector?

Future funding of palliative care is certainly one issue which must be addressed. The most recent estimates suggest that 71% of inpatient hospice care is provided by independent charities, and organisations such as Macmillan Cancer Support and Marie Curie Cancer Care remain dependent on legacies and fundraising practice points for the bulk of their operating costs (Help the Hospices 2005). There is evidence from the US that some hospices are responding to financial pressures by introducing more efficient and innovative business practices (Kirby et al. 2007). However, this is only part of the answer, and government commitments in terms of partial funding may have to grow if current service levels are to continue or increase.

Another challenge in contemporary palliative care is the maintenance of quality. Palliative care is highly labour intensive and, consequently, a relatively expensive model of care delivery. Funding bodies, whether statutory or voluntary, must be assured that they are receiving value for money. Measuring outcomes in palliative care is fraught with difficulties, not least because relief of suffering is a highly subjective concept and potential respondents are frequently too ill or too upset to comment on their experiences. However, systematic quality improvement in palliative care is achievable and sustainable if supported by policy reforms and local practice initiatives (Lynn et al. 2008).

And what will palliative care look like in another 40 years? Some important groups apparently continue to define palliative care in terms of cancer services (e.g. National Institute for Health and Clinical Excellence 2004; Ahmedzai et al. 2004) in spite of the momentum of the non-malignant agenda. There are calls for greater use of invasive interventions, but counter claims that the speciality is becoming over-medicalised (Clark 2002). The current proliferation of cancer support services in UK hospices suggests a move to the inclusion of palliation earlier in the disease process, but where does that leave the trend towards end of life initiatives? Finally, there is the issue of physician-assisted suicide – clearly rising up the political agenda with a bill before the House of Lords in 2006 (and a palliative care bill the same year) and a consultation before the Scottish Executive in 2005 (Finlay 2006; Joffe 2006; Purvis 2005). Perhaps, the way palliative care responds to this particular issue will define, more than any other factor, its future direction and values.

References

Ahmedzai SH, Costa A, Blengini C, Bosch A, Sanz-Ortiz J, Ventafridda V and Verhagen SC, on behalf of the international working group convened by the European School of Oncology (2004) A new international framework for palliative care. *European Journal of Cancer Care*. 40(15):2192–2200.

Bailey M (1959) A survey of the social needs of patients with incurable lung cancer. *Almoner*. 11:379–397.

Booth C (2002) The Daily Telegraph (London), September 5, 2002.

Clark D (2002) Between hope and acceptance: the medicalisation of dying. *British Medical Journal*. 324(7342):905–907.

Clark D (2007) From margins to centre: a review of the history of palliative care in cancer. *The Lancet Oncology*. 8(5):430–438.

Clark D, Small N, Wright M, Winslow M and Hughes N (2005) *A Bit of Heaven for the Few? An Oral History of the Modern Hospice Movement in the United Kingdom*. Lancaster: Observatory Publications.

Cooley C (2007) Equality and choice in palliative care (editorial). *International Journal of Palliative Nursing*. 13(5):204.

Costello J (2005) Palliative care for all: a global challenge. *International Journal of Palliative Nursing*. 11(10):540.

Department of Health (2007) *End of Life Care Strategy: Letter from Professor Mike Richards, Chair of End of Life Care Strategy Advisory Board.* London: Department of Health.

Doyle D, Hanks G, Cherny N and Calman K (Eds) (2005) *The Oxford Textbook of Palliative Medicine.* Oxford: Oxford University Press.

Ellershaw J and Wilkinson S (2003) *Care for the Dying: A Pathway to Excellence.* Oxford: Oxford University Press.

Finlay IG (2006) *A Bill to Make Provision for Palliative Care for Persons Who Are Suffering from a Terminal Illness; and for Connected Purposes.* London: House of Lords.

Glynn Hughes HL (1960) *Peace at the Last: A Survey of Terminal Care in the United Kingdom.* London: The Calouste Gulbenkian Foundation.

Gold Standards Framework Scotland Project Team (2007) Gold Standards Framework Scotland final report. Available at http://www.gsfs.scot.nhs.uk/documents/GSFS%20Final%20Report.pdf. Accessed on 22 November 2008.

Gomes B and Higginson IJ (2004) Home or hospital? Choices at the end of life. *Journal of the Royal Society of Medicine.* 97(9):413–414.

Help the Hospices (2005) *Hospice and Palliative Care Facts and Figures 2005.* London: Hospice Information.

Help the Hospices (2008) Who we are. Available at http://www.helpthehospices.org.uk/whoweare/index.asp. Accessed on 31 August 2008.

Hinton J (1964) Problems in the care of the dying. *Journal of Chronic Diseases.* 17:201–205.

Hoffmann RL (2005) The evolution of hospice in America: nursing's role in the movement. *Journal of Gerontological Nursing.* 31(7):26–34.

Hospice History Project (2001) Balfour Mount [Interview Two]. Recorded 14 March 2001. Available at http://www.hospice-history.org.uk/byoralsurname?id=0077&search=m&page=0. Accessed on 22 November 2008.

Hospice Information Service (2008) *Hospice and Palliative Care Directory United Kingdom and Ireland 2008.* London: HIS.

House of Commons Select Committee on Health (2004) *Palliative Care: Fourth Report of Session 2003–2004.* London: The Stationary Office Limited.

Joffe J (2006) *A Bill to Enable an Adult Who Has Capacity and Who Is Suffering Unbearably as a Result of a Terminal Illness to Receive Medical Assistance to Die at His Own Considered and Persistent Request; and for Connected Purposes.* London: House of Lords.

Kearney M (1996) *Mortally Wounded: Stories of Soul Pain, Death and Healing.* New York: Touchstone/Simon and Schuster.

Kirby EG, Keeffe MJ and Nicols KMA (2007) A study of the effects of innovative and efficient practices on the performance of hospice care organizations. *Health Care Management Review.* 32(4):352–359.

Kubler-Ross E (1970) *On Death and Dying.* London: Routledge.

Lancashire and South Cumbria Cancer Services Network Project Team (2004) The preferred place of care explained. Leaflet available at http://www.cancerlancashire.org.uk/leaflet.pdf. Accessed on 22 November 2008.

Lloyd-Williams M (Ed.) (2003) *Psychosocial Issues in Palliative Care.* Oxford: Oxford University Press.

Lynn J, Murray S and Sheikh A (2008) Palliative care beyond cancer: reliable comfort and meaningfulness. *British Medical Journal.* 336(7650):958–959.

Macmillan Cancer Support (2006) Our history. Available at http://www.macmillan.org.uk/About_Us/Our_ambition/Our_history.aspx. Accessed on 22 November 2008.

Macmillan Cancer Support (2007) *Annual Review 2006.* London: Macmillan Cancer Support.

Marie Curie Palliative Care Institute Liverpool (2008) Liverpool Care Pathway for the dying patient (LCP). Available at http://www.mcpcil.org.uk/liverpool_care_pathway. Accessed on 22 November 2008.

Matthew A, Cowley S, Bliss J and Thistlewood G (2003) The development of palliative care in national government policy in England, 1986–2000. *Palliative Medicine.* 17(3):43270–43282.

Milicevic N (2002) The hospice movement: history and current worldwide situation. *Archive of Oncology.* 10(1):29–32.

National Council for Hospice and Specialist Palliative Care Services (1995) *Specialist Palliative Care: A Statement of Definitions.* London: NCHSPCS.

National Council for Hospice and Specialist Palliative Care Services (1998) *Reaching Out: Specialist Palliative Care for Adults with Non-Malignant Diseases.* Occasional Paper 14, London: NCHSPCS.

National Council for Hospice and Specialist Palliative Care Services (2003) *Palliative Care for Adults with Non-Malignant Diseases: Developing a National Policy.* Briefing Bulletin 12. London: NCHSPCS.

National Council for Palliative Care (2006) *End of Life Care Strategy: The National Council for Palliative Care Submission.* London: NCHSPCS.

National Health Service Executive (1996) *A Policy Framework for Commissioning Cancer Services: Palliative Care Services EL (96)85.* London: NHS Executive.

National Health Service Quality Improvement Scotland (2004) *Specialist Palliative Care: National Overview – January 2004.* Edinburgh: NHSQIS.

National Institute for Health and Clinical Excellence (2004) *Supportive and Palliative Care: Improving Supportive and Palliative Care for Adults with Cancer.* London: NICE.

National Preferred Priorities of Care Team (2007) Preferred priorities of care. Available at http://www.endoflifecareforadults.nhs.uk/eolc/files/F2110-Preferred_Priorities_for_Care_V2_Dec2007.pdf. Accessed on 22 November 2008.

Newman L (2004) Obituary: Elizabeth Kubler-Ross. *British Medical Journal.* 329(7466):627.

Potts S (2005) *Everylife: Death, Bereavement and Life through the Eyes of Children, Parents and Practitioners.* Wiltshire: APS books.

Prail D and Pahl N (2007) The worldwide palliative care alliance: networking national associations. *Journal of Pain and Symptom Management.* 33(5):506–508.

Purvis J (2005) Dying with dignity: a consultation by Jeremy Purvis MSP. Edinburgh: The Scottish Parliament. Available at http://www.scottish.parliament.uk/business/bills/pdfs/mb-consultations/Dying%20with%20Dignity%20Consultation%20paper.pdf. Accessed on 22 November 2008.

Roscoe LA and Schonwetter RS (2006) Improving access to hospice and palliative care for patients near the end of life: present status and future direction. *Journal of Palliative Care.* 22(1):46–50.

Saunders C (Ed.) (1978) *The Management of Terminal Disease.* London: Edward Arnold.

Saunders C (1993) Introduction – history and challenge. In: Saunders C and Sykes N (Eds), *The Management of Terminal Malignant Disease.* London: Edward Arnold, pp. 1–14.

Saunders C (2000) The evolution of palliative care. *Patient Education and Counselling.* 41(1):7–13.

Scottish Partnership Agency and the Clinical Resource and Audit Group (1994) *Palliative Cancer Care Guidelines.* Edinburgh: HMSO Scotland.

Scottish Partnership Agency for Palliative and Cancer Care (2000) *A Framework for the Operation of Managed Clinical Networks in Palliative Care: Report of a Working Party.* Edinburgh: SPA.

Scottish Partnership for Palliative Care (2006) *Joined Up Thinking, Joined Up Care: Increasing Access to Palliative Care for People with Life Threatening Conditions Other than Cancer.* Edinburgh: SPPC.

Scottish Partnership for Palliative Care (2007) *Palliative and End of Life Care in Scotland: The Case for a Cohesive Approach.* Edinburgh: SPPC.

Scottish Partnership for Palliative Care (2008) *Update*, Issue 54, p. 1. Edinburgh: SPPC.

Seale C and Kelly M (1997) A comparison of hospice and hospital care for people who die: views of the surviving spouse. *Palliative Medicine.* 11(2):93–100.

Sepulveda C, Marlin A, Yoshida T and Ullrich A (2002) Palliative care: the World Health Organization's global perspective. *Journal of Pain and Symptom Management.* 24(2):91–96.

Standing Medical Advisory Committee and the Standing Nursing and Midwifery Advisory Committee (1993) *The Principles and Provision of Palliative Care.* London: HMSO.

Thompson G (2002) *God Knows Caregiving Can Pull You Apart: 12 Ways to Keep It All Together.* Notre Dame, IN: Sorin Books.

Wright M (2007) *Victor Zorza: A Life amid Loss.* Lancaster: Observatory Publications.

Chapter 2

Definitions and aims of palliative care

Elaine Stevens

Introduction

This chapter is going to investigate the definitions and aims of palliative care and begins by providing the current definitions of terms used within the palliative care arena. Then, using the aims of palliative care as defined by the World Health Organization (2002), the chapter reviews the main principles of palliative care, discussing the implications these have when providing nursing care to dying people and their families.

Learning outcomes

Once you have read this chapter and completed the associated reflective practice points, you will be able to:

- Discuss the meaning of the types of palliative care that are currently available
- Describe the components of holistic palliative care
- Illustrate how optimal palliative care can be provided within your own clinical area

Definitions and terminology

The first global definition of palliative care was issued by The World Health Organization (WHO) in 1990. This was to ensure all those diagnosed with advanced cancer received holistic, individualised care that focused on quality of life. Over the coming years there was recognition within the UK that palliative care was evolving into two distinct levels, as the 'specialism' of palliative care emerged (Ford 1995). Although still firmly rooted in the care of advanced cancer patients, The National Council for Hospices and Specialist Palliative Care Services (NCHSPCS 1997) provided definitions to differentiate specialist palliative care from general palliative care. They stated that specialist palliative care:

> 'is that provided in units and services with palliative care as their core speciality and where all senior members of professional staff are accredited

specialists, having undertaken the requisite training required by their respective professional body.' (NCHSPCS 1997, p. 8)

Since this definition emerged, there is now a firm belief that palliative care within the UK is provided at two levels, namely, general palliative care and specialist palliative care (National Council for Palliative Care 2008).

In 2002 the WHO updated its 1990 definition of palliative care in response to the acknowledgement that palliative care should be available, when required, to everyone with a life-limiting illness, regardless of place of care or diagnosis. As previously noted, before this their definition focused on the care of people who had advanced cancer and required palliative care (WHO 1990), which was also the main focus of the hospice movement until fairly recently. The current WHO definition is as follows:

'Palliative care is an approach that improves the quality of life of patients and their families facing the problems associated with life-threatening illness, through the prevention and relief of suffering by means of early identification and impeccable assessment and treatment of pain and other problems, physical, psychosocial and spiritual.' (WHO 2002)

This supports the principles of the modern hospice movement that palliative care should be a holistic, individualised approach to the care for people who have been diagnosed with an illness that cannot be cured or is no longer curable. However, the new definition moves away from the notion that palliative care is exclusively for those diagnosed with cancer.

The National Institute of Clinical Excellence (2004) suggests that this general level of palliative care should be an integral clinical skill for all caring professionals, as the majority of palliative care will be provided by the dying person's day-to-day professional carers. Some reports also refer to the 'palliative care approach' which is defined by the Scottish Partnership for Palliative Care as:

'a basic approach to caring for people as individuals which emphasises the importance of good communication and of respect for individual autonomy and dignity. It recognises that people may have needs which are physical, social, psychological or spiritual, or a combination of these. Such an approach is particularly appropriate when dealing with those who have long-term progressive conditions and should be adopted by anyone in a caring role, whether health and social care professionals, volunteers, family or friends.'
(Scottish Partnership for Palliative Care 2006, p. 3)

This definition not only includes the aspects of general palliative care, reviewed above, but it also acknowledges that this approach involves the ill person's family and friends as well as professional carers. Both the term general palliative care and the term the palliative care approach are often used interchangeably and as such have come to mean the same thing within the health care arena.

However, even though we now have quite clear definitions of this level of palliative care, professional carers continue to equate it with terminal care, that is the care provided to a person in the last days or hour of life (Scottish Executive Health Department 2001). This prevents the application of the palliative care ethos to those who would benefit from its holistic, person-centred approach at an earlier point in their illness. This is further compounded by the notion that the general public has little idea of what palliative care could offer them at the end of life (Wallace 2003). Therefore, many people are unaware of how palliative care may help them, if diagnosed with a life-limiting illness, by relieving physical or other symptoms or indeed supporting them and those closest to them during their illness and during their loved ones' bereavement.

The term specialist palliative care was redefined in the NICE (2004) strategy, and is described as the same holistic palliative care discussed above but which is provided by professionals with specialist training. NICE (2004) suggests that this care is required by patients and carers who experience:

• Unresolved symptoms and complex psychosocial issues in advanced disease
• Complex end of life issues
• Complex bereavement issues

(NICE 2004, p. 21)

This is the type of care now provided by the majority of hospices and specialist palliative care teams across a number of care settings in the UK, although it is recognised that only 20% of dying people will need this type of specialist care (Doyle 2008). Both, Scotland and Wales have developed standards in to ensure these services can provide this higher level of care to an acceptable quality (Clinical Standards Board for Scotland 2002; Welsh Assembly Government 2005).

Another term that has come to the fore recently is that of supportive care. This is defined in the NICE (2004) guidance as care that:

'... helps the patient and their family to cope with cancer and treatment of it – from pre-diagnosis, through the process of diagnosis and treatment, to cure, continuing illness or death and into bereavement. It helps the patient to maximise the benefits of treatment and to live as well as possible with the effects of the disease. It is given equal priority alongside diagnosis and treatment.' (NICE 2004, p. 18)

Although this definition is described here in relation to cancer care, it can be adapted to meet the needs of people with other life-threatening illnesses (National Council for Palliative Care 2008). NICE (2004) suggests that supportive care is an overarching expression for a type of care that includes:

• self-help and support
• user involvement
• information giving
• psychological support

- symptom control
- social support
- rehabilitation
- complementary therapies
- spiritual support
- palliative care
- end of life and bereavement care

(NICE 2004, p. 18)

From this it can be seen that palliative care can be a part of supportive care, but they are not the same thing.

The End of Life Programme (2008), the newest palliative care initiative to be developed in NHS England, uses the terminology that seeks to confuse many people across the country, both in health care and in the general population. They use the term 'End of Life' in their programme in the same way other documents, services and professionals would use palliative care. However, until this programme began the term end of life care was equated with terminal care, that is care of the dying person in the last few days or hours of life. Indeed, the tools that this programme suggests ensure good 'end of life' care come from well-known palliative care providers and are not exclusively for the final days or hours of life (End of Life Programme 2008). We are now left wondering if this new term will replace palliative care or will it just confuse the public and professionals further, as it has already been shown that both groups currently have a poor understanding of the terminology associated with palliative and hospice care.

Practice Point 2.1

Review the above definitions – which levels and types of palliative care do the patients you look after require?

Commentary:

This section has shown that there are distinct levels in palliative care provision in the UK, and you will probably find that, as an illness advances, individual patients will require a number of different types of care. However, the same terminology needs to be used across the UK so that both the general public and care providers know what is meant by the terms used and the type of care provided. In addition, it has been acknowledged that many professionals who should theoretically provide general palliative care do not have the knowledge and skills to do so (NICE 2004). However, the idea that the upsurge in the number of specialist nursing posts may deskill the general palliative care provider (Open University 2004) suggests that many of those who require general palliative care are not receiving it. Finally, there is the suggestion that Specialist Palliative Care

(SPC) services are becoming elitist by focusing their efforts on dying people with moderate-to-complex needs as this only affects a small number of the dying population. As such many dying patients do not receive SPC, as they do not fit the NICE (2004) criteria.

So, in conclusion, nurses need to be aware of the different levels and type of care that may be available to dying people, and they should ensure that each dying patient receives the care required to allow them to live as actively as possible while ill and to die in a peaceful, dignified manner.

The next section shows the aims of palliative care that would help nurses working in all settings to provide the palliative care to all dying patients when required.

The aims of palliative care

In 2001, when discussing the evolution of palliative care Cicely Saunders wrote:

> 'Palliative Care is a philosophy based not on physical facilities but on attitudes and skills, as the many interpretations around the industrialised and developing world show forcefully.' (Saunders 2001, p. 432)

This is reflected in the general aims of palliative care provided by the WHO (2002) which states that palliative care:

- provides relief from pain and other distressing symptoms
- affirms life and regards dying as a normal process
- intends neither to hasten or postpone death
- integrates the psychological and spiritual aspects of patient care
- offers a support system to help patients live as actively as possible until death
- offers a support system to help the family cope during the patients illness and in their own bereavement
- uses a team approach to address the needs of patients and their families, including bereavement counselling, if indicated
- will enhance quality of life, and may also positively influence the course of illness
- is applicable early in the course of illness, in conjunction with other therapies that are intended to prolong life, such as chemotherapy or radiation therapy, and includes those investigations needed to better understand and manage distressing clinical complications

(WHO 2002).

Using these broad aims, which can be applied across all care settings and diagnoses, this chapter now investigates the philosophy of palliative care in more depth.

Provides relief from pain and other distressing symptoms

It is imperative that good physical symptom management is an integral part of the care of the person with advanced disease, and before the opening of the first hospice Cicely Saunders intimated that there was a connection between physical problems and psychological, spiritual and social issues (Clark 1999). She spoke of the concept of 'total pain' which was described as a myriad of physical, psychological, social and spiritual needs that would be different in every dying individual (Saunders 1996). She also recognised that each of these facets would impact on another, citing the comments of one patient who said, 'It was all pain but now it is gone and I am free' (Saunders 2001). This concept has become one of the cornerstones of the palliative care philosophy which recognises the importance of an individualistic, rigorous approach to the management of all symptoms experienced by each dying person. Indeed, the principles of physical symptom management in palliative care have been well documented (Doyle et al. 2005a; Twycross and Wilcock 2002; Faull and Woof 2002), and are summarised using the following acronym by Twycross and Wilcock (2002):

- **E** – Evaluation – make a clear and accurate assessment of each symptom
- **E** – Explanation – to the patient and/or the family on the cause and possible treatments
- **M** – Management – an individual treatment plan should be formulated in consultation with the patient and/or the family
- **M** – Monitoring – each symptom should be continuously reviewed and adjustments to treatments made
- **A** – Attention to detail – never say there is nothing more we can do. Make use of all available resources, treatments and expertise

(Twycross and Wilcock 2002, p. 6)

Using this simple method, in a logical stepwise way, will help to ensure the symptom is relieved to each dying person's satisfaction.

One of the most common physical symptoms experienced by people with advanced disease is pain (Faull and Woof 2002). Although much of the work in pain management has focused on advanced cancer patients, there is now recognition that chronic pain in non-malignant conditions should be managed in the same rigorous way (British Pain Society 2005). The current gold standard method of managing chronic pain is by utilising the World Health Organization's (1996) guidelines which was revised edition for its earlier 1990 guidance. Chapter 8 on palliative care in heart failure discusses the use of this framework which aims to ensure pain is correctly managed.

Other common physical symptoms of advanced disease are dyspnoea, fatigue and constipation (Faull and Woof 2002), while nausea and/or vomiting are also recognised as symptoms that occur in many people with advanced cancer (Twycross and Wilcock 2002). Therefore, every person with advanced disease should be assessed for multiple symptoms, recognising that each symptom will impact one another, newer information on symptom clusters in advanced cancer suggests some physical symptoms appear together specifically because they have the same physiological mechanisms (Lacasse and Beck 2007). Good physical symptom management, however, should not be at the expense of symptoms within the other three domains of total pain; each should be regarded with equal importance, and assessed accordingly, or optimal palliative care cannot be provided.

Affirms life and regards dying as a normal process

It can be difficult for both lay people and caring professionals to subscribe to these proposals for a number of reasons. Most of us in the Western World live in a society that does not like to think about death; indeed, some writers suggest that we deny that death exists (Zimmermann and Rodin 2004). This idea has come about because we are now living to a much older age and the death of an elderly person, who is seen not to have a role within society, makes death almost invisible (Walter 1992). This compounded with the fact that the majority of the British population die in hospital (Gomes and Higginson 2008) adds to the lack of experience that the general public has in dealing with dying and death. Society's exposure to death is further complicated by the media who tend to glorify the death of younger people and those who have died violently, while only covering the death of an older person if they are of celebrity status. All these factors reinforce the notion that death can be conquered, so when dying and death come into a person's life they believe that it is something that can be conquered and as such not the natural end of physical life at all.

The birth of the biomedical model of care, in which disease was to be eradicated, led to death being seen as a failure within health care organisations (Middlewood et al. 2001). Although this biomedical model has been criticised for not taking a holistic view of patients (Wade and Halligan 2004), many continue to be offered treatments that could be classed as futile in the name of 'not giving up', as this would be considered as failure. As such quantity of life within the biomedical model is often seen as the goal of care, which makes it more difficult to provide good palliative care within acute care where this view can still be held quite strongly (Beckstrand et al. 2006). It is therefore recognised that a lot still needs to be done to help some professionals understand that death is the natural conclusion to life and that a good quality of life and death is more important to dying patients (Vig and Pearlman 2003) and families than an extended quantity of life which is painful and distressing (Beckstrand et al. 2006).

Intends neither to hasten nor postpone death

Good palliative care aims, as the WHO (2002) states, to improve the quality of life of patients through the prevention and relief of suffering. However, this may be more difficult to achieve than it first appears. There are many interventions that can be employed in palliative care to relieve suffering, whether it is physical, psychological, social or spiritual pain, which could be deemed to either hasten or postpone death.

Practice Point 2.2

Think about some of the interventions that may be offered to dying patients in your area? Could they be seen to hasten or postpone death?

Commentary:

Some of those treatments on your list may include artificial nutrition, artificial hydration, cardiopulmonary resuscitation, courses of antibiotics and chemotherapy. This list is not exhaustive and is given merely to show the array of interventions available.

It is important, however, for nurses working with dying patients to be able to judge which treatments and interventions are in the patient's best interests, thus promoting quality of life. This helps to ensure that treatments deemed to be futile are not offered or indeed assures that treatments are not withheld or withdrawn if they potentially have a therapeutic effect. This brings to the fore the concept of ethical decision-making, and in palliative care it is important for all nurses to participate in ethical decision-making in partnership with the patient and the professional care team. Indeed, nurses are often seen as the patient's advocate (Odom 2002), so it is useful to have a sound knowledge of the ethical principles that support good palliative care. The four main ethical principles utilised in health care were developed by Beauchamp and Childress (2001): these are autonomy, beneficence, non-maleficence and justice.

In palliative care the creation of and respect for autonomy is a central tenet, underpinning the recognition that the patient is in the best position to say how specific treatments and interventions will affect themselves and their families. However, it has to be recognised that not all dying people can make autonomous decisions, and when this occurs the nurse needs then, in consultation with the rest of the care team, to decide what treatments are in the patient's best interests. The principles of non-maleficence and beneficence are helpful here, as they help the professional to decide whether the proposed plan of care would do the person more harm than good (Seedhouse 1998). It is a good practice to keep family members of all patients, including those who cannot make their own decisions, fully informed of what is happening and why and also to allow them to take part in the decision-making process where this is appropriate. However, Twycross (2003) notes that in order to discuss the patient's issues with the family the patient should have consented to this. This reinforces the importance of forward planning in palliative care so that the care team knows what a patient would want should they no longer be able to make decisions for themselves. Seedhouse (1998) suggests that part of the principle of providing care that is just and fair is that professionals need to know the effectiveness and efficiency of actions they are intending and also have knowledge of the underpinning evidence to support their stance. In conclusion, it can be seen that to ensure dying people are offered treatments and interventions that are seen to be in their best interests, which neither hasten nor postpone death, nurses need to be able to make ethically sound decisions, in partnership with the patient, family and care team. Indeed, Odom (2002) suggests that for nurses to act as a patient advocate they need to be competent and well educated to make decisions about their care.

Integrates the psychological and spiritual aspects of patient care

Earlier in this section the importance of good physical symptom management was shown to be integral to the provision of good-quality palliative care. Although physical symptoms may be well managed, the psychological and spiritual facets of total pain may not be addressed so well, and as such these aspects of palliative care may require more attention from nurses. This may be because it is much easier to manage physical symptoms, utilising the plethora of research conducted in this area. Also, many professionals are fearful of engaging with dying people at a deeper level, as they feel they do not know what to do if psychological or spiritual issues are disclosed. However, to ensure a holistic approach to care, these sometimes intangible concepts need to be understood. This section reviews both concepts to show what they encompass and why they are important for good palliative care provision.

Psychological well-being

There are a number of areas that need to be considered to ensure that good psychological care is provided within palliative care. In 1989, Ryff suggested that psychological well-being had a number of dimensions which encapsulated the concept. These are:

- Self-acceptance – this is related to feelings of own personal worth and of a good past life
- The establishment of quality ties to other – this is concerned with the quality of relationships and concern about others
- A sense of autonomy in thought and action – this is related to independence, being a burden and being able to make one's own decisions without submitting to outside pressures
- The ability to manage complex environments to suit personal needs and values – this is concerned with the ability to manage one's everyday affairs and of the feelings of control over one's world
- The pursuit of meaningful goals and a sense of purpose in life – this is related to the ability to achieve life goals and have a sense of purpose and motivation in life

- Continued growth and development as a person – this is concerned with how one views one's own potential within life and how to mature and develop through experiences

(Adapted from Ryff and Keyes 1995).

To provide good psychological care, professionals working in palliative care need to ensure they support the dying person within all these domains. However, it has been reported that there is high incidence of anxiety (Jackson and Lipman 2004) and depression (Smitz and Woods 2006) in dying patients, which suggests that they may not indeed by receiving adequate psychological support. Therefore, a more proactive approach is required to ensure that this aim of palliative care is met within all care settings. NICE (2004) provides a framework of four levels of psychological care for dying people and suggests that all professional should be able to identify psychological issues and provide a basic form of psychological care and know when to refer patients on to those with further expertise.

Spirituality

There is recognition that spirituality is as subjective an experience as physical pain. However, in order to incorporate good spiritual care into palliative care, it is helpful to try and define the concept. Spirituality was defined by Murray and Zenter in 1989 as:

> 'A Quality that goes beyond religious affiliation, that strives for inspiration, reverence, awe, meaning and purpose, even in those that do not believe in any God. The spiritual dimension tries to be in harmony with the universe, strives for answers about the infinite and comes into focus when the person faces emotional stress, physical illness and death.'

Although nearly 20 years old, this definition still reflects the current thinking of what spirituality means, in that it includes not only religious issues but also existential questions. In addition to this, it is recognised that when a person is diagnosed with a life-limiting illness there are a number of spiritual issues that may come to the fore. These are:

- disorganisation and disruption of life
- search for meaning
- reliance on hope, inner strength and the love of others
- reliance on other spiritual resources

(Narayanasamy 2004)

There has been much debate around who should provide the care required to address the dying person's spiritual concerns (Tan et al. 2005), and many different professionals purport to provide spiritual care within their role. However, regardless of which team member provides the spiritual support, McSherry and Cash (2004) suggest that all spiritual issues need to be addressed within people's cultural frameworks. Nevertheless, there is evidence to suggest that although nurses see the provision of spiritual care in palliative care important, they find it difficult to both identify these needs and meet them (Milligan 2004). Indeed, Gilliat-Ray (2001) also recognised that nurses needed education in this area to allow them to provide effective spiritual care. It can therefore be seen that spiritual care is integral to the provision of good-quality palliative care; however, work still needs to be done to ensure effective spiritual care is available to all dying patients.

Offers a support system to help patients live as actively as possible until death

The process of helping dying patients to remain as active as possible is often seen as impossible to achieve in the face of advancing illness. However, the concept is not new, with Dietz defining palliative rehabilitation within the sphere of cancer care in 1981. This concept suggested that rehabilitation in advanced cancer should focus on limiting the effects of the illness and promoting independence where achievable (Dietz 1981). The WHO (1990) then introduced this as one of the main aims of palliative while the Calman–Hine (Calman and Hine 1995) report suggested that rehabilitation was an integral part of cancer care from diagnosis onwards. However, it is now also recognised that focused rehabilitation within incurable non-malignant illness, such as chronic obstructive pulmonary disease and motor neurone disease, also has a positive impact on the quality of life (McCluskey 2007; Harris 2007).

So, as the concept has evolved it has been proved that rehabilitation in palliative care can, through good multi-professional team working, provide a system that supports dying people to keep as well as possible. This led the NCHSPCS in 2006 to state that:

> 'a rehabilitative approach can help people with advancing, life-threatening disease lead fulfilling lives within the constraints of their illness; and that the approach should be an integral part of palliative care.'
> (National Council for Hospices and Specialist Palliative Care Services 2006)

Therefore, the goal of rehabilitation in palliative care is not always to improve function but to help dying people to maintain as much independence for as long as possible. This is described by Pearson et al. (2007) as a compensatory approach which aims to adjust functional ability in response to the patient's aims and objectives. Therefore, the rehabilitation process takes into account the ever-changing needs of people with advanced, progressive disease and central to this is the ability of the care team to set mutually acceptable goals with the dying person (Tookman et al. 2005). This in turn improves feelings of control and helps dying people feel less of a burden on others (Kim et al. 2005). However, it can be difficult to help dying people to maintain their independence, as rehabilitation is often not seen as important as other aspects of care and poor function and fatigue are seen as a normal part of advanced illness (Doyle et al. 2005b; Ream 2008). This combined with the idea that many professionals do not understand the benefits of rehabilitation for this group means that referrals to occupational or physiotherapy are not made in a timely fashion. In particular, the availability of rehabilitation services to support patients with a non-cancer diagnosis remains poor (Tookman et al. 2005). It can therefore be deduced that although rehabilitation in advanced illness is known to have a positive impact on dying people, it is not always recognised as an intervention that should be employed and therefore more work needs to be done to educate nurses of its benefits in palliative care.

Offers a support system to help the family cope during the patient's illness and in their own bereavement

The impact of the impending and actual death of a loved one often disables families and prevents them caring for each other effectively. It has also been long recognised that the family members of dying patients often have similar or more distressing physical, psychological, social or spiritual issues that need to be addressed to maintain their quality of life while their loved one is ill (Northhouse 1984; Doyle 1996; NICE 2004). Family issues may include change of role, the burden of care giving, frailty, distress, and the need to attend church. These are further compounded by the social isolation that is related to a full-time caring role or a role which entails visiting a care organisation a number of times per week. Many of these concerns do not surface until the patient has died, resulting in a poorer bereavement outcome as the family member may have ill health and exhaustion that prevents them reintegrating back into their social group. Indeed, poor social support is recognised as a determinant to a poorer grief reaction (Matheson 2003). Therefore, professionals who provide care to dying patients should ensure that each family, which is as unique as their dying member, is supported and cared for to ensure their needs are addressed.

However, NICE (2004) suggests that currently within the UK the support for relatives before and after the death of their loved one is often substandard. Their report also acknowledges that professionals are not always good at assessing, predicting or responding to families needs and that better systems need to be developed to ensure all the organisations involved in the patient's care communicate well with each other to remedy this current situation (NICE 2004). NICE (2004) provide a comprehensive, three level, model of bereavement support that may be required by families, noting that all care organisations should be able to achieve the first level which is that:

> 'All bereaved people should be offered information about the experience of bereavement and how to access other forms of support.'
>
> (NICE 2004, p. 161)

In order to do this effectively, each care team then requires the expertise to do this, and as such professional carers need education on family and bereavement care.

> **Practice Point 2.3**
>
> Does your clinical area have information to give to families following bereavement?

Commentary:

It may be of use to know where to find information that is suitable for family members. Perhaps, if you have a chaplain or social worker in your team, they may be able to direct you to this type of information. There are also booklets such as:

'At the End of Life' –
  http://www.cancerbackup.org.uk/Resourcessupport/Advancedcancer/
    Dyingwithcancer/Attheendoflife

'What to do After a Death in England and Wales' –
  http://www.dwp.gov.uk/publications/dwp/2006/d49_april06.pdf

'What to do After a Death in Scotland' –
  http://www.scotland.gov.uk/Resource/Doc/47133/0025575.pdf

These may help to begin conversations with bereaved relatives.

Uses a team approach to address the needs of patients and their families, including bereavement counselling, if indicated

It has been recognised that each dying individual and their family has a unique mix of physical, psychological, social and spiritual needs. Therefore, it is acknowledged that no one professional will have the all the skills to address every problem that arises. The central aim of palliative care is then to ensure that each dying person is afforded the expertise of a multi-professional team (Lickiss et al. 2005). However, it has been shown that many dying patients do not have their needs addressed due to poor communication between professionals either within one care team or indeed across different agencies. Crawford and Price (2003) exemplify poor team working by describing professionals as 'wedges in a pie'. In this model of care there are clearly demarked roles and the skills required to meet patient's needs, but these are provided in virtual isolation, with little communication between professional groups involved in the person's care. Indeed, on reviewing the list of the professionals NICE (2004) suggests may be required to ensure the needs of the dying person are met, it can be seen that maintaining effective communication in palliative care is a challenge in itself. NICE (2004) suggests the following should be part of the team supporting dying people and their families:

- GPs and other members of primary care teams
- community nurses

- care home staff
- doctors and nurses in hospitals
- allied health professionals in the community and in
- hospitals
- social workers
- general and community dental practitioners
- participants and facilitators in self-help and support groups

(NICE 2004, p. 105)

This list is not exhaustive and NICE (2004) suggests that the core care team should also be able to refer the patient and family to other teams or professionals as necessary to ensure their needs are addressed. This may include referral to the Specialist Palliative Care Team. The list, however, does not show that the most important members of the team are the patient and the family, or that they are central to all decisions that the team makes (Crawford and Price 2003).

Therefore, to make the best of each team member's expertise, there needs to be a coordinated approach to the patient's care, which involves good planning and communication within organisations and across all care agencies (Yuen et al. 2003). The aim of this is to provide seamless continuity of care throughout the dying person's journey from diagnosis to death.

Will enhance quality of life, and may also positively influence the course of illness

Although the WHO (2002) definition of palliative care states that promotion of quality of life is central to the well-being of dying patients, it can be a difficult concept to quantify. Therefore, in order to promote quality of life in people who have a life-limiting illness, it needs to be recognised that this is subjective, meaning different things to different people (Kaasa 2000). Twycross (2003) agrees and states that quality of life is:

'an individual's subjective satisfaction with life and is influenced by all aspects of personhood: physical, psychological, social and spiritual.'

Twycross (2003) goes on to say that in palliative care it is the mismatch between the dying individual's ambitions and their ability to achieve these that causes poor quality of life. This situation can lead to feelings of poor self-esteem, which may in turn result in anxiety and depression. Indeed, hope and 'fighting spirit' have been correlated with a higher quality of life and the ability to adjust to one's situation (O'Connor et al. 2007). Therefore, Kim et al. (2005) suggest that quality of life can be improved in dying people by treating them holistically and ensuring their symptoms are managed, thus allowing the patients precious time with family and friends. This chapter has already discussed the principles of physical, psychological and spiritual care and also support of the family. How well these techniques can be employed within different care settings determines whether or not they have a positive or negative impact on the patients' and families' quality of life.

Is applicable early in the course of illness, in conjunction with other therapies that are intended to prolong life, such as chemotherapy or radiation therapy, and includes those investigations needed to better understand and manage distressing clinical complications

Many illnesses are incurable from diagnosis but may have a long disease trajectory. This includes dementia, chronic pulmonary disease, multiple sclerosis and some of the cancers. However, not all those diagnosed with these illnesses will require continuous care throughout their illness. What is required is a seamless multi-agency approach to each person's care that is flexible and which can call on the appropriate personnel in a timely fashion. Loftus (2000) suggests the solution to this is that each dying patient should have a nurse specialist, who acts as a key worker and has the ability to refer the patient to any services required during their illness. This would mean patients receiving the care and support they require in a timely fashion, which is not happening in the current health care arena. Indeed, Doyle (2008) suggests that palliative care provision for people who are dying of illnesses other than cancer remains poor as health care providers lack the confidence to provide palliative care to this group.

This WHO (2002) aim also suggests that when someone is receiving treatments early in an illness that is potentially curable, for example cancer, palliative care should be offered to alleviate current symptoms or to support the patient and family with other issues. However, this may be short-term involvement, until the symptom or crisis has resolved. Indeed, many palliative day services will support people undergoing chemotherapy or radiotherapy to prevent them from becoming isolated in the community (Stevens 2004).

The main issues with the utilisation of palliative interventions, as previously discussed, centres on ethical decision-making, in that all treatments offered at the end of life should be done so in the patient's best interests. This may include treatments such as chemotherapy, radiotherapy and the use of invasive investigations.

Practice Point 2.4

Having read this section, reflect on the barriers that prevent optimal palliative care being delivered in your clinical area.
   Are there any that could be easily remedied?

Commentary:

From this chapter it can be seen that there are many barriers to the provision of good palliative care, but many of these can be overcome using some of the guidance in this section. It is important for nurses to have in-depth under-standing of how palliative care can improve the quality of life of those with life-limiting illness and also promote a peaceful death. This is especially true given that it is nurses who spend most time with dying patients and their families.

References

Beauchamp TL and Childress JF (2001) *Principles of Biomedical Ethics*. Oxford: Oxford University Press.

Beckstrand RL, Clark-Callister L and Kirchhoff KT (2006) Providing a good death: critical care nurses suggestions for improving end of life care. *American Journal of Critical Care*. 15(1):38–45.

British Pain Society (2005) *Recommendations for the Appropriate Use of Opioids for Persistent Non-Cancer Pain*. London: BPS.

Calman K and Hine D (1995) *A Policy Framework for Commissioning Cancer Services*. London: Department of Health.

Clark D (1999) 'Total pain' disciplinary power and the body in the work of Cicely Saunders, 1958–1967. *Social Science and Medicine*. 49:727–736.

Clinical Standards Board for Scotland (2002). *Clinical Standards for Specialist Palliative Care*. Edinburgh: CSBS.

Crawford GB and Price SD (2003) Team working: palliative care as a model of interdisciplinary practice. *Medical Journal of Australia*. 176(Suppl 6): S32–S34.

Dietz JH (1981) *Rehabilitation Oncology*. New York: John Wiley.

Doyle D (1996) *Domiciliary Palliative Care: A Guide for the Primary Care Team*. Oxford: Oxford University Press.

Doyle D (2008) Palliative medicine in Britain. *Omega*. 56(1):77–88.

Doyle, D, Hanks G, Cherny N and Calman K (2005a) Introduction. In: Doyle D, Hanks G, Cherny N and Calman K (Eds), *Oxford Textbook of Palliative Medicine* (3rd edition). Oxford: Oxford University Press.

Doyle L, McClure J and Fisher S (2005b) The contribution of physiotherapy to palliative medicine. In Doyle D, Hanks G, Cherny N and Calman K (Eds), *Oxford Textbook of Palliative Medicine* (3rd edition). Oxford: Oxford University Press.

End of Life Programme (2008) Available at http://www.endoflifecare.nhs.uk/eolc. Accessed at 28 April 2008.

Faull C and Woof R (2002) *Palliative Care: An Oxford Core Text*. Oxford: Oxford University Press.

Ford G (1995) For Working Party on Clinical Guidelines in Palliative Care. *Information for Purchasers: Background to Available Specialist Palliative Care Services*. London: NCHSPCS.

Gilliat-Ray S (2001) Sociological perspectives on the pastoral care of minority faiths in hospital. In: Orchard H (Ed), *Spirituality in Health Care Contexts*. London: Jessica Kingsley, pp. 135–146.

Gomes B and Higginson IH (2008) Where people die (1974 – 2030): past trends, future projections and implications for care. Palliative Medicine. 22(1):33–41.

Harris S (2007) COPD and coping with breathlessness at home: a review of the literature. *British Journal of Community Nursing*. 12(9)411–412.

Jackson KC and Lipman AG (2004) Drug therapy for anxiety in palliative care. *Cochrane Database of Systematic Reviews*. Issue 1, Art No. CD004596.

Kaasa S (2000) Assessment of quality of life in palliative care. *Innovations in End of Life Care*. 2(6)12–14.

Kim A, Fall P and Wang D (2005) Palliative care: optimising quality of life. *Journal of the American Osteopathic Association*. 105(Suppl 5):9–14.

Lacasse C and Beck SL (2007) Clinical assessment of symptom clusters. *Seminars in Oncology Nursing*. 23(2):106–112.

Lickiss JN, Turner KS and Ploock ML (2005) The interdisciplinary team. In: Doyle D, Hanks G, Cherny N and Calman K (Eds), *Oxford Textbook of Palliative Medicine* (3rd edition). Oxford: Oxford University Press.

Loftus L (2000) A collaborative nursing model for advanced non-malignant disease. *International Journal of Palliative Nursing*. 6(9):454–458.

Matheson KW (2003) *Understanding and Resolving Grief*. Utah: Brigham University.

McCluskey L (2007) Palliative rehabilitation and amyotrophic lateral sclerosis: a perfect match. *Neurorehabilitation*. 22(6):407–408.

McSherry W and Cash K (2004) The language of spirituality: an emerging taxonomy. *International Journal of Nursing Studies*. 41(2):151–161.

Middlewood S, Gardner G and Gardner A (2001) Dying in hospital: Medical failure or natural outcome? *Journal of Pain and Symptom Management*. 22(6):1035–1041.

Milligan S (2004) Perceptions of spiritual care among nurses undertaking post-registration education. *International Journal of Palliative Nursing*. 10(4):162–171.

Murray RB and Zenter JB (1989) *Nursing Concepts for Health Promotion*. London: Prentice-Hall.

Narayanasamy A (2004) The puzzle of spirituality for nursing: a guide to practical assessment. *British Journal of Nursing*. 13(9):1140–1144.

National Council for Hospices and Specialist Palliative Care Services (1997) Dilemmas and directions: The future of specialist palliative care. A discussion paper. Occasional paper 11. London: NCHSPCS.

National Council for Hospices and Specialist Palliative Care Services (2006) *Fulfilling Lives: Rehabilitation in Palliative Care* (2nd edition). London: NCHSPCS.

National Council for Palliative Care (2008) Palliative care defined. Available at http://www.ncpc.org.uk/palliative_care.html. Accessed at 10 May 2008.

National Institute for Clinical Excellence (NICE) (2004) *Improving Supportive and Palliative Care for Adults with Cancer*. London: NICE.

Northhouse L (1984) The impact of cancer on the family: an overview. *International Journal of Psychiatry in Medicine*. 14(3):215–242.

O'Connor M, Guilfoyle A, Breen L, Mukhardt F, Fisher C (2007) Relationships between quality of life, spiritual well-being, and psychological adjustment styles for people living with leukaemia: an exploratory study. *Mental Health, Religion and Culture*. 10(6):631–647.

Odom J (2002) The nurse as patient advocate. *Journal of Perianaesthesia Nursing*. 17(2):75076.

Open University (2004) *K260 Death and Dying. Workbook 2: Caring for Dying People*. Milton Keynes: Open University.

Pearson EJM, Todd JG and Futcher JM (2007) How can occupational therapists measure outcomes in palliative care? *Palliative Medicine*. 21:477–485.

Ream E (2008) Fatigue. In: Stevens E and Edwards J. (Eds), *Palliative Care: Learning in Practice*. Exeter: Reflect Press.

Ryff C (1989) Happiness is everything, or is it? Explorations on the meaning of psychological well-being. *Journal of Personality and Social Psychology*. 57:1069–1081.

Ryff C and Keyes C (1995) The structure of psychological well-being revisited. *Journal of Personality and Social Psychology*. 69:719–727.

Saunders C (1996) Into the valley of the shadow of death. *British Medical Journal*. 313:1599–1601.

Saunders C (2001) The evolution of palliative care. *Journal of the Royal College of Medicine*. 94:430–432.

Scottish Executive Health Department (2001) *Cancer in Scotland – Action for Change*. Edinburgh: SEHD.

Scottish Partnership for Palliative Care (2006) *Joined up Thinking, Joined up Care*. Edinburgh: SPPC.

Seedhouse D (1998) *Ethics the Heart of Healthcare* (2nd edition). Chichester: Wiley.

Smitz LL and Woods AB (2006) Prevalence, severity and correlates of depressive symptoms on admission to inpatient hospice. *Journal of Hospice and Palliative Nursing*. 8(2):86–91.

Stevens E (2004) Palliative day care – more than tea and sympathy – Workshop 63: 15th International Congress on Care of the Terminally Ill. *Journal of Palliative Care*. 20(3):243.

Tan HM, Braunack-Mayer A and Beilby J (2005) The impact of the hospice environment on patient spiritual expression. *Oncology Nursing Forum*. 32(5):1049–1055.

Tookman A, Hopkins K and Scharpen-van-Heussen K (2005) Rehabilitation in palliative medicine. In: Doyle D, Hanks G, Cherny N and Calman K (Eds), *Oxford Textbook of Palliative Medicine* (3rd edition). Oxford: Oxford University Press.

Twycross R (2003) *Introducing Palliative Care* (4th edition). Oxford: Radcliffe Medical Publishing.

Twycross R and Wilcock A (2002) *Symptom Management in Advanced Cancer* (3rd edition). Oxford: Radcliffe Medical Press.

Vig EK and Pearlman RA (2003) Quality of life while dying: A qualitative study of older terminally ill men. *Journal of American Geriatric Society*. 51(11):1595–1601.

Wade DT and Halligan PW (2004) Do biomedical models of illness make good healthcare systems. *British Medical Journal*. 329:1398–1401.

Wallace J (2003) *Public Awareness of Palliative Care*. Edinburgh: SPPC.

Walter T (1992) Modern death – taboo or not taboo? *Sociology*. 25(2):293–310.

Welsh Assembly Government (2005) National Standards for Specialist Palliative Care Cancer Services. Wales Cancer Services Co-ordinating Group.

World Health Organization (1990) Cancer pain relief and palliative care. Report of an expert WHO committee. *Technical Support Series 804*. Geneva: WHO.

World Health Organization (1996) *Cancer Pain Relief* (2nd edition). Geneva: WHO.

World Health Organization (2002) WHO definition of palliative care. Available at http://www.who.int/cancer/palliative/definition/en/. Accessed on 29 April 2008.

Yuen KJ, Behrndt MM, Jacklyn C and Mitchell GK (2003) Palliative Care at home: General Practitioners working with palliative care teams. *Medical Journal of Australia*. 179(Suppl 6):S38–S40.

Zimmermann C and Rodin G (2004) The denial of death thesis: sociological critique and implications for palliative care. *Palliative Medicine*. 18(2):121–128.

Chapter 3

Providing palliative care for marginalised and disenfranchised people

John Atkinson

Introduction

Although currently an academic, my experience has emerged through clinical and management practice points. Specifically I nursed homeless men in Glasgow as a District Nurse and, undertaking my PhD with this group, subsequently published (Atkinson 2000). I was a member of the first HIV/AIDS community team in Scotland (Atkinson 2006). During this period, I was assisting a project in the early 1990s, caring for 200 children with HIV in Romania (Atkinson 1993). Before coming into academic life, I was the Health Care Manager in HM Prison Barlinnie. Finally, a profound influence has been the journey with my son who has a severe language and communication disability. Our family engages in activity with the AFASIC charity, which supports families with children with communication difficulties (Atkinson and Atkinson 2008). In recent years, I have also been influenced by friendship with Dr Paul Keeley, Palliative Care Consultant at Glasgow Royal Infirmary.

The readers will see that this is an assortment of experience. For this reason, therefore, my contribution is not written as an academic thesis or a mainstream assertion of being representative. It is presented as a reflection from a traveller and imperfect witness with some signposts to assist the readers. The overarching themes in the journey are:

- How contextually specific palliative care is in practice
- The limitations of being without autonomy and financial and/or social resource
- The burden of moral worthiness and patient conformity
- The curse of an evidence base
- The use of public money and distributive versus social justice

These themes combine with underlying non-clinical (but perhaps the central) features currently being discussed in the 'palliative care' field. Specifically, how do we address loss of identity, disengagement from social context and exile, or loss of meaning? Referring to Coyle's (2004) work *The Existential Slap*, Duncan Forbes, Chief Executive of the Shakespeare Hospice, has described the objective, measurable nature of these elements (Forbes 2007). My journey often takes place in a non-medical world where clinical care appears peripheral. This resonates with the debate regarding the medicalising of death and palliative care (Clark 2002).

Learning outcomes

Once you have read this chapter and completed the associated practice points, you will be able to:

- Discuss what is meant by the term marginalised and disenfranchised people
- Describe the place where marginalised and disenfranchised people can be found
- Discuss the impact of marginalisation and disenfranchisement on the provision of palliative care.

Where are they?

HM Prison Barlinnie is one of the busiest prisons in Europe with 16 000–18 000 admissions a year, all of whom have to be assessed and monitored by health care staff; a great many of the prisoners have enduring mental and physical health problems. During my time there, I was asked to come and speak to a nursing interest group about palliative care in prisons. At first, my intended response was simple – there wasn't any – therefore, I would write a polite letter of refusal.

On brief reflection, however, some questions emerged. These combined with experience with homeless people in hostels and sleeping rough, also adults and children with HIV. Other marginalised people met while a community nurse such as the isolated elderly – whether in their own or nursing homes – also resonated. The most obvious answer regarding prisons was that most of the prisoners were under 35 years of age. Although many of them had ill health, very few had cancer or were dying. Nevertheless, the consideration of these practical issues did reveal some of the fundamental barriers and pathways to resolution of the provision of palliative care to marginalised and disenfranchised people. I gave the presentation and began a continuing journey of discovery and reflection. The rest of this contribution will highlight these features. They do not pretend to be the truth, merely observations which may be useful.

Overview and context

The idea of 'marginalised' people can be seen throughout the non-specialist and professional literature. For the purposes of this contribution, it simply means individuals and groups who are considered by society to be outside the mainstream. This may stem from ethnic or cultural difference, contrast in moral values, different social and domestic structure, all of which are often associated with conflicting or aberrant behavioural norms. An associated theme is a lack of voice or influence – the disenfranchised – with a concomitant lack of access to succour and advocacy. Individuals and groups often cited are the homeless, those with self-inflicted diseases; prisoners; ethnic minorities; vulnerable children and the elderly.

In relation to palliative care, provision also means those considered 'difficult to reach'. This concept has wide and unfocused boundaries. Those of us who assist the marginalised may sometimes wryly think or remark:

> *'Yes, the homeless are difficult to reach in a hospital or health centre, but considerably less so if you actually go and speak to them on the street or in a hostel.'*

The package versus active ingredients

In relation to many forms of professional care, these contextual issues are important when providing a service. If I set up a prisoner or homeless person in a cell or hostel with a syringe driver, am I giving palliative care? If not, how much intervention by designated professionals and other parts of the 'package' would constitute palliative care?

There is an old story from the Jewish tradition of a dying elder who had managed to keep his people safe. Passing on the secret, he told his successor a precise place in the wood, and then asked him to build a special fire, say a particular prayer and pass the secret on to future generations. The first generation eventually forgot where the place was, the next forgot how to build the fire and the third forgot the prayer. Worried, the fourth generation elder looked heavenwards and said 'I've forgotten the place, the fire and the prayer – but I remember the story, does this count?'

If I care for someone in a 'palliative way' without diagnosis or formal recognition, is it still palliative care? Do outsiders have to recognise what you are doing for it to be palliative care?

Bioethical principles

Returning to my own journey, I began to consider 'what are the objective, rather than perspective, challenges to the provision of palliative care to marginalised people?' A good seam of insight came by considering the well-known 'Georgetown School' bioethical principles: autonomy, beneficence, non-malfeasance and justice (Gillon 1994). These principles echo the older precepts found in most ancient religions and cultures, in particular the ethic of reciprocity, 'The Golden Rule'. That is to treat your neighbour as you would like to be treated (Fredriksson and Eriksson 2003).

Autonomy and non-malfeasance

During my period of office in the prison service, there was a spate of trials of elderly men for sexual crimes they had committed some decades before. Special provision was made for them. Part of the clinical discussion was the procedures to be enacted in case of cardiac arrest and other circumstances where resuscitation was required. Legal and other advice was sought. It was decided that assertive intervention must always be practised to demonstrate that the prisoner was given the same service available to any citizen regardless of context.

Allied to this judgement was the recognition of an unequal power relationship with the prisoner/patient who had been deprived of his liberty. In cases like these, it is difficult to demonstrate freedom, lack of coercion and informed consent. As with many other marginalised individuals, there is often a fine line between accounting for an individual's wishes for autonomous action or inaction and malfeasant negligence. Such defensive practice, while necessary, strikes at an important precept of palliation.

The nature of good palliative care is a contract between equals. The helper should not be in authority over the helped. However, this 'clean' position is often compromised if the individuals have difficulty in communicating, or cannot communicate, their wishes. The practitioner with relatives and other members of the team may then be in the position of enacting what they think would be in the best interests of the patient – benign paternalism.

Autonomy and resource

Another aspect of autonomy, the authority over financial and social resource, is not generally part of an ethics discussion. It may be seen with individuals living in limited or dangerous circumstances. When planning any package of care, severe financial and social limitations, for example housing and family, restrict the ability of the individual to access the broad range of care. That is, one requires a certain amount of financial or collateral social resource to 'buy' one's space and room to operate. Even in a social medicine model, like the UK National Health Service, freedom of choice is often severely curtailed by lack of resource. Those without social or family resource can find themselves in desperate and straitened circumstances, despite relative monetary afflu-ence. The elderly persons living alone in their family house is an often-seen example.

Precipitate illness careers

The effect of restricted social and financial resource can have a devastating clinical impact. This derives from the lack of ability to self-care and the limitation of the ability to improve the environment or increase support. Some examples exemplify these issues.

Example one

During the study of homeless men in hostels (Atkinson 2000), a battery of assessments was administered including the Barthel Index of Physical Function which marks the individual out of 100 (Mahoney and Barthel 1965). In a well-equipped and -serviced council-run hostel, a variety of ability and disability scores were recorded. In the ill-equipped, minimally serviced private hostel, the pattern was completely different and disturbing. The scores tended to be in the 90s until an individual had a calamitous downturn to 0–10, at which stage he would have to go to hospital. Many would never return and die.

On further investigation it was found that the score actually gave more information about the facilities than about the individual. The individual would be in physical decline for some time. Because the toilet, or other feature, was up two flights of stairs, for example, he would score highly because he could achieve the task, but the tool did not record that it took half an hour to accomplish it. Eventually, the individual can no longer achieve these tasks and 'crashes'.

Example two

In places like prisons the limitations on personal freedom exacerbate seemingly minor problems. Examples such as septic fingers, small injuries and dehydration can often result in serious illness because of the individual's inability to enact minor restorative interventions. This also applies to people with mental health problems and is commonly seen when there is a combination of marginalising factors. In hospitals it may be witnessed when, for example a disabled or mentally ill person is admitted with an acute event like a fracture. The new incapacity destroys the individuals', sometimes fragile, ability to deal with their other problems. In the care of patients with diseases like cancer, this situation is often compounded by the physical deterioration of the individual's health.

Example three

In the project looking after 200 HIV positive children in institutions in Romania (Atkinson 1993), the first impression was one of high mortality. On further investigation, however, it was discovered that the children were not dying from HIV/AIDS but from malnutrition and dehydration. Enough food and fluid was available, but it was not being taken by all the children. The children were in large wards and were literally lost. Nobody knew who they were, whether they were better or worse than last week or whether they had eaten or not. The stronger, more resourceful, children would steal the milk bottles from other cots where they were lying unattended. A simple programme of identification (names on plastic bibs), progress/centile and feeding charts was enacted with dramatic results.

It may be seen from these examples that the 'space' where one might normally find palliative care was missing entirely. The inability of the individual to impact on their context – self-agency – curtailed access to care and a positive outcome.

The lie of consent?

In these circumstances the very idea of choice and consent is compromised. There is also the attitude of the outsider or carer looking in. Using a quasi non-judgemental approach, the onlookers shake their head and may say 'what can be done? It's his choice'. This is stated as though the homeless man has experienced the same decision-making journey as, say, a large middle-aged comfortable academic.

In the same way, as patients, our actual choice would be not to have the cancer or illness. Given that this is not possible, we are given the imperfect choices with which to consent. However, these come with several terms, conditions, behaviours and other strings. That is not to say they are wrong, but we should, perhaps, recognise more robustly what they really are – compromises and trade-offs.

Practice Point 3.1

Consider the place of care and its impact on palliative care provision. How do you think palliative care could be provided to this group?

Commentary:

The place of care has a huge impact on the provision of palliative care as seen in this account. This combined with the issues of being a prisoner where liberty and choice are affected means that palliative care provision can be difficult to access. Read Shaw's (2007) report into the death of a prisoner at MHP Norwich. It gives some insight into the challenges of providing good care to prisoners at the end of life in the prison environment. It can be accessed at http://www.ppo.gov.uk/download/fatal-incident-reports/B081.06%20Death%20of%20a%20Male%20Prisoner.pdf.

Beneficence and the curse of evidence base

The idea of beneficence – doing good – at first appears to be the least complicated ethical principle to undertake. And yet in areas like palliative care and assisting those in marginalised positions, the experience of doing good things can be thorny. There is sometimes a dissonant interaction between the principal of ensuring autonomy – the right to free action – and beneficence, doing good. Autonomy is only of value if the proposed action produces benefit, for example if an individual demands treatment which the practitioner thinks will do them harm. In a professional, public service context, the difficulty often arises in the interpretation of the universally accepted definitions of 'evidence-based care'.

This is not as heretical as it sounds. In the pure, abstract sense it can only be 'good' if we care for others using practice points which have been demonstrated or measured to be effective. The difficulty arises in how and what we measure.

What are the active ingredients? Are we trying to measure or enact a specific intervention or, conversely, create a generally conducive environment?

Coming from a family of caterers, I can feel the frowns of my much missed English chef father and Italian hotelier forbears as I sit here eating my lunch and writing this. The meal is very healthy with lots of fruit, oatcakes, humus, fluid, etc. However, there is no event, meal or ritual, no companionship – literally there is no sharing of bread. It is a functional fuel stop. Conversely, would one look at the menu, nutritional value and cooking *or* the human interaction if one were to measure the efficacy of a conference dinner or wedding? In clinical care we tend to examine the content of the activity rather than its human context and impact.

As with many aspects of care there is a long history in the spiritual and religious literature connecting the efficacy of the deed with 'sacramental' impact on the 'soul' or well-being and the demonstration of the great agape or love. (McCabe 1986).

A more worldly, but nevertheless poignant, example was witnessed by my family with my son and his friend in their first year of school in a language unit. Both had only a few words between them, so to converse they would sit together, pointing and speaking the names of the items in each other's lunch boxes to each other in companionship.

The importance of impact rather than content in areas such as palliation or the care of marginalised people with deep and complex problems comes into relief if we add the words 'effective' and 'value for money'. These terms are inextricably linked in the public service discourse with any notion of doing good.

What is effective and valuable?

As my wife, daughter and I have accompanied my son through his journey with a severe language and communication disability, several examples have emerged (Atkinson and Atkinson 2008). He was not able to speak at all until he was seven and now at 12 he is gaining in articulacy and fluency. We can itemise certain active ingredients to this progress: the correct professional help, domestic strategy, tactics for encouraging positive interaction, etc. However, having set up a few important principles, there have been long hours and days of not much happening.

In my case this has been characterised by constant physical presence, literally following him, looking out for danger as he walked, quartered and discovered the world, without language at first, but gradually mapping and making sense of it. This has been highly successful, but it would be difficult to measure just how many hours and days walking and wandering in the wilderness was effective. As to value for money, we were unpaid informal carers for these practice points, but the whole situation had considerable impact on our family's earning capacity. It is difficult to set up a professional service of this kind. They are expensive and time-consuming.

Another simple example of the difficulty of achieving evidence-based, effective value for money 'good' came in a study undertaken examining patients' cancer journeys in Kintyre, where individuals had to travel 120 miles to receive their treatment in Glasgow (Atkinson et al. 2002). A small but key feature that improved patients' experience was if they had a contact living in the Glasgow area. Regular short visits and the ability to undertake small services, such as washing clothes, made a great difference. When the study team and professional carers came together, we were struck by the complexity of trying to professionally replicate these small but important informal interventions. This included a hilarious conversation. The possibilities of 'laundry liaison operatives', with Control of Substances Hazardous to Health committees and other bureaucratic considerations were absurdly deliberated.

Social and distributive justice

Once an intervention or service is professionalised, it can become a blunt and time-limited weapon. Having to demonstrate that all highly paid (compared to informal care) time is effective provides challenges. Clinical rather than social interventions are often easier to measure and justify, with their firm causal links. Presence, expert monitoring, improving the general situation and seeming inaction are all difficult to advocate, even if they are recognised as good and just.

The difficulties in translating notions of good are reflected in the delivery of justice – doing the right thing. Evidence and financial probity tend to drive us towards distributive justice – providing tangible, effective intervention to the most needy – rather than the more rights-based precepts of social justice. The term 'effective' takes on another dimension when considering distribution of resource or service within any population. It ceases to mean the content of the intervention 'does it work?' and becomes the measurement of positive uptake 'how many hits?' It is here that the individual and groups' compliance or concordance to the intervention and programme become part of the efficacy equation. This is compounded in many countries with the consideration of the individuals' personal resources and their ability to sustain an expensive programme of care. Transplant and associated therapy are a good example.

It may therefore be seen that delivering highly measurable, clinically based interventions to individuals and groups who are well behaved, obedient, reliable and able to take forward the programme in a stable environment is *actually* the more effective pathway. It is rationally the most just thing to do and fits the philosophical utilitarian principle of 'the greatest good for the greatest number'. It also has an extreme effect on others – it marginalises, not least because we may also be delivering the right care but to those who need it least.

Time limitations – cancer, non-malignancy and lifestyle

Distributive justice is often well served by the life-limiting aspects of cancer disease. It compartmentalises events to a particular time and place in an individual's life. It can have the effect of, perhaps conveniently, helping practitioners to focus on the immediate and short-term illness, rather than have to engage with the complexity of an ongoing life. This has profoundly marginalising consequences.

Through the looking glass – the after and secondary cancer marginalised

The marginalising effects of distribution have been a part of the personal journey. This has been seen both as a parent and as a 50 something adult. There are now considerable numbers of the population, including close family and friends, who have survived the first onslaught of cancer but have now gone into another world of either secondary cancer or non-malignant, debilitating consequences of malignant disease and its treatment.

BBC Radio 4 *Woman's Hour* recently had a series where women described their experience of cancer. A recurring theme was the isolation, loss of friends and community experienced, especially in secondary and post-cancer illness. Having been through their first 'war', where those around engaged in supportive actions and attitudes, subsequent malignant and non-malignant illness was met with avoidance, horror and sometimes ostracisation. Here was a new marginalised group. Again the non-clinical themes of existence, loss of place and meaning were central.

Practice Point 3.2

Think about the patients in your care. How does their diagnosis marginalise them in health care and in society?

Commentary:

You may see patients who have illnesses such as HIV shunned as there is still stigma around this illness. Those with chronic obstructive pulmonary disease are denied access to public areas because of the safety factors associated with oxygen. People with dementia in general wards may be classed as disruptive and not receive the care they deserve as they are unable to express their choices and needs. There are many more examples, but is it fair to say may be that at some point in time we be marginalised when we are ill?

Non-malignant long-term illness

The problem of 'existing beyond' goes further. For the purposes of this contribution the debate regarding non-malignant palliative care is not concerned with methodology – how it can be achieved in various taxonomies of disease. Rather it is the fascinating realisation that more of us, if not everyone, can benefit from palliative care. This immediately raises the practical and conceptual difficulties of the movement and practice not being special anymore if it is for everyone. Where does palliative care end and 'ordinary' care begin?

Of interest is that this consideration brings us back to the ideas of the founders of terminal and palliative care. A BBC Radio interview several years ago described the mission of taking care out of the mainstream and improving it, before taking it back. We have seen this develop over the years, so that some practices, considered specialist previously, may be observed in general situations.

In terms of addressing the dilemma of social versus distributive justice, it may be said that part of the energy must be used to generalise, if not industrialise, the bespoke specialist to the mainstream ready to wear.

Culture and moral worthiness

Another, often-criticised but well-grounded utilitarian principle is seeking the happiness of the majority and avoiding their unhappiness or discomfort, which may place further restrictions. Firstly, ideas of the public comfort can appear- and be experienced-as unbalanced and capricious. Tolerance of situations and behaviour is often culturally or familiarity, not evidence, based. For example, in the area I live, I have never seen a drunken person thrown off a bus, but my son and I have been when, aged about seven, he became upset. We have also been asked on occasion, when interacting with public institutions, to consider whether his presence would be wise given that his possible behaviour may upset people. Smiling outwardly, but in despair and rage internally, we have sometimes considered it better to withdraw.

The esteem of cancer and the undeserving – existential assumptions

When people are at the end of their life, especially if they are considered blameless, they must be protected even more than most. The more limited and sheltered an individual's life has been, the more protection they must receive. This is not an argument against these standpoints, but it may be seen that if one takes them as principles for what is acceptable or not, severe restrictions are placed on a service which purports to be inclusive.

Combined with this approach is often the existential assumption that it is somehow more tragic when a young and gifted musician dies of cancer than a young drug user of AIDS. It is more tragic because one person was seen to be 'going' somewhere. The esteem in which cancer is held and the moral worthiness bestowed on cancer 'victims' as they 'battle' their way through their journey have a marginalising effect on the patients themselves as well as those with less worthy diseases. The late John Diamond's *Because Cowards Get Cancer Too* (1999) is a highly recommended reading as is Ruth Picardie's *Before I Say Goodbye* (1998) and Jonathan Wilson's *Deadman Writing* (2002).

Another example was a man I cared for who had received HIV-infected blood while being treated for leukaemia. The attitude towards him, in many quarters, changed dramatically as someone with AIDS rather than someone with cancer.

The religion, language and ritual of hospice

Perhaps in consequence to its special place of moral worthiness, the practice of caring for people with cancer and palliative needs has taken on a ritual observance ethos, outside strictly spiritual considerations. From the outside this is dramatic for patients and others alike.

'The hospice movement is too good to be true and too small to be useful' (Douglas 1992) In the nearly 5 years spent in the prison service, our health centre received one or two 'thank you' letters. In the ribald way that nurses do, colleagues would mercilessly take the rise out of workmates leaving to work with children or palliative care: 'Send us some of the chocolates!' 'You won't need all those presents!' and other remarks. The palliative workers are put in a special place of respect.

The activity of physically caring for dying or distressed people is also special. When I first worked with homeless men, I engaged in many clinics and physical care. I would wash and bind wounded legs and feet. I felt truly good, like Jesus. My proudest day occurred when a man returned to me after about 3 months. My bandage was still intact. By some miracle it had also done him no harm. More importantly, the event made me change the course of my actions. Instead of concentrating on hands-on care, I engaged more in advocacy, registering individuals with GPs and other services – recruiting more help from more people. I was not at the centre of the activity any more. In my present position I continue this underground 'pushing pennies up the board' approach, helping students, colleagues and groups. There are fewer big hits but many minor victories. The shift is to make a change in the environment not just the individual, so that he or she and others would not necessarily need you in the future. This links with the ideas seen in health and overseas development education: 'If you teach a man to fish he can feed himself for the rest of his life'.

Cinderella practitioners

To deliver care effectively, the practitioner must also have place, identity, purpose and meaning. When people are on the edge and in distress, their problems, behaviour and situation are often perceived as negative and a malign influence. They upset the calm and do not sit well in nice surroundings. Their problems are messy and intractable; there is often no 'closure' or satisfactory outcome. The only justification or satisfaction gained is often abstract: That one did one's duty. Examples may be found:

In De la Mare's poem *The Listeners*
'Tell them I came, and no one answered, that I kept my word;'

From principles of shared exile and humanity from a religious perspective – as in the *Conversations and Exhortations of Father Zossima* in Dostoevsky's *The Brother's Karamazov*:

> 'Lord, have mercy on all who appear before Thee today. For every hour and every moment thousands of men leave life on this earth, and their souls appear before God. And how many of them depart in solitude, unknown, sad, dejected that no one mourns for them or even knows whether they have lived or not!' (From *Of Prayer, of Love, and of Contact with other Worlds*)

From a secular existentialist standpoint, as with Dr Rieux in Albert Camus's *The Plague*:

> 'Following the dictates of his heart, he has deliberately taken the victim's side and tried to share with his fellow-citizens the only certitudes they have in common – love, suffering and exile.' (From Part V Chapter 7)

Although these motivations are easily recognised, they do not always sit easily with a highly focused clinical approach. Perhaps there needs to be a mixture of focus and 'embracing the mess'.

Pathways to resolution – clinical and restorative palliative care

To conclude this contribution, there follows some synthesis of the observations into possibilities for action. Over the time of this journey I have been constantly amazed how much real change can be implemented by looking at the 'problem' differently. This combines with the more obvious elements of new evidence and good planning. There is evidence that all of these possibilities are being practised, some more than others.

Self-inflicted? We are all marginalised

Over the last few years the demarcation between innocent victims and self-inflicted pariahs is becoming blurred. As each scientific insight emerges it appears that all of our behaviours, positive and negative, can influence our sickness and wellness journeys and trajectories. For those of us who have engaged in most of them this is all very alarming! There is a growing need, therefore, to strive to enable access to appropriate care for all, without discrimination.

The mental shift is, perhaps, to recognise that – instead of marginalised groups – we all become marginalised at periods in our life. This may be precipitated by illness, change of circumstances or disastrous event. If that principle is accepted, it is probably also logical that a variety of delivery methods and contexts is likely as a consequence. The emphasis becomes on recognising the effective active ingredients, not only on how they are delivered.

Use of non-clinical evidence and criteria – changing the stated aims

If we absorb the existential, non-clinical, but measurable impacts of cancer/ disability/long-term illness discussed by Clark (2002), Coyle (2004), Forbes (2007) and others, it is possible to improve and change the stated aims of care 'packages'. These include the loss of identity, place in community, purpose and meaning. This widens the variety of inputs, outputs and outcomes and enables appropriate evaluation. It also stamps on some nonsensical red herrings, such as using randomised controlled trials as the only proof of evidence.

For example, if a formal stated aim is to encourage practice points and interventions to restore an individual's sense of identity and community, then the focus of evaluation would perhaps focus on the impact of the event rather than its content, not whether tai chi or bingo was most effective.

Assisting non-professional approaches

The just distribution of resources can also be achieved if the practitioner/ clinical setting stops being the centre of intervention and become the advocate and commissioner of a variety of community-based approaches. Clinical practitioners, hospices, and others command great respect. Spreading the message and practice through committees and other minimal intervention community strategies – the organisation of focused voluntary activity for example – is an effective way of reaching those in marginalised circumstances.

The judicious and subtle involvement of palliative care practitioners and institutions as integrated in their mainstream and outcast communities may strengthen identity and community and affirm shared humanity. This is practical not ethereal, just as the great cities of California are named after the Franciscan missionary outposts which embedded in their communities. Sometimes a telephone call or short show of presence from a respected professional or institution can make all the difference to a marginal cause.

Sometimes the clinician's skill is not the most important. A patient with AIDS our team was looking after had a distressing skin condition. This was in the early days of the HIV phenomena. How could we assist while keeping his confidentiality? The nurses and social workers cogitated and deliberated specialist laundry and other ideas.

'Why don't I organise a washing machine?' said the colleague from Housing.

'Of course!' we exclaimed. In Scotland many elderly people's lives have been improved dramatically by the government scheme to upgrade people's heating with new systems. It enables their homes to be fully functional and good to visit, apart from benefiting health. The job here is to connect the individual with the right assistance. Sometimes I need a radiator not a nurse. The lesson is to have a wide variety of professional input – and possibly, always have someone from Housing on your team!

Focus on outcome rather than method

The encouragement of variety also enables a less field-dependent approach to clinical and non-clinical intervention. Caring for someone in a prison or hostel is different than in a hospice, but satisfactory outcomes may be achieved nonetheless.

Conclusion – the palliative approach

The reason, in my analysis, why positive outcomes are possible in a variety of good and bad environments is that individuals all respond to interaction which seeks to support and restore identity, community, meaning and purpose. The bestowal of these precepts of shared humanity makes the literal difference between life and death and of a life worth living. It is strange to use a term like 'love' in reference to places like prisons, hostels, dark orphanages and streets, unless one has witnessed it and its lack. It is not sentimental and can be described by observing quantitative aspects of health, function and reciprocity. There are also elements of mutual self-interest.

However, in the homeless study several relationships were recorded of younger residents assisting older, infirm men for specific tasks, building up small therapeutic regimes. Similarly, in prisons and elsewhere, relationships and actions beyond survival encourage life and restore. When in situations which are stripped out of other features, these elements are seen clear. Perhaps, these are the centre of the 'palliative approach'.

If asked what are the most useful tools learned and used, repeated experience has shown three.

Bearing witness

Accompany the individual into the desert, literally or metaphorically. Make it plain that their story is not forgotten. It will be recorded, told and action advocated and undertaken. Assist an individual stabilise and come to a realisation that life can go on even when everything held dear appears to be smashed. That it is possible to proceed without a previous identity and perhaps find a new one or return after a period in the wilderness, as in the old anonymous song.

> 'Farewell my friends I'm bound for Canaan
> I'm traveling through the wilderness
> Your company has been delightful
> You who doth leave my mind distressed
> I go away behind to leave you

Perhaps never to meet again
But if we never have the pleasure
I hope we'll meet on Canaan's land'

Assertive beneficence

There is a diplomatic position associated with witness and action enshrined in the Scottish Crown and Black Watch motto 'Nemo me impune lacessit' meaning 'No one provokes me with impunity'. It can be a war cry, but it also means that one advocates and stands with an individual, group or cause so that it must be taken into account. In clinical practice terms this means having the personal and professional confidence, and sometimes status, to advocate for an intervention or action.

The grace of disgrace

A disturbing part of 'professionalism' can be the need for the professional to look good, at the centre of their competent world, and not to engage in practice points where they cannot shine. It is often argued that this is essential to instil public confidence. When assisting those in marginalised circumstances this can be a serious barrier. Sometimes the best outcome is achieved and the practitioner or service does *not* appear to come out well, going in 'under fire' and without all the answers.

Perhaps we did forget the precise place, how to build the special fire, say the particular prayer, but we saved the patient and remembered the story.

References

Atkinson J (1993) When somebody knows my name – report on a care project for care of 200 HIV positive children in Romania. *Radix Journal* 7, October San Francisco.

Atkinson J (2000) *Nursing Homeless Men – A Study of Proactive Intervention.* London: Whurr Publishers.

Atkinson J (2006) The person with HIV/AIDS, Chapter 37. In: Alexander MF, Fawcett JN and Runciman PJ (Eds), *Nursing Practice – Hospital and Home, The Adult.* Edinburgh: Elsevier Health Sciences, pp. 1169–1190.

Atkinson P and Atkinson J (2008). It's just the words are stuck in his heart. *AFASIC Magazine* Spring: 4:10–12.

Atkinson J, Kennedy E, Goldworthy S and Drummond S (2002) Patients' cancer journeys in Kintyre – a qualitative study of the care, support and information needs of people with cancer and their carers. *European Journal of Oncology Nursing.* 6(2):85–92.

Clark D (2002) Between hope and dying: the medicalisation of dying. *British Medical Journal.* 324:905–907.

Coyle N (2004) The existential slap – a crisis of disclosure. *International Journal of Palliative Nursing.* 10:520.

Diamond J (1999) *Because Cowards Get Cancer Too – A Hypochondriac Confronts His Nemesis*. London: Crown Publishers.

Douglas C (1992) For all the saints. *British Medical Journal*. 304:579.

Forbes D (2007) Conference presentation. Association of Palliative Day Care Leaders Annual Conference, 12 September Birmingham.

Fredriksson L and Eriksson K (2003) The ethics of the caring conversation. *Nursing Ethics*. 10(2):138–148.

Gillon R (1994) Medical ethics: four principles plus attention to scope. *British Medical Journal*. 309:184–188.

Mahoney FI and Barthel D (1965). Functional evaluation: the barthel index. *Maryland State Medical Journal*. 14:56–61.

McCabe H (1986) A long sermon for Holy Week Part 1. Holy Thursday: the mystery of unity. *New Blackfriars*. 67:59–69.

Picardie R (1998) *Before I Say Goodbye*. Harmondsworth: Penguin.

Shaw S (2007) Investigation into the circumstances surrounding the death of a man who was a prisoner at MHP Norwich in September 2006: Report by the Prisoners and Probation Ombudsman for England and Wales. Available at http://www.ppo. gov.uk/download/fatal-incident-reports/B081.06%20Death%20of%20a%20Male% 20Prisoner.pdf. Accessed on 28 April 2008.

Wilson J (2002) *Deadman Writing*. Ayrhsire: Deadman Publishers.

Section Two

Palliative Nursing Across Care Settings

Chapter 4

Palliative nursing care in the acute hospital

Philip Saltmarsh

Introduction

The aim of this chapter is to discuss the provision of palliative nursing care in the acute hospital setting. It begins by examining the demographics relating to dying in hospital before reviewing the identified barriers that prevent the provision of optimal palliative nursing care within the hospital setting. The chapter then proceeds to show how good palliative care can be provided in the hospital setting.

Learning outcomes

Once you have read this chapter and completed the associated practice points, you will be able to:

- Discuss the different settings where people die within the acute hospital
- Describe the process of accessing a specialist palliative care team within your own clinical area
- Give examples of the barriers to the provision of optimal palliative care within the hospital setting
- Illustrate the benefits of the Liverpool Care Pathway (LCP) for your own clinical area

Background

Over 500 000 adults die in England each year (Office of National Statistics 2005) and although over 50% of people say they would like to be cared for and die at home if they were terminally ill, at present only 20% of people die at home (DoH 2006). The choice to die at home is also a priority for those dying in other countries of the UK (Scottish Partnership for Palliative Care 2007; Thomas 2007; Tiernan et al. 2002), although the guidance from the DoH (2006) recognises this and is working towards improving choice for all patients, through initiatives such as The End of Life Programme (www.endoflifecare.nhs.uk). However, as in England the majority of deaths in the UK continue to take place in hospitals which is not only expensive but also affects the quality of the dying experience (Thomas 2007). Indeed there are reports that dying in hospital can be a distressing experience for both patients and families, with reports from relatives such as:

> 'My husband died without a shred of dignity. His nursing care was shamefully poor. The communication from the nurses was minimal, grudging and curt.'
> (Robinson 2007).

The National Institute of Clinical Excellence (2004) suggests that there are two levels of palliative care, generalist palliative care and specialist palliative care, and that all those with a life-limiting illness should receive the level of palliative care required regardless of place of care. This poses two challenges for hospital nurses in that first and foremost they should have the knowledge and skills to provide general palliative care when it is required but secondly they should know when they have exhausted their expertise and have the ability to call in a specialist palliative care team. Indeed, Scott (2005) suggests that nurses, no matter the area of their expertise, should have the skills to care for dying patients and that these skills are essential to the provision of individualised, holistic palliative care.

Practice Point 4.1

In the last month how many patients died in your clinical area? Of these how many died from a degenerative condition such as cancer, heart failure or a neurological condition? Do you know if hospital was their preferred place of death?

Commentary:

What you will probably find is that the number of deaths in your area rises and falls within any monthly period unless you work in an area that is dedicated to the care of people at the end of life. However, it is likely that in most ward areas the majority of the deaths occurred in older adults who had been diagnosed with a life-limiting illness. However, there are specific issues relating to death in intensive care units (ICU) and accident and emergency (A & E), which will be reviewed later in the chapter. If you look at the figures for deaths in your unit over a year, you could calculate the percentage of annual deaths and this would give the nursing team an idea of how many people would require palliative or end of life care in the future. In relation to preferred place of care, unless the patient has been referred to a specialist palliative care team these wishes may not be known. The guidance from the DoH (2006) recognises and is working towards improving choice for all patients. However, there is also recognition that wherever we care for people all staff should have the necessary skills to meet the needs of patients and carers.

The next section looks at the barriers that exist in hospitals that prevent the provision of the best possible palliative care regardless of the level required.

Barriers to palliative care provision in hospital

It is important to understand how institutions dominated by a scientific medical model of care manage the process of death and dying amidst the work of sustaining life. There is a conflict between the stated professional ambition to heal and restore (British Medical Association 1999) and the reality of human mortality. This combined with the notion that society celebrates the healthy, the beautiful and the living (Walter 2004) makes it difficult for professionals to acknowledge that death is the final part of life. Therefore, without the correct knowledge and skill nurses can act like much of the rest of society and simply look the other way when faced with loss and death (Robinson 2007).

It is known that palliative care is only a small part of the remit in some hospital areas and as such nurses may not have access to the education and training required to provide optimal palliative care. This is especially true of the availability and attendance at communication skills courses which can help nurses to offer effective palliative care by providing them with the skills to do so (Jarrett and Maslin-Prothero 2004). The need to have adequately trained nurses has also been identified within national guidance (DoH 2006). Nurses need to be able to assess and manage the palliative care needs for their patients within their skill base, as a fundamental part of their practice (Scott 2005). However, they also need to know when to refer patients to a specialist team when their skills are exhausted. Indeed, the National Institute of Clinical Excellence (NICE) (2004) suggests that where the general palliative care providers have not received adequate training they should refer all patients at the end of life to the specialist team.

Dying in a hospital ward

When a patient dies in a general ward the conflict between cure and care may result in awkwardness and embarrassment and attempts to conceal death from other patients (Bryan 2007). Also within this ethos many professionals working in hospitals feel they have failed patients if they cannot cure them (Smith 2000). These feelings of failure lead to the dying feeling alone and isolated as staff may distance themselves from such patients. However, Middlewood et al. (2001) suggest that professionals frequently feel they need to keep treating patients to prolong life, often at the expense of the quality of such life. While often this is done to maintain hope within the patient and family, it prevents them from making decisions about the life they have left together.

The majority of people with life-limiting illnesses die on wards within acute hospitals where the care is geared to managing acutely unwell patients who require intensive, curative treatments which are time orientated. This inevitably means that dying patients not always afforded the time to form relationships with the nursing team and as such feelings of loneliness and abandonment are compounded. The Audit Commission (2003) also suggests that many patients do not receive a bed on the ward that was most suitable for them and that this could have a negative impact on the care they receive. Indeed elderly patients who have life-limiting conditions often fair worst within the acute sector and are often referred to as 'bed blockers'. Bates (2004) suggests that political pressures have replaced compassionate care when patients are at their most vulnerable and that they are no longer afforded the dignity and care they deserve when they have nowhere to go. This ultimately affects their feelings of well-being and we know that anxiety and depression cause more suffering in the dying person than physical symptomology.

Dying in hospital, however, does not just happen in ward areas but also in areas such as A & E departments and intensive care units. This chapter now reviews the barriers identified in the literature that may prevent the provision of good palliative care within these areas.

Dying in Accident and Emergency

Accident and Emergency (A & E) units have to prioritise the care they provide to ensure those suffering acute illness, that is stroke and myocardial infarction, and accidental injury are seen and treated first (Quigley and Burton 2003). However, NICE (2004) suggests that because of poor out-of-hours or uncoordinated care in the community 50% of people end up dying in hospital, often admitted to A & E during the night or at a weekend because of a crisis or increased symptoms (Thomas 2001). Unfortunately, because dying people do not require urgent life-saving interventions they can be left lying on a trolley for some time, without any privacy (Speirs 2006). The development of the 4-hour maximum waiting time for those waiting on trolleys in England has allowed more patients to be seen and moved out more quickly (McClelland 2003), although some patients are now admitted to a clinical area that does not meet their needs. Good practice is evident in A & E departments where patients who are obviously terminally ill can be admitted in short-stay wards where they are given privacy and professional support during the terminal phase (Pedley and Johnston 2001). However, these seem to be pockets of good practice as we continue to hear of dying people in A & E in fear and with no privacy as staff try to deal with other, often disruptive, patients (BBC 2007). Consequently, we can see that this care environment combined with the ethos of cure versus care that permeates acute care settings leads to the idea that dying in A & E is not peaceful for the patient and family and therefore not in keeping with the philosophy of good palliative care.

Dying in intensive care units

As well as the general barriers that affect palliative care provision in hospitals, there are some that only apply to ICU. Indeed, the sterility of the environment leads Smith (2000) to suggest that a soulless death in ICU is the most modern of deaths. While Dawson (2008) suggests that critical care teams are inadequately prepared to deliver palliative care although many patients with life-limiting illnesses are admitted to ICU if they have acute exacerbations of symptoms (Sibbald et al. 2008). It is noted however that few of this type of patient survive little more than a few weeks after this admission (Sibbald et al. 2008). It has also has been proposed that ICU devotes a great deal of time and effort in providing 'intensive rescue' interventions such as artificial ventilation and resuscitation (Faber-Langendoen and Lanken 2000). This combined with the notion that ICU often provides futile treatment where there is little hope of recovery (Sibbald et al. 2008) inevitably means that people dying in this setting do so in an undignified manner (Hadders 2007). It has also been suggested that care in ICU may violate personal integrity as patients often have little or no control in the decisions that are made, especially if they are ventilated. Also they have no control of their bodily functions and they may have little dignity as they are often only covered by a small sheet (Lock 2002). There is also evidence of poor support for families of dying patients in ICU (Kirchhoff et al. 2002) and often they are not fully involved in treatment decisions. This returns us to the beginning of this section where the communication skills of staff working in acute care are known to be poor and that they dread any direct communication with the patient or the family about death (Mandeep 2007).

In conclusion, the evidence suggests that Smith (2000) is correct in the assumption that those who die in hospital die badly. However, death cannot ultimately be avoided, even in hospital. In fact, 350 520 deaths occurred in hospitals in England and Wales in 2004, 68.38% of the total number of deaths during that period (Bryan 2007), and although the advent of specialist palliative care teams has gone some way to alleviating some of the issues reviewed, Kinder and Ellershaw (2003) suggest that staffing and monetary issues make it idealistic to expect specialist palliative care services could be involved with every dying patient, especially within bigger hospitals.

The next section discusses some specific barriers to the provision of good palliative nursing care before reviewing how good palliative nursing care can improve the quality of dying within the hospital setting.

Palliative nursing care in hospital – redressing the balance

There may be a number of reasons why nurses more recently appear to be less confident and less able to deliver good palliative care, including working in a climate of cure mentioned above. The development of Clinical Nurse Specialist role has had its criticism for potentially deskilling general nurses (Gibson and Bamford 2001), while the current notion that the 'science' of nursing, that is the technical skills, attracts more kudos from other members of the multi-professional team seems to prevail in modern nursing. As such the 'art' of caring which invests heavily in being with patients has become less glamorous and many of the traditional tasks of the nurse have been devolved to support workers. However, to ensure that patients and their families receive the palliative care they require, nurses need to overcome the divide between these two cultures (Derbyshire 1999).

So, while we acknowledge that there are barriers to providing good palliative nursing care in hospitals, such as poor communication, lack of education, and working in an environment where the drive is primarily 'cure' focused, there is much to be positive about in empowering nurses to provide the optimal level of nursing care for patients and families.

The recognition that all nurses need to be trained to care for patients who are dying is a significant step towards addressing these weaknesses (National Institute for Clinical Excellence 2004; West of Scotland Managed Clinical Network for Palliative Care 2006). While Palliative Care Services have strived to educate fellow health care professionals that the service offered goes beyond terminal care in the last hours and days of life, it is perhaps ironic that the end of life care tools have been a significant lever for education and change in practice around broader palliative care issues.

Palliative medicine is a relatively modern recognised specialty; however, health care professionals and especially nurses have always cared for people at every stage of their illness. Nurses often use the intuitive skills developed when being alongside patients and their families, thus allowing them to remain the patient's advocate from cradle to the grave. Indeed, The Royal College of Nursing began as a specialist interest group for nurses interested in care of the dying in 1982 to acknowledge this role (Royal College of Nursing 1994).

We have to acknowledge that more people die in hospitals than anywhere else in the UK, and although there may be a drive to allow more people to die at home, we, as nurses, have a duty to provide the best care now for the people who do die in hospital. As nurses we should also understand how we can help facilitate people's wishes to be cared for and die in their preferred place. The distinction between general and specialist palliative care may have gone some way to bring some clarity in the differences in the role of the general nurse and the role of the specialist, but this needs to be treated with the recognition that there needs to be sensitivity in relation to each individual nurse's level of confidence when dealing with issues.

Table 4.1 shows the referral criteria to a specialist palliative care service and may give a more clear distinction between generic and specialist roles and allow nurses to have more confidence in the provision of palliative care within the hospital setting. As Hansford et al. (2007) state:

> 'Care of the dying is not an option, it is a nursing necessity. It is where nursing and nurses can excel.' (Hansford et al. 2007)

Practice Point 4.2

How well does you own clinical area provide palliative care? Do you recognise any of the barriers discussed here? How will your team be able to overcome these barriers?

Table 4.1 Referral criteria to a specialist palliative care service.

Reason for referral	A: Ward team with support from Specialist Palliative Care Team	B: Specialist Palliative Care Team in conjunction with ward team
1. Pain	Assessment of pain and documentation of site(s) and severity. Appropriate investigation of cause of pain. Commence regular analgesia as per hospital formulary. Increase analgesia as appropriate. Review and document outcome daily.	Symptoms not fully controlled despite appropriate use of analgesia OR medication resulting in unacceptable side effects.
2. Any other symptoms	Assessment of symptoms and appropriate investigation of causes. Initiate treatment as per hospital formulary guidelines. Review and document outcome daily.	Symptoms not fully controlled despite appropriate use of medications OR medication resulting in unacceptable side effects. Complex multiple symptom control problems.
3. Psychological support for patient/family	Make assessment of psychological and spiritual support needs. Initiate basic support and reassess as necessary.	Psychological and spiritual support needs cannot be met by ward staff.
4. Patient is dying/ distressed	Following discussions with multi-professional team, family and possibly patient, it is identified that the patient is dying. Commence Liverpool Care of the Dying Pathway (LCP) and prescribe as per guidelines.	Uncertainty around diagnosis of dying. When specialist support is required to control physical, psychological or spiritual distress.
5. Insight of patient/family	Assess and document information needs of patient and family. Ensure appropriate information is given to enable informed decision-making. Reassess regularly.	Management or placement decisions are impaired by issues of denial or collusion. Complex family dynamics, e.g. young children.
6. Placement	Discuss placement with patient and relatives and contact CAT according to hospital policy.	Assessment required of whether hospice transfer appropriate. Complex circumstances requiring coordination of multiple teams across care sectors.

Adapted and reproduced with permission of the Hospital Palliative Care Team, Royal Liverpool and Broadgreen University Hospitals NHS Trust.

Commentary:

You may have recognised that some barriers exist in your area. You could overcome a number of these by ensuring the nursing team of all grades have access to palliative care education. Hansford et al. (2007) suggest that providing nurses with evidence-based, practical information on the management of difficult and psychologically demanding situations will increase the nurse's confidence. This in turn will allow them to be more involved in the care of future dying patients. The type and content of education provision required to ensure that the nursing team has all the knowledge and skills to effectively care for each individual person with a life-limiting illness will be discussed in more depth in Chapter 18 of this book.

The next section of this chapter discusses the nursing management of the person diagnosed with a life-limiting condition who requires palliative care while in the acute hospital.

Palliative nursing care in the acute hospital

In this section we review current best practice in assessing pain and symptoms, the use of syringe pumps, the provision of end of life (terminal) care and the management of discharging someone who wished to go home to die. It is the responsibility of all nurses to assess, document and act upon symptoms expressed by a patient. Identifying and treating a symptom appropriately may reduce the risk of escalation or further complications and does not always require the intervention of a specialist. However, remember that if there is not a suitable qualified nurse who has the knowledge and skills to put these practices into place, then the patient should be referred to the specialist palliative care team (NICE 2004).

It is important to recognise the many factors that may affect a person's actual or perceived symptoms and their willingness to disclose the symptom or its true severity. Some of these factors may be coming to terms with their diagnosis and prognosis, loss of role within society and the effects of the progressive disease on other personal relationships. There may be cultural or generational impacts on how symptoms are reported complicated by societal and health care professionals' misconceptions of the use of drugs such as morphine or administration of drugs via a syringe pump. Fear of admission to hospitals or extended inpatient admissions may also add to a lack of willingness to fully disclose symptoms. All these factors are included in what Cicely Saunders referred to as total pain (Clark 1999), which is why holistic care that responds to each unique individual is of the utmost importance in the care of dying people.

Assessing pain and symptoms

The complexity of each individual adds to the importance of a good nursing assessment. However, it is known that people who are in the advanced stages of illness have a number of common symptoms which impact markedly on the quality of a person's life. These include:

- Pain
- Dyspnoea
- Fatigue
- Anxiety and/or depression

(Stevens and Edwards 2008)

There are a number different models for assessing symptoms but most have common themes. Therefore, it is of use to consider a short reliable way of objectively assessing symptoms so that the patient is not burdened by too many questions. Remember that the ethos of palliative care is to improve the quality of life of patients.

O'Connor and Aranda (2003) suggest the 'PQRST' model as an objective and reliable way of assessing any of a patient's symptoms. It is as follows:

Provoke
Ask what provokes the symptoms, what makes them better or worse?
Quality
What is the quality of the symptoms being experienced? What words does the person use to describe the symptom?
Regional
Is the symptom regional, general or local?
Severity
On an agreed scale how severe does the person rate each symptom?
Timing
What is the timing of the symptoms?

In addition to generic symptom assessment tools there are many pain assessment tools within the literature such as the Memorial Pain Assessment Card (Fishman et al. 1987), but some simple measures such as asking whether the pain is mild, moderate or severe can be used as part of any nursing assessment. Indeed, the Modified Early Warning System (Subbe et al. 2001), used in many acute hospitals, uses this system and may be a good tool to use as it covers a number of symptoms. Whichever tool you decide to use it is a good practice to assess pain using the following:

- Ask the patient to identify where the pain is?
- Is it in more than one site?
- Can you describe it? (Acknowledge that this might be difficult for some people.) Consider prompts without putting words in people's mouth, that is burning, shooting, aches, sharp, gripey or cramps.
- Ask what brings the pain on?
- Is it cyclical?

- What makes it better? If anything.
- Document the sites and descriptions of the individual pain sites.

(Scottish Intercollegiate Guidelines 2000)

Knowledge and use of the WHO (1996) analgesic step ladder offers a firm foundation for understanding the appropriate titration and escalation of analgesia, but more importantly in assessment of the pain as the words mild, moderate and severe relate directly across to the steps on the ladder. Consider use of language as there may be generational or cultural perceptions of the word pain. It is not infrequent for some patients to 'put up' with or expect pain. Consider the use of words such as 'discomfort' or 'aches' in an attempt to ascertain the level of pain a patient may be in. Further reading on pain management can be found at http://www.sign.ac.uk/guidelines/fulltext/44/index.html.

Syringe pumps/drivers – continuous subcutaneous infusion (CSCI)

A syringe pump/driver is just an alternative route for drug delivery – it is not a method of pain or symptom control in itself. A continuous subcutaneous infusion is an effective method of drug administration that is particularly suited to palliative care. Administration via the oral route should be maintained for as long as practical although a patient's condition is likely to deteriorate as their disease progresses so that it is no longer possible to administer drugs this way. In such cases the use of a CSCI is the preferred method of drug administration to maintain symptom control; rectal administration is not always practical, or acceptable; intravenous injections or infusions should be avoided, particularly as CSCIs are less invasive and as effective, intramuscular administration would be painful, especially if the patient is cachectic (Dickman et al. 2005). The use of a CSCI is often wrongly associated with imminent death, not just by the patient and carer but by health care professionals as well. It should be understood that the use of a syringe driver can be for a multitude of reasons and that its use does not always mean that the end of life is approaching; for example, a CSCI can be employed to control the symptoms of intractable nausea and vomiting.

In the following circumstances and with the consent of the patient a CSCI should be considered:

- Where there is persistent nausea/vomiting
- Where there is severe dysphagia
- Where the amount of tablets or liquid medicines is of a quantity unacceptable for the patient to swallow
- When oral medication is not being absorbed, for example severe diarrhoea or bowel obstruction

- In the dying phase when injections become necessary and/or the patient has been taking regular medication by mouth and a conversion to a syringe driver has to be made

(Dickman et al. 2005)

When converting a patient from a modified release preparation of an oral opioid (e.g. morphine, hydromorphone or oxycodone) to a CSCI, there is no need for a crossover period; it may be started at the time of the next dosage. In other words you can start the CSCI at the same time you give the last dose of the oral medication. For practical purposes, this is often the best method. However, in order to achieve or maintain adequate analgesia, it may be necessary to administer a suitable 'rescue' dose of subcutaneous opioid until the medication being administered by CSCI reaches a therapeutic limit.

When considering administration of medication via a CSCI the nurse must select a suitable infusion site. This may be the:

- Anterior aspect of upper arm
- Anterior aspect of the thighs
- Anterior chest wall
- Anterior abdominal wall
- Scapula region (confused patients)

(Dickman et al. 2005)

Areas of oedema or ascites should be avoided, as drug absorption may not be effective. Bony prominences should also be avoided as this would cause pain if the patient were to lie on the area.

What can be done if a syringe driver is unavailable?

This is a fairly common problem in the UK. As a short-term measure a butterfly needle may be sited subcutaneously and bolus injections given, as necessary, to cover the period until a pump/driver becomes available. It would be wise to check with a Palliative Care Specialist for advice.

End of life care

It has been acknowledged that most people still die in hospital despite indicating that they would choose to die at home. The reasons for this may be multi-factorial despite efforts to impact on the equity of care regardless of setting. Murphy et al. (2004) suggest that end of life programmes are intended to span the health, social care and voluntary sector, although there continues to be inequality in care provision across sectors for a number of reasons. These may be because of family and/or carer fatigue, lack of monetary resources or professional input or poorly coordinated multi-agency care. Patients may also change their minds in relation to their preferred place of death as their illness progresses, meaning that the end of life decisions may change as time goes on. However, in all locations, the particular needs of patients who are dying from cancer or other life-limiting illness should be identified and addressed. The LCP for the Dying Patient provides one mechanism for achieving this within the hospital setting. Indeed, the use of this tool has been recommended by NICE (2004) as good practice in all care settings where end of life care is provided.

The LCP was developed to take the best of hospice care into hospitals and other settings. It is used to care for patients in the last days or hours of life once it is known that they are dying. The LCP involves prompting good communication with the patient and family, anticipatory planning including psychosocial and spiritual needs, symptom control (pain, agitation and respiratory tract secretions) and care after death. The LCP has accompanying symptom control guidelines and information leaflets for relatives (DoH 2006; Marie Curie Palliative Care Institute Liverpool (MCPCIL) 2008).

When considering the use of the LCP a team approach to diagnosis should be used, as this unites the care given and avoids giving conflicting information to the family (Kinder and Ellershaw 2003).

Diagnosing dying

A diagnosis of dying is made when the multi-professional team agrees the patient is dying and two of the following may apply:

- The patient is bed bound
- The patient is semi-comatosed
- The patient is only able to take sips of fluid
- The patient is no longer able to take tablets

(MCPCIL 2008)

However, there are barriers to diagnosing dying and it is acknowledged that identifying when patient has entered the dying phase is difficult (Higgs 1999). There can be nothing more frustrating for a nurse than to recognise that a patient is dying and yet be frustrated in giving the best and most appropriate care because of a number of possible barriers created by other health care staff, families and patients. Some barriers may include the hope that the patient may improve, that there is no authoritative diagnosis or where pointless treatments continue to be given (Ellershaw and Ward 2003). These authors also suggest that there may be different points of view within the team as to the patients' condition and that they may fail to distinguish the signs of impeding death and the families' cultural requirements. Little knowledge of how to prescribe in the terminal phase or how to communicate with patients and families also hinder good end of life care as do professional and family concerns of withdrawing or withholding interventions that may lead to a dread that a patient's life will be cut short (Ellershaw and Ward 2003).

The effects on patient and family if the diagnosis of dying is not made

Failure to recognise that a patient is dying may have a detrimental impact on both the patient and family. Ellershaw and Ward (2003) suggest the following effects can occur.

The patient and family may be unaware that death is imminent and as such the patient may lose trust in the doctor as his or her condition deteriorates without acknowledgment that this is happening. This may lead to both the patient and family feeling dissatisfied with care provision. The patient and relatives may also get conflicting messages from the multi-professional team and the patient may die with uncontrolled symptoms, leading to a distressing and undignified death. Or in another scenario at the point of death, cardiopulmonary resuscitation may be inappropriately initiated. All these issues may ultimately mean that the patient's and family's cultural and spiritual needs are not met and can result in complex bereavement problems and formal complaints about care. Some practical objectives identified by Ellershaw and Ward (2003) to help the care team reduce the barriers may be to:

- Communicate sensitively on issues related to death and dying
- Work as a member of a multi-professional team
- Prescribe appropriately for dying patients to:
  - discontinue inappropriate drugs
  - convert oral to subcutaneous drugs
- Prescribe drugs appropriately as required, including for pain and agitation
- Prescribe subcutaneous drugs for delivery by a syringe driver if needed
- Use a syringe pump/driver competently
- Recognise key signs and symptoms of the dying patient
- Describe an ethical framework that deals with issues related to the dying patient, including resuscitation, withholding and withdrawing treatment, foreshortening life, and futility
- Appreciate cultural and religious traditions related to the dying phase
- Be aware of medicolegal issues
- Refer appropriately to a specialist palliative care team

(Ellershaw and Ward 2003)

How to use the LCP

The LCP replaces all other forms of documentation when the patient has been diagnosed as dying. Many nurses feel it makes documentation more accurate and less time-consuming, and so means more time can be spent with patients and families. The LCP is a legal document that every member of the multi-professional team works with, and as such should be treated in the same way as other legal documentation. The LCP can be discontinued, for example if a dying patient improves. The care team would then revert back to using the care plans and other documentation, such as prescription charts, as per the ward policies.

The LCP is presented as a series of goals and prompts to act as a guide for all care provision in the patients' last hours or days of life. An initial assessment is completed only once and ongoing care is then assessed at least four-hourly. If a goal is not achieved or the pathway is not followed, then the health professional documents the reason for this as a 'variance'.

The series of seven sets of goals of care for patients in the dying phase are outlined below to allow you to gain further insight into how the pathway helps to ensure the patient has the good death that palliative care strives for. Each goal contains the rationale for the goal as well as the behaviours required to achieve the goal (MCPCIL 2008). An example of the LCP for the hospital setting can be viewed at http://www.mcpcil.org.uk/files/LCPHOSPITALVERSION printableversion.pdf.

Set 1. Comfort measures

Goal 1 – Current medication is assessed and nonessentials discontinued

Goal 2 – As required subcutaneous drugs prescribed according to protocol (pain, agitation, respiratory tract secretions, nausea, vomiting)

Goal 3 – Discontinue inappropriate interventions (blood tests, antibiotics, intravenous fluids or drugs, turning regimens, vital signs); document not for cardiopulmonary resuscitation (having discussed this with the patient and family)

Set 2. Psychological and insight issues

Goal 4 – Ability to communicate in English is assessed as adequate (translator not needed)

Goal 5 – Insight into condition assessed (both patient and family)

Set 3. Religious and spiritual support

Goal 6 – Religious and spiritual needs assessed with patient and family

Set 4. Communication with family or others

Goal 7 – Identify how the family or other people involved are to be informed of patient's impending death

Goal 8 – Family or other people involved are given relevant hospital information

Set 5. Communication with primary healthcare team

Goal 9 – General practitioner is made aware of the patient's condition

Set 6. Summary

Goal 10 – Plan of care is explained and discussed with patient and family
Goal 11 – Family or other people involved are able to express an understanding
of plan of care.

(MCPCIL 2005)

Set 7. Care after death

Goal 12 – GP contacted re patient's death
Goal 13 – Procedures for laying out followed according to hospital policy
Goal 14 – Procedures following death discussed or carried out
Goal 15 – Family/other given information on hospital procedures
Goal 16 – Hospital policy followed for collection of patient's valuables and
belongings
Goal 17 – Necessary documentation and advice given to the appropriate person
Goal 18 – Bereavement leaflet given

(MCPCIL 2005)

So it can be seen that the use of the LCP within a general hospital team can create the knowledge, skills and confidence to provide good care so that the last few hours or days of life can be managed well and patients die in peace and with dignity. In reality:

'Results from interviews suggest that the nurses using the LCP perceived it to have a positive impact on the care of dying patients, their relatives and medical and nursing staff.' (Jack et al. 2003).

Rapid discharge pathway home to die

NICE (2004) recommends that people with incurable illnesses should be able to make choices relating to end of life care, including where to die. Therefore, as hospital nurses we are provided with a unique opportunity to empower people to have their choice met, and by engaging with patients and carers in an open and sensitive way we can better understand their wishes and work towards helping them achieve these. It can seem easy for policy makers to suggest this is what we must achieve without ever having thought through the complexity of making goals happen at the clinical level. In reality this desire to enable rapid discharge of a patient home to die is often thought of as unworkable and there-fore unfeasible (Murphy et al. 2004); however, there are increasing examples of making these often-complex tasks more achievable and thus increasing choice (Marie Curie Cancer Care 2006; Northumbria Care NHS Foundation Trust 2008).

The LCP for the Rapid Discharge Home of the Dying Patient is one such tool. It was designed to support the transfer from hospital to home of a dying patient, who was not expected to survive more than a few hours or days. Feedback from ward and community staff indicated that the process provided a clear framework during what is often a most distressing time reflecting complex concerns from all parties. Family and carer informal feedback demonstrated that despite the risks and complex nature of this often-distressing time, all patients discharged remained at home until their death, which the families considered dignified and peaceful, with the majority of patients dying within three days as expected. (Murphy et al. 2004). You can view the pathway document by logging onto http://www.mcpcil.org.uk/frontpage.

Conclusion

Palliative care today seeks to integrate curing with caring, improve quality of life and support the patients view of a 'good death,' one that is free from avoidable distress and suffering for patients, families and caregivers – in accordance with the wishes of the patients and families and consistent with clinical, cultural, and ethical standards. (Coyle, cited by Rushton et al. 2004, p. 36). Yet, palliative care nursing in hospital is faced with contradictions. We are told that more people want to die at home, and although we are uniquely placed to impact on this, we know that more people continue to die in hospital than anywhere else in the UK.

Although we have seen that there are barriers to ensuring that all people receive the best level of care in hospitals, there has never been a better time for nurses to impact on this. However, to achieve these changes nurses need to act as the patients advocate and to champion their cause. This is summed up by Rushton et al. (2004) who say that to improve the palliative care in hospitals we need:

'nursing leadership from the bedside to the boardroom.'

When we put this suggestion into practice, the palliative care we provide transforms behaviours, ending the tradition that physicians 'do things *to* patients' and nurses 'do things *for* patients.' A new pattern of behaviour evolves across disciplines and results in medical professionals planning, providing and 'being with patients'. This appears to fit in more with the vision Dame Cecily Saunders advocated for palliative care, as she proposed that:

'If we can come not only in our professional capacity but in our common, vulnerable humanity there may be no need of words on our part, only of concerned listening. For those who do not wish to share their deepest needs, the way care is given can reach the most hidden places. Feelings of fear and guilt may seem inconsolable, but many of us have sensed that an inner journey has taken place and that a person nearing the end of life has found peace. Important relationships may be developed or reconciled at this time and a new sense of self worth develop.' (Saunders 1996, p. 1559)

Therefore, if we are to continue to move palliative care nursing in hospitals forward, there is still a lot to do and this will not happen unless we, as nurses, educate ourselves, unite, organise and help build an health care system that will sustain our focus on the individualised, holistic care of patients and their families and the supports the art of humane caring.

Finally, nurses can be powerful messengers.

'If we embody one vision and speak with one voice, we can bring palliative care nursing out of the shadows and into the light.' (Rushton et al. 2004, p. 37).

References

Audit Commission (2003) *Bed Management – Review of National Findings*. London: Audit Commission.

Bates J (2004) One day it could be you. Why Jane Bates hates the term bed blocker. *Nursing Standard*. 18(38):24.

BBC (2007) Dying woman's family hear tirade. Available at http://news.bbc.co.uk/2/hi/uk_news/scotland/south_of_scotland/7091130.stm. Accessed on 15 April 2008.

British Medical Association (1999) *Withdrawing and Withholding Life Prolonging Treatment: Guidance for Decision Making*. London: BMJ Books.

Bryan L (2007) Should ward nurses hide death from other patients? *End of Life Care*. 1:1–79.

Clark D (1999) Total pain, disciplinary power and the body in the work of Cicely Saunders 1958–1967. *Social Science and Medicine*. 49:727–736.

Dawson (2008) Palliative care for critically ill older adults: dimensions of nursing advocacy. *Critical Care Nursing Quarterly*. 31(1):19–23.

Department of Health (2006a) *Our Health, Our Care, Our Say: A New Direction for Community Services*. London: DoH.

Department of Health. (2006b). *NHS End of Life Care Programme Progress Report*. London: DoH.

Derbyshire P (1999) Nursing, art and science: revisiting the two cultures. *International Journal of Nursing Practice*. 5(3):123–131.

Dickman A, Schneider S and Varga J (Eds) (2005) *The Syringe Driver – Continuous Subcutaneous Infusions in Palliative Care* (2nd edition). Oxford: Oxford University Press.

Ellershaw J and Ward C (2003) Care of the dying patient: in the last hours or days of life. *British Medical Journal*. 326:30–34.

Faber-Langendoen K and Lanken P (2000) Dying patients in the intensive care unit: forgoing treatment, maintaining care. *Annals of Internal Medicine*. 133(11):886–893.

Fishman B, Pasternak S, Wallenstein SL, Houde RW, Holland JC and Foley KM. (1987) The memorial pain assessment card. A valid instrument for the evaluation of cancer pain. *Cancer*. 60:1151–1158.

Gibson F and Bamford O (2001) Focus group interview to examine the role and development of the Clinical Nurse Specialist. *The Journal of Nurse Management*. 9(6):331–342.

Hadders H (2007) Relatives presence in connection with cardiopulmonary resuscitation and sudden death in the intensive care unit. *Nursing Enquiry*. 14(3):224–232.

Hansford P, Robinson V and Scott H (2007) Care of the dying is not an option but a nursing necessity. *End of Life Care*. 1:1–6.

Higgs R (1999) The diagnosing of dying. *Journal of Royal College of Physicians.* 33(2):110–112.

Jack B, Gambles M, Murphy D and Ellershaw JE (2003) Nurses' perceptions of the Liverpool Care Pathway for the dying patient in the acute hospital setting. *International Journal of Palliative Nursing.* 9(9):375–381.

Jarrett N and Maslin-Prothero S (2004) Communication, the patient and the palliative care team. In: Payne S, Seymour J and Ingleton C (Eds), *Palliative Care Nursing: Principles and Evidence for Practice.* Maidenhead: Open University Press.

Kinder C and Ellershaw JE (2003) How to use the Liverpool Pathway for the dying patient. In: Ellershaw JE and Wilkinson S (Eds), *A Pathway to Excellence.* Oxford: Oxford University Press, pp. 11–41.

Kirchhoff KT, Walker L, Vaughn Cole B and Clemmer T (2002) The Vortex: family experiences with death in the intensive care unit. *American Journal of Critical Care.* 11:200–209.

Lock M (2002) *Twice Dead: Organ Transplantation and the Reinvention of Death.* Berkley: University of California Press.

Mandeep MR (2007) Mixed messages. *British Medical Journal.* 335(7633):1296–1297.

Marie Curie Palliative Care Institute Liverpool (2005) Care of the dying Patient (LCP): Hospital version 11. Available at http://www.mcpcil.org.uk/files/LCPHOSPITALVERSION printableversion.pdf. Accessed on 27 April 2008.

Marie Curie Cancer Care (2006) Evaluation of the Marie Curie Nursing Service in Lanarkshire. Available at http://www.palliativecareglasgow.info/pdf/MCNS_Discussion_Paper_%20Sept_2006.doc. Accessed on 19 November 2008.

Marie Curie Palliative Care Institute Liverpool (2008) Available at www.mcpcil.org.uk/liverpool_ care_pathway. Accessed on 27 April 2008.

McClelland H (2003) What a difference a month makes. *Accident and Emergency Nursing.* 11(3):129–130.

Middlewood S, Gardner G and Gardner A (2001) Dying in hospital: medical failure or natural outcome. *Journal of Pain and Symptom Management.* 22:(6):1035–1041.

Murphy D, Ellershaw JE, Jack B, Gambles M and Saltmarsh P (2004) The Liverpool Care Pathway for the rapid discharge home of the dying patient. *Journal of Integrated Care Pathways.* 8:127–128.

National Institute for Clinical Excellence (2004) *Improving Supportive and Palliative Care for Adults with Cancer.* London: NICE.

Northumbria Care NHS Foundation Trust (2008) Palliative Care Northumbria: Standards for practice. Available at http://www.northumbria.nhs.uk/page.asp?id=252980. Accessed on 19 November 2008.

O'Connor M and Aranda S (Eds) (2003) *Palliative Care Nursing – A Guide to Practice* (2nd edition). Oxon: Radcliffe Medical Press.

Office of National Statistics (2005) Deaths in England and Wales 2004. Available at http://www.statistics.gov.uk/default.asp. Accessed on 15 April 2008.

Pedley DK and Johnston M (2001) Death with dignity in the accident and emergency department. *Emergency Medicine Journal.* 18:76–77.

Quigley M and Burton J (2003) Evidence of cause of death in patients dying in an accident and emergency department. *Emergency Medicine Journal.* 20(4):349–351.

Robinson V (2007) Dying without dignity: my husband's story. *End of Life Care.* 1(1):88–90.

Royal College of Nursing (1994) *Palliative Nursing Forum Information Leaflet.* London: RCN.

Rushton CH, Spencer KL and Johanson W (2004) Bringing end of life care out of the shadows. *Nursing Management.* 4(35):34–40.

Saunders C (1996) Into the valley of the shadow of death – a personal therapeutic journey. *British Medical Journal*. 313:1599–1601.

Scott H (2005) Nurses should become more skilled in palliative care. *British Journal of Nursing*. 14(12):631.

Scottish Intercollegiate Guidelines (SIGN) (2000) *The Management of Chronic Cancer Pain in Patients with Cancer*. Edinburgh: SIGN.

Scottish Partnership for Palliative Care (2007) *Palliative and End of Life Care in Scotland: The Case for a Cohesive Approach*. Edinburgh: SPPC.

Sibbald R, Downar J and Hawryluck L (2008) Perceptions of the futile care among caregivers in intensive care units. *Canadian Medical Association Journal*. 177(10):1201–1208.

Smith R (2000) A good death? *British Medical Journal*. 320:129–130.

Speirs M (2006) Message from a trolley. *World of Irish Nurses*. 14(3):18.

Stevens E, Edwards J (Eds) (2008) *Palliative Care in Clinical Practice*. Dorset: Reflect Press.

Subbe CP, Kruger M and Ritherford P (2001) Validation of a modified early warning score in medical admissions. *QJM: An International Journal of Medicine*. 94(10):521–526.

Thomas K (2001) *Out-of-Hours Palliative Care in the Community: Continuing Care of the Dying at Home*. London: Macmillan Cancer Relief.

Thomas K (2007) Living and dying at home – challenges and successes. End of life care in Wales. Available at https://www.rcgp.org.uk/pdf/wales_Living%20and%20Dying%20at%20home%20Keri%20Thomas.pdf. Accessed on 15 April 2008.

Tiernan E, O'Connor M, O'Siorain L and Kearney M (2002) A Prospective study of preferred vs actual place of death among patients referred to a palliative care home care service. *Irish Medical Journal*. 95(8):232–235.

Walter T (2004) Historical and cultural variants on a good death. *British Medical Journal*. 327:218–220.

West of Scotland Managed Clinical Network for Palliative Care (2006) *Palliative Care Educational Core Competencies Framework*. Glasgow: WoSMCNPC/NHS Scotland.

World Health Organization (1996) *WHO Guidelines: Cancer Pain Relief* (2nd edition). Geneva: World Health Organization.

Chapter 5
Palliative nursing care in the community
Wendy Wesson

Introduction

The aim of this chapter is to outline the issues, priorities and direction in the UK of palliative care services in the community. Using the patient priorities identified in the Cancer Plan (Department of Health (DoH) 2000) professional and nursing roles in community palliative care are explored, taking into account the impact of government policy, new initiatives and demographic changes which impact on care delivery. The chapter ends by reviewing the Gold Standards Framework (GSF) to show how it can help to ensure that high-quality palliative care is available to those dying at home.

Learning outcomes

Once you have read this chapter and completed the associated practice points, you will be able to:

- Recognise drivers which influence community palliative care delivery, including policy directives and patient preference
- Appreciate the importance of coordinated services in the delivery of community palliative care accessible to all, regardless of diagnosis or illness trajectory
- Understand the internal and external factors which impact the effectiveness of palliative care delivery, thereby influencing the patient's journey

Background

Palliative care provision in any setting should recognise and respond to the needs of family and carers, as well as those of the patients themselves. This is especially relevant in the community setting, where the inherent problems and issues in the home are highlighted and have a direct impact on care delivery. Most dying people would prefer to remain at home, but most of them die in institutions. (Thorpe 1993). In spite of the expressed wishes of patients, carers and health and social care professionals, this lamentable situation continues to occur, with only 23% of patients with cancer dying at home, and even less – 20%, of all deaths from a terminal illness occurring in the patients own home (DoH 2006; Watson et al. 2005).

Clarke (2002) highlights that with an increasing focus on cure and rehabilitation in the mid-twentieth century a sense of failure for the carers of those patients recognised as dying from their illness or condition has resulted. Consequently, care has become medicalised, the goal being cure rather than alleviation of symptoms. This approach does nothing to promote the plight of the patient with palliative needs, and it was not until the development of the hospice movement in the 1960s, a leading proponent of which was Dame Cicely Saunders, that interest in effective pain and symptom management prior to and at the end of life was re-evaluated (Addington-Hall 2004).

This shift in priorities, alongside a desire to enhance and improve the support offered to patients and carers to enable the patient to remain in their preferred place of care, has further augmented the need to focus on care delivery in the community setting.

Good-quality domiciliary palliative care, available to all, is essential if we are to meet the needs and grant the wishes of the majority of patients with a life-limiting illness. In England, the White Paper, *Our Health, Our Care, Our Say* (DoH 2006) states that the government is committed to doubling its investment in palliative care services to enable more people to die at home if they express the wish to do so. Investment in support for carers is also identified in the White Paper, under the New Deal for Carers initiative (DoH 2006). This type of financial commitment is vital if palliative care in the community is to be improved. In Scotland the government paper *Building a Health Service Fit for the Future* also acknowledges the importance of providing more services in the community and that a priority in this is to redesign health care services to meet local needs, although palliative care is not individually mentioned within the report (Scottish Executive 2005). However, the importance of promoting greater access to information regarding funding and available services cannot be underestimated. Caring for a person with palliative needs, although often very rewarding, can be challenging and exhausting, both physically and mentally. Unless services such as out-of-hours provision are clearly explained and easily accessible, the provision and quality of palliative care in the community will not be improved.

It is a testament to the advances in clinical care and treatment that people with serious illnesses are now living longer, and, as recognised by Watson et al. (2005), 90% of the patient's final year of life is spent at home. It is a tragedy, therefore that in many cases we stumble at the last hurdle, unable to maintain this support and sustain the patient and carers at home at the end of life.

The onus for delivery of palliative care in the community tends to fall to the GP and District Nursing services, whose roles are to coordinate care packages and manage care delivery. This type of care is recognised by these professionals as being a challenging, central aspect of their role, requiring a holistic, patient-centred approach to ensure individual, personalised planning and delivery, from referral and throughout the episode of care.

Dy and Lynn (2007) anticipate, in the next two decades, that the number of elderly people living with a serious chronic condition is set to double in the US, with similar trends occurring in other countries. Given the movement towards community-based care, the impact of this demographic change on community services will be considerable.

With a reduction in length of stay in hospice care in the UK to an average of two weeks, and 50% of the patients discharged from hospice being returned to community care, there is naturally a greater emphasis on an improvement and increased focus on community palliative care services. In England, the NHS Cancer Plan (DoH 2000) recognises the need to raise the standard of care of the dying to the best it can be. This recognition is also apparent in *Cancer in Scotland – Action for Change* (Scottish Executive Health Department 2001). *The National Service Framework for Long Term Conditions* (DoH 2005) stresses the importance of patients with long-term conditions being able to exercise choice as to where they wish to die, and states that with a coordinated approach, care for these patients can be effectively provided in the home. Yet inequalities in palliative care provision still exist between patients with a cancer or non-cancer diagnosis (Connolly 2000; McIlfatrick 2007). This problem is compounded by lack of knowledge regarding the remit of the available community palliative care services. Many hospice and specialist palliative care services have traditionally been accessible only to patients with a cancer diagnosis, although this situation is gradually changing. Communication regarding these changes and clear criteria for referral are necessary to enable health and social care professionals to refer on promptly and appropriately (Shipman et al. 2000).

The Cancer Plan (DoH 2000) identifies patient priorities in supportive and palliative care as shown in Box 5.1:

Box 5.1 Patient priorities in supportive and palliative care.

1. Being treated with humanity, dignity and respect
2. Good communication
3. Clear information giving
4. Symptom control
5. Psychological support

(Adapted from DoH 2000)

These priorities could easily be applied to patients with life-limiting illnesses other than cancer – illnesses which may be far less predictable, requiring flexible levels of support which respond promptly to fluctuating levels of need.

Practice Point 5.1

With reference to your own area of practice, examine the priorities of The Cancer Plan in England for palliative care delivery. Are these priorities reflected in the care provided to all patients with palliative care needs in your area?

Identify good practice and any shortfalls, and consider the means to address the shortfalls to improve palliative care delivery.

(If you work in Scotland you may also wish to review your service against the recommendations of *Cancer in Scotland – Action for Change*)

Commentary:

This activity should have raised some salient points in relation to the links between patients, health and social care staff and carers in palliative care delivery in the community. The role of the family caregiver in supporting and maintaining the patient at home cannot be underestimated. The role is often acquired rather than sought and can therefore transform the caring role into an obligation rather than a choice (Lawton 2000). Consequently, shortfalls in current delivery should be considered in relation to the impact on family carers. Disease trajectory, regardless of diagnosis, is unpredictable. Unless agencies work together to develop a community care package which reflects individual need and incorporates the above priorities, sufficient support will not be made available to maintain the patient and carer(s) at home at the end of life.

The provision of palliative nursing care in the community

Recognising the applicability of the priorities listed in Box 5.1 to all patients with a life-limiting illness, regardless of country of care and diagnosis, the following discussion will relate these priorities to the provision of good-quality palliative nursing care in the community.

Priority 1 – humanity, dignity and respect

Any one of us, facing a life-limiting illness, would expect that the basic human rights of dignity and respect will be upheld in the care we receive. Yet perhaps it is a sad reflection on current services that patients feel it necessary to identify these areas as specific priorities. Positive patient outcomes may be severely compromised if care does not reflect the expectations of the patient.

Luker et al. (2000) recognise the importance of knowing the patient to ensure that the quality of palliative care provision is maintained. This assertion is set in the context of a health service which on occasion relies upon fragmented care from a variety of agencies. In recent years health services have to some extent moved away from the principles of holistic, patient-centred care towards task-orientated allocation of responsibility. This is partly as a result of funding issues and changes to care delivery initiated in the UK by the Community Care Act in 1990 (DoH 1999). This is in direct opposition to the ethos of palliative care, which promotes coordination of services (Thomas 2003) and a cooperative approach to care delivery (DoH 2006). The district nurses studied by Luker et al. (2000) felt that early referral resulted in greater continuity of care. They valued the opportunity to spend time with the patient, providing support beyond the most easily quantifiable physical aspects of care

The delivery of palliative care in the community should reflect a holistic, patient-centred approach, thereby enhancing the ability to promote the principles of dignity and respect, which should be afforded to all. Provision of a seamless service should be achievable if the extra resources recognised as being required are forthcoming. A health or social care professional is required who can take the lead and facilitate liaison between those delivering care, ensuring the maintenance of optimal provision, whilst maintaining confidentiality and recognising patient choices as the driver for delivery. In reality this is a role most likely to be part of the District Nurse's remit.

Priority 2 – good communication

'Different disciplines need to maintain clear channels of communication to acknowledge difficulties and reach a consensus rather than perceiving one discipline as being critical of another.' (Doyle and Jeffrey 2000)

A coordinated approach to care is vital if the needs of the individual patient are to be met effectively. Care coordination promotes an effective interface between all community agencies involved in the provision of palliative care. Munday and Dale (2007) recognise that primary care professionals have a central role in optimising the care available to meet the patient's palliative needs at home, yet this is often hampered by a lack of clear processes and accessible resources (Thomas 2003). Fragmented care can result in duplication of care delivery, misunderstandings and gaps in the service. Indeed McIlfatrick (2007) suggests that communication problems and lack of coordination of services are regularly reported by patients and carers in palliative care situations. Within the community setting this problem is further complicated by professionals being based in diverse locations, having to rely on telephone, email, fax and so on to communicate with each other. Partnership working is therefore required to ensure the provision of optimal palliative care, ensuring that patients are at the centre of this care, having informed choices and their wishes being respected (Doyle and Jeffrey 2000).

Late referrals to District Nurses often result in a reactive service which, whilst prioritising need, may be unable to provide the level of support required to maintain the patient at home. Implementation of the Gold Standards Framework (Thomas 2003), which is discussed in depth later in the chapter, affords health professionals in the community early identification of patients with palliative care needs. This allows them to develop a supportive relationship and anticipate their requirements from the service over a longer period.

The care coordinators for community palliative care services, most often the District Nursing services, recognise their responsibility for sharing information and maintaining good communication links with all care providers. This is a pivotal role in care management (DoH 2006). Prompt, early referral is essential if the District Nursing services are to be successful in maintaining frank communication with the patient. It is important for the health professional to recognise at an early stage the patient's knowledge of their illness if communication is to be effective (Lawton and Carroll 2005). The opportunity to anticipate concerns and problems is greatly enhanced, which enables the community nurse to develop a trusting, therapeutic relationship with the patient and their carers. The issues that surround and impact upon the patient experience can be recognised, incorporating the assessment of body, mind and spirit. From here the nurse can make contact with other community services that are most likely to be able to meet the patient and family's needs.

Priority 3 – clear information giving

'When people are considering their choices about end of life issues, it is essential that information to support their decision making is conveyed with sensitivity.' (DoH 2005).

In recent years, professionals have adopted a far less paternalistic attitude towards information giving, and as a result patients are generally better informed regarding the nature and treatment of their condition. This situation is recognised by Jarrett and Maslin-Prothero (2004) who acknowledge, however, that the skill of the nurse lies in their ability to assess the most appropriate level and means of delivering the required information. This ensures that the patient absorbs and processes the knowledge to best effect, thus allowing them to make an informed choice.

When involved in palliative care in the community, the professional, through their privileged access to the patient's home, can often develop a clear understanding of the individual context and circumstances, and build up close relationships with both the patient and their carers. It is important in this situation that the nurse remains aware of the need to maintain confidentiality, and obtain consent from the patient for information sharing, for example with the family or close friends.

Practice Point 5.2

Consider the following scenario, making notes based on the questions included:
You have been asked to visit Joe, a 72-year-old gentleman who, after a protracted period of illness due to chronic obstructive pulmonary disease, requires end of life care at his home.
    On previous visits, the gentleman has repeatedly asked you whether he is going to get better. He has not been directly given his prognosis at the express request of the family.

How might you handle this situation?
What ethical dilemmas are presented here?
What might the outcome of your actions be?

Refer to your professional Code of Conduct in formulating your response.

Commentary:

This scenario raises clear issues of accountability, confidentiality, autonomy and advocacy. In this case, the patient's relatives have made the decision not to share information with the patient, which directly affects his ability to make decisions and limits his access to choices in care. This 'conspiracy of silence', also known as collusion (Vivian 2006), also limits the care delivery options open to the family and community care team. For example, referral to specialist palliative care services, such as Macmillan Nurses and Hospice at Home teams, to support the patient and family may not be an option, due to the perceived link between these services and terminal illness. The relatives' actions could also be seen as being paternalistic, that is acting on what they perceive to be in the dying person's best interests, without allowing them to make an autonomous choice.

Woods (2007) refers to respect for autonomy as an important moral principle that requires the palliative care patient the ability to think and reflect, then decide for themselves. However, many external influences impact on autonomy and the subsequent choices made, for instance the wishes of the family, feeling a burden, past experiences and future goals. The nurse, respecting the patient's right to decision-making, must ensure that sufficient information and advice has been given to enable informed choices to be made.

Priority 4 – symptom control

Where symptom control in relation to palliative care is concerned, pain is often the primary concern. There are, however, numerous symptoms which may need to be considered when providing palliation for the patient, such as dyspnoea, constipation, fatigue and depression. However, control of symptoms may not always be reliant upon medication, and the source of the symptom needs to be established before it can be managed.

In relation to pain, the cause may be physical or emotional, or a combination of the two – one often impacting on the other (Penson and Fisher 2002). For instance, anxiety and depression may cause worsening of pain experienced. The treatment therefore should attempt to address issues such as these and should consider offering alternative and complementary therapies alongside, or instead of, traditional pharmacological treatments.

The assessing nurse should employ skills in active listening and reflection to evaluate the patient's symptoms in the context which the patient experiences them. Recognising and respecting the social network, informal support mechanisms, relationships and priorities of the patient in relation to their care is important if positive patient outcomes are to be achieved. This is particularly pertinent in light of the fact that pain is overall one of the most common reasons for unplanned hospital admission at the end of life (McLean et al. 2004). Recognising predisposing factors, such as lack of adequate emotional support or inappropriate treatment regimes, is a vital part of a comprehensive assessment in the community, to avoid emergency admissions or inappropriate treatment. After initially addressing or ruling out external influences on symptom control, the assessing nurse should be prepared to manage the symptoms by providing the means of addressing these symptoms, such as ensuring the provision of anticipatory medication or instigating referral to the Specialist Palliative Care team.

A 24-hour community service is often required, leading up to and during the physically and mentally draining period of the terminal phase, in order to adequately support the patient and carers to maintain the patient at home. In a study by Shipman et al. (2000), GPs and District Nurses identified that problems associated with poor 24-hour community service provision were the main reason for inappropriate hospital admissions for their palliative care patients. Integrated services, resulting in coordinated care across settings, are vital to avoid these admissions and prevent a revolving door scenario for care delivery.

Consultation with Specialist Palliative Care Teams and the implementation of a care pathway for the terminal phase, such as the Liverpool Care Pathway (LCP) (Ellershaw and Wilkinson 2003), will assist in addressing symptom management through advice, support and anticipatory treatment regimes.

Priority 5 – psychological support

Box 5.2 Quote from Cicely Saunders.

> You matter because you are you.
> You matter to the last moment of your life
> And we will do what we can,
> Not only to help you die peacefully,
> But to live until you die.
>
> (Saunders, cited in Twycross 1986, p. 19)

The above quote from Dame Cicely Saunders (Box 5.2) recognises the importance of maintaining quality of life for those living with a terminal illness. As alluded to in Practice Point 5.2, it is everyone's right to be informed of the nature of their illness. How they react to that information will be as individual as the patients themselves.

Receiving bad news of any kind is a traumatic event, often stimulating a response of shock or disbelief (Fig. 5.1). To be informed that you have a life-limiting illness would be likely to provoke such a response. Given this type of initial reaction, the importance of psychological assessment is immeasurable in

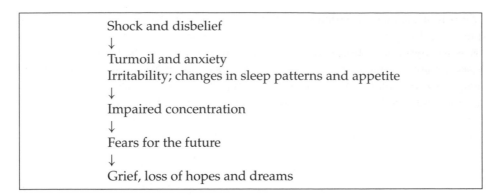

Shock and disbelief
↓
Turmoil and anxiety
Irritability; changes in sleep patterns and appetite
↓
Impaired concentration
↓
Fears for the future
↓
Grief, loss of hopes and dreams

Fig. 5.1 Example of an initial response to bad news (Adapted from Lloyd-Williams et al. 2001.)

reassuring the patient that they will receive the support and care required to avoid pain and distress at the end of life.

This type of care once again requires the professional to display excellent communication skills, and as necessary, recognise when the extent of these skills has been reached. On occasion, the initial reaction to the bad news may develop into a longer term anxiety or depression, which would certainly necessitate referral to an expert in psychological care. The unpredictability of disease progression, particularly for patients with one or multiple long-term conditions, may lead to a roller coaster of emotions for the patient and their family, who may all need a high level of psychological support. Therefore, acknowledgement of one's own limitations in providing psychological support should result in appropriate referral to other agencies, such as clinical nurse specialists in palliative care or specialists in psychosocial care, such as a spiritual advisor, psychotherapist or social worker.

Specialist Palliative Care Teams are a vital resource in community care. They enable GPs, District Nurses and other health and social care professionals to identify the point at which they require assistance in supporting the patient. The clinician may then either access this resource for themselves, in the form of information and advice and to gain a fresh perspective on patient care, or refer to the team to directly provide a greater depth of psychological support for the patient and carers (Lloyd-Williams et al. 2004).

Hospice at Home teams are also crucial in assisting to provide the 24-hour care required in the terminal phase of illness, often providing the respite and overnight nursing care which enables the patient and carers to continue to cope at home. The benefits of hospice at home teams are reviewed in more depth in the chapter covering palliative care in hospices.

Having discussed each of the priorities from the Cancer Plan to show how community palliative care services can ensure that palliative care meets the needs of the patient and family, the chapter now reviews the use of care pathways that can further enhance the quality of palliative care provision in the community.

The use of care pathways in the community

Two relatively new initiatives have recently been incorporated into palliative care delivery in primary care settings care in the UK. These initiatives, namely the Gold Standard Framework (GSF) (Thomas 2003) and the Liverpool Care Pathway (LCP) (Ellershaw and Wilkinson 2003), have been employed to great effect in the community to ensure the provision of good quality palliative care. This chapter reviews in depth the GSF while Chapter 4 discusses the use of the LCP in more detail.

Dr Keri Thomas, a practicing GP for over 20 years, developed the GSF with colleagues in response to an organisational aspiration for best practice in palliative care in the community (Thomas 2003). She identifies that the aim of the GSF is to develop community care at the end of life by improving both the quality and organisation of care for patients in the last stages of life.

The Gold Standards Framework has attracted international interest, as it enables care providers in the community, such as District Nurses and GPs, to implement effective processes which enhance community palliative care (Munday and Dale 2007). A GP or District Nurse is identified as the lead for each patient with palliative care needs. It is this professional who identifies and coordinates services and establishes multi-agency communication channels between professional teams, the patient and the family.

This advanced planning and coordination of services is particularly pertinent and useful in the identification and development of out-of-hours service provision. As pointed out earlier in this chapter, effective and sufficient round-the-clock care can be problematic, often resulting in unplanned admission to hospital. Therefore, anticipating and establishing the need for out-of-hours care as part of the GSF planning process is a major step forward in maintaining the patient at home.

Box 5.3 illustrates ways in which the GSF assists in enabling the movement from reactive to proactive care.

Box 5.3 Elements of the GSF which contribute to a more proactive approach to community palliative care.

- Development of a register; identifying patients who require support and palliative care in their final year of life. (See Prognostic Indicator Guidance paper at www.goldstandardsframework.nhs.uk.)
- Assessment of the needs of these patients and their carers
- Planning in anticipation of problems, through 24-hour care provision.

(Adapted from Thomas 2003)

The intention is for the GSF to address the needs of patients approximately in the final year of life, which can be difficult to recognise. However, it has been suggested that the professionals should ask themselves 'would I be surprised if this patient dies within the next year?' (Gomm 2007). If the answer to this rhetorical question is no, then the patient should be on the GSF register.

Practice Point 5.3

Go to the Gold Standards Framework website (www.goldstandardsframework.nhs.uk).
  Click on link, 2 (GSF in practice). Identify and familiarise yourself with the three processes and the seven C's of the GSF.

Commentary:

Box 5.4 lists the three processes of the GSF which need to be put into place by the community team. It clearly shows that in order to provide the best quality

---

Box 5.4 The GSF planning process.

1. **Identify** patients in need of palliative/supportive care towards the end of life
2. **Assess** their needs, symptoms, preferences and any issues important to them
3. **Plan** care around patient's needs and preferences and enable these to be fulfilled, in particular allow patients to live and die where they choose

   (http://www.goldstandardsframework.nhs.uk/gsf_in_practice.php)

---

of palliative care to dying patients in their own homes, a stepwise process is needed. Indeed, it has been previously noted in this chapter that optimal palliative care can only be provided where everyone involved in the patient's care communicates effectively. The use of the GSF can ensure this happens in practice.

The seven Cs of good practice are shown in Box 5.5. Communication and co-ordination are clearly central to the successful implementation of the GSF and to

---

Box 5.5 The 7 Key Tasks or standards to aim for – the 7 Cs

C1 – Communication
C2 – Coordination
C3 – Control of symptoms
C4 – Continuity including out of hours
C5 – Continued learning
C6 – Carer support
C7 – Care in the dying phase

   (http://www.goldstandardsframework.nhs.uk/gsf_in_practice.php)

improved palliative care in the community. The coordination of services which are sufficiently flexible to meet the ongoing needs of patients and their families, including out-of-hours care, are also essential for the provision of optimal care. Good symptom management and carer support will reduce the anxieties already discussed within this chapter, while community professionals need continued learning to ensure that they are able to provide the best level of care that is current and evidence based. The GSF priorities for good community palliative care mirror those shown in The Cancer Plan (DoH 2000) and previously discussed. The GSF has now become one of the three recommended pathways to ensure that patients can be cared for in the community if this is their choice (www.endoflifecare.nhs.uk). Results from evaluations of the GSF indicate that it has considerably improved the patient and primary health care team experience (King et al. 2005). This is also evident from the positive responses from health professionals consulted (Thomas 2003). However, the full impact on community palliative care across all life-limiting illnesses remains to be seen.

Summary

- This chapter has discussed the issues and priorities in community palliative care delivery using the priorities of the NHS Cancer Plan.
- Palliative care in the community is the preference of the majority of patients. This has been recognised by government in the UK and many other countries.
- The reader should have gained a greater insight into community care for life-limiting illness, and appreciate the impact of policy and standard setting on the patient experience.
- It is imperative that we strive to make these services the best that they can be, and provide a real choice for terminally ill patients, regardless of their diagnosis.

References

Addington-Hall J (2004) Referral patterns and access to specialist palliative care. In: Payne S , Seymour J and Ingleton C (Eds), *Palliative Care Nursing: Principles and Evidence for Practice.* Oxford: Oxford University Press, pp. 142–162.

Clarke D (2002) Between hope and acceptance: the medicalisation of dying. *British Medical Journal.* 324:904–907.

Connolly M (2000) Patients with non-malignant disease deserve an equitable service. *International Journal of Palliative Nursing.* 6(2):91–93

Department of Health (1999) *National Health Service and Care in the Community Act.* London: Department of Health.

Department of Health (2000) *The NHS Cancer Plan: A Plan for Investment, A Plan for Reform.* London: Department of Health.

Department of Health (2005) *The National Service Framework for Long Term Conditions.* London: Department of Health.

Department of Health (2006) *Our Health, Our Care, Our Say: A New Direction for Community Services*. London: Department of Health.

Doyle D and Jeffrey D (2000) *Palliative Care in the Home* (2nd edition). Oxford: Oxford University Press.

Dy S and Lynn S (2007) Getting services right for those sick enough to die. *British Medical Journal*. 334(7592):511–513.

Ellershaw JC and Wilkinson S (2003) *Care of the Dying: A Pathway to Excellence*. Oxford: Oxford University Press.

Gomm S (2007) Primary and palliative care: end of life care meeting the challenge. Available at www.gmccn.nhs.uk/hp/portal_repository/files/StephGommPres.Mar07.pdf. Accessed on 25 April 2008.

Jarrett N and Maslin-Prothero S (2004) Communication, the patient and the palliative care team. In: Payne S , Seymour J and Ingleton C (Eds), *Palliative Care Nursing: Principles and Evidence for Practice*. Oxford: Oxford University Press, pp. 90–107.

King N, Thomas K, Martin N, Bell D and Farrell S (2005) 'Now nobody falls through the net': practitioners' perspectives on the Gold Standards Framework for community palliative care. *Palliative Medicine*. 19(8):619–627.

Lawton J (2000) *The Dying Process: Patients' Experiences of Palliative care*. London: Routledge.

Lawton S and Carroll D (2005) Communication skills and district nurses: examples in palliative care. *British Journal of Community Nursing*. 10(3):134–136.

Lloyd-Williams M, Dennis M and Taylor F (2004) A prospective study to determine the association between physical symptoms and depression in patients with advanced cancer. *Palliative Medicine*. 18(6):558–563.

Lloyd-Williams M, Friedman T and Rudd N (2001) An analysis of the validity of the Hospital Anxiety and Depression scale as a screening tool in patients with advanced metastatic cancer. *Journal of Pain and Symptom Management*. 22:990–996.

Luker KA, Austin L, Caress A and Hallett CE (2000) The importance of 'knowing the patient': community nurses' constructions of quality in providing palliative care. *Journal of Advanced Nursing*. 31(4):775–782.

McIlfatrick S (2007) Assessing palliative care needs: views of patients, informal carers and healthcare professionals. *Journal of Advanced Nursing*. 57(1):77–86.

McLean S, Domeier R, Hill E, Maio R and Frederiksen S (2004) The epidemiology of pain in the prehospital setting. *Prehospital Emergency Care*. 6(4):402–405.

Munday D and Dale J (2007) Editorial: palliative care in the community. *British Medical Journal*. 334(7598):809–810.

Penson J and Fisher RA (2002) *Palliative Care for People with Cancer* (3rd edition). London: Arnold.

Scottish Executive (2005) *Building a Health Service Fit for the Future*. Edinburgh: Scottish Government.

Scottish Executive Health Department (2001) *Cancer in Scotland – Action for Change*. Edinburgh: SEHD.

Shipman C, Addington-Hall J and Barclay S (2000) Palliative care in primary care: how satisfied are GPs and District Nurses with current out of hours arrangements. *British Journal of General Practice*. 50:477–479.

Thomas K (2003) *Caring for the Dying at Home: Companions on the Journey*. Oxford: Radcliffe Medical Press.

Thorpe G (1993) Enabling more dying people to remain at home. *British Medical Journal*. 307:915–918.

Twycross R (1986) *A Time to Die*. London: Christian Medical Fellowship.

Vivian RJ (2006) Truth telling in palliative care: the dilemmas of collusion. *International Journal of Palliative Nursing*. 12(7):341–348.

Watson M, Lucas C, Hoy A and Back I (2005) *Oxford Handbook of Palliative Care*. Oxford: Oxford University Press.

Woods S (2007) *Death's Dominion: Ethics at the End of Life*. Maidenhead: Oxford University Press.

Chapter 6

Palliative nursing care in nursing and residential care homes

Carol Komaromy

Introduction

This chapter is concerned with issues relating to the provision of palliative nursing care in care homes. Under current legislation the distinction between nursing and residential care homes has disappeared. In England the National Care Standards Commission holds registration and enforcement powers that encompass not only care homes but also independent hospitals and other forms of social care; likewise responsibility lies with the National Assembly for Wales, and the Scottish Commission for the Regulation of Care.

This chapter begins with an overview of where older people die before it reviews the policy background to the provision of care in care homes. The chapter then discusses dying in homes and end of life policies before focusing on the challenges of providing palliative care in this setting. This will include reviewing issues such as training needs of care home staff, end of life care and the implication this has for nursing practice.

Learning outcomes

Once you have read this chapter and completed the associated practice points, you will be able to:

- Appreciate some of the key concerns and constraints associated with the delivery of end of life care in care homes for older people
- Recognise the extent to which education and training might impact upon the quality of that care
- Appreciate the extent to which rehabilitation has framed the dying trajectory and limited the time in which end of life care can be delivered

Demographic information

Over half a million deaths (557 789) take place in England and Wales each year (ONS 2002). While in the United Kingdom over the past century there have been dramatic demographic changes that are reflected in age-specific death rates; for example, at the beginning of the twentieth century 24% of deaths occurred in people over the age of 65 compared with 83% by the end of the century (ONS 1999).

In 2002 institutional deaths accounted for over 400 000 per year of the total deaths across all ages in England and Wales, and of these, over 300 000 took place in NHS hospitals (ONS 2005). Deaths in people over 65 accounted for nearly 250 000 of all deaths in hospital. Twenty-three per cent of deaths took place in care homes, the majority of whom were women over 85 (ONS 2000). The number of people who die in their own home each year is proportionately low, for example typically twice as many people died in 1998 in psychiatric hospitals as at home (ONS 2005). As well as age, place of death needs to be taken into account in exploring how death and dying is experienced and managed. For example, the way in which death and dying is situated in institutional spaces might suggest that there are reasons to conceal or in some way to contain the event.

Policy background

The 1990 NHS and Community Care Act (Department of Health 1990), which was implemented in 1993, had a dramatic impact on the care of dying older people. One of the effects of the Act was the decrease in NHS long-stay care. Statistics show that between 1970 and 1998 the number of long-stay NHS beds fell by 54% (ONS 2002). With the burden of care previously absorbed by the NHS, now relocated to the community, difficult decisions had to be made in the face of finite resources. One of the consequences of the increase in need for care of older people in the community was that the available money was targeted at a small group of people considered to be most in need of care. For example, the intensity of home help increased while the numbers of households in receipt of this help decreased (Department of Health 1999). In other words local authorities provided more intensive services to a smaller number of service users. Added to this is the reality that twice as much money was spent on residential care as on non-residential care for older people (Department of Health 2000). Furthermore, Peace (2003) argues that the post-Thatcher financial changes since 1979 were fundamental to the increase in private sector provision of the then nursing/residential home placements. One of the consequences has been that the profile of older people in care homes has changed to one of greater needs. According to a study by Bajekal and Purdons (2003) and Bajekal et al. (2003), in English care nursing/residential homes three in four of all residents were severely disabled. While the main contributing factor to this disability was dementia, and while most were in nursing homes, the physical incapacity of residents contributed significantly to their state of well-being. There is more likelihood that residents will suffer from chronic conditions associated with ageing, who will be further along the illness trajectory to dying and death.

The state of death in care homes

Mozley et al. (2004) make the point that reliable data on the causes of death are difficult to acquire, both because they are incomplete and information on residents in care homes for older people is not available separately. Having made these qualifications, their study findings from physical health comparisons between 300 residents showed a death rate of 30% in a 9-month period. This echoed the findings of a Department of Health study (Sidell et al. 1997), explored in more detail below, which revealed that death and dying is a regular event in care homes for older people. Occurring at the end of a long life, death in old age could be considered to be more 'normal' and, therefore, acceptable than deaths that occur in younger people. Furthermore, it is argued that Western cultures youth is privileged over old age (Timmermans 1998; Tulle-Winton 2000). Therefore, in care homes for older people, it might be reasonable to expect that there would be an acceptance of death that reflected a wider social view. However, the Sidell et al. (1997, 1999) study findings revealed that this did not seem to be the case and the extent to which death was not treated as 'normal', but rather as something separate from life and something that seemed to require special management. The extent to which death requires special management is a continuing tension with the institutional care of older people.

End of life care policy

The delivery of palliative care as part of end of life care is no longer the sole domain of hospice teams. At the time of writing, policy changes have meant that there are increasing expectations about the delivery of care to care home residents. The Department of Health (2003) end of life care initiative extends the rights to supportive and palliative care to all dying people and includes an expectation that care will be delivered through the Gold Standards Framework and the Liverpool Care Pathway, and take account of the preferred place of care. In Scotland the development of Palliative Care Standards for Nursing Homes (Scottish Partnership for Palliative Care 2006) also suggest it is best practice to utilise these integrated pathways. However, in practice the delivery of this care is dependent on a range of resources including the skills of the staff at the frontline of care delivery.

While policy demands and any resources and care delivery infrastructure are in place to support the delivery of care, there are other internal factors that influence practice. A review of the challenges to providing this care by Wowchunk et al. (2007) highlights what they call the internal factors that impact upon care delivery and include lack of care provider knowledge, care provider attitudes and beliefs about death and dying, lack of privacy, family expectations and insufficient time as a direct correlation of insufficient available care staff. The next section explores some of the detail of similar findings and highlights constraints that continue to impact upon the delivery of care.

Table 6.1 Stages of commissioned research.

Stage 1	A postal survey of 1000 homes in three geographical areas in England.
Stage 2	Tape-recorded interviews with 100 heads of homes, sample from stage 1.
Stage 3	Participant observation in 12 homes selected from stage 2.

Adapted from Komaromy (2002).

Exploring the case for palliative care

The data that underpins this section is taken from a wider Department of Health investigation into the case for palliative care in care homes for older people and a later study into the training needs for care workers, also commissioned by the Department of Health. These two studies took place over a 5-year period. The first (Sidell et al. 1997) was a multi-method investigation into the need for palliative care in nursing and residential homes in England. It was conducted over a period of two and a half years. The first 6 months of Stage 1 comprised a postal survey questionnaire and, for the next 2 years, I was in the field, first, interviewing heads of homes for Stage 2, and second, for Stage 3, as a participant observer in care homes. It was while I was conducting and analysing the Stage 2 interviews that I began to formulate questions that arose from the tensions and contradictions that I perceived in what people were telling me about death and dying.

Table 6.1 summarises the commissioned study that took place between November 1994 and July 1997.

Constraints and challenges

Institutional life as part of dying presents many challenges. Home as the preferred place of death does not necessarily provide the comforts that are associated with domestic spaces, although care home staff portray the care home as the residents' home. The tensions between the response to the series of losses that result from being admitted into institutional care and through intense rehabilitation and the reality that residents are likely to be much closer to death, as a consequence of delayed admission to a home, makes the role of the institution highly relevant. According to Goffman (1961), people suffer a series of mortifications of the self on admission to total institutions. The series of practice points that 'rob' people of their role(s), and instil in them a belief that institutional life is forever. The way in which Townsend (1986, p. 15) presents his form of 'structured dependency' suggests that the dependency is more symbolic than real and serves a purpose of legitimating a lack of access to equality of status. This is a more subtle form of criticism of the quality of life for older people in institutions and raises questions about the symbolic elements of the quality of dying. Goffman (1961) places the admission to institutions as a rite of passage into a world in which the process of social control and restrictions remove people's self-determination, autonomy and 'adult competency'. Goffman (1961) goes on to note that as 'inmates' become increasingly institutionalised they begin to regulate themselves and their own behaviour. The similarity between this and Bentham's (1995) notion of the panopticon is striking. The concept of the panoptical prison building is that it allows all prisoners to be observed without knowing whether or not they are being watched, and thus they have to assume that they are being observed and behave accordingly.

Goffman's (1961) study of institutions complements Townsend's (1962) seminal study and provides an explanation of what happens to people when they enter such places. He argues that the main features of social life that produce and sustain people's identity are lost when they enter 'total' institutions in that 'social arrangements regulate, under one roof and according to one rational plan, all spheres of institutional life' (Townsend 1962, p. 18). Wilcocks et al. (1987) discuss the degree to which institutional living structures the routines of daily life and argue that any adaptations which residents make to residential life will be varied and multi-faceted because of the functional, personal and symbolic impact of environment on quality of life.

Glaser and Strauss (1976) highlight the importance of being able to make temporal predictions of death for those people who work in the area of death and dying. They claim that this is explained by the need to reduce the uncertainty associated with death, and thus 'temporal predictions of dying trajectories' enabled staff to prepare for death and, in care homes, this included the expressed aim of affording residents the benefit of terminal care. While staff often speculated about the significance of particular signs of dying, this dying status had to be confirmed, or conferred onto specific residents by a doctor, most often the resident's GP. GPs might also decide to transfer residents if it was agreed that it was beyond the home's capacity to care for them in this terminal phase. Therefore, despite the fact that it was usually the resident's GP who made any formal diagnosis of dying, the senior staff members were the people who orchestrated the management of death and dying. A senior staff member or head of home would summon a doctor and request his or her opinion and, once confirmed would draw up a plan for terminal care and notify any close family members.

The privileged status of dying afforded a routine of care that was distinct from other forms of care. By setting up a routine of terminal care, usually through a care plan, staff differentiated dying care from that given to living residents. This involved residents being nursed in the private space of their own bedroom and no longer sharing the communal spaces of the home. But if the status of dying was one of privilege, what was the material benefit which that status bestowed? The rhetoric of a good death was not always the reality. My observations revealed that the main focus of end of life care was on the physical needs of residents. In particular, keeping residents clean and free from pressure sores was the main aspect of this care. Furthermore, staff to whom I talked to expressed the aim of avoiding a lonely death by sitting with dying residents, but this seemed to be compromised by staff shortages and different priorities. If relatives were not available to keep a bedside vigil, then staff would visit on a regular basis. All of the focus on the last days or weeks at the end of the life of a resident placed a high premium on the care that was given in this period.

I noted that the members of staff of care homes were generally concerned that residents should achieve a 'good death'. While the change from 'living' to 'dying' was marked by the change of routine where features of 'living', such as being got out of bed, dressed and fed, were no longer required, the continued focus on the residents' bodies through their intensity of care and the addition of pain relief marked a difference, even though pain relief might be more symbolic than instrumental.

Drawing on Goffman's (1959/1990) notion of performativity, I argue that the performance at the time of death might have served several purposes. First, the performance of terminal care provided staff with the means by which to manage the tensions around the boundaries between life and death. This was because, despite the emphasis on living, the day-to-day reality for care staff was one of the constant management of the slowly disintegrating bodies of residents who were washed, cleaned, fed and presented as living. Having a distinct form of care for dying residents enabled this boundary to be better maintained. Second, it seemed to be likely that providing more intense care near the end of life conferred significance upon a life, when that significance had been eroded or lost. By foregrounding death-bed scenes as performances, I inevitably drew upon the ideas of Goffman (1959/1990). The dramaturgy in which care staff, visitors, dying and surviving residents presented themselves in everyday life was dependent on convincing the 'audience' that their actions were authentic. Senior care staff directed the drama and 'caring' relatives who kept a bedside vigil were significant actors in this drama. The successful outcome of a 'good death' required that everyone should be convinced of the performance.

I would argue that, in a spiral of gradual but highly uneven decline, which was the case for many older and frail residents, the boundary between living and dying was not easily demarcated, and therefore, predictions were difficult to make. Keeping death concealed as part of the focus on life resulted in seemingly inherent contradictory performances around dying and living residents. Furthermore, I argue that separating dying residents from those who were living was problematic in settings where death was viewed as the 'natural and timely' outcome of a long life. It would appear that one of the strategies to cope with this ambiguity and the blurred boundary was to keep living and dying residents physically apart, not into dying spaces but into the private spaces of the home; usually the resident's bedroom transformed into a sick room.

Practice Point 6.1

End of life care and resources: Make notes on the factors that influence the quality of end of life care that are resource dependent. What factors are not dependent upon resources but are more related to a lack of needs awareness?

Commentary:

Whatever the resource demands, it is clear from research into end of life care in care homes for older people that the needs for training and development are ongoing. This is the subject of the next section.

Training needs for end of life care in care homes

Population projections suggest that the proportion of people living into extreme old age in the UK is set to increase. 15% of the deaths that occur in England and Wales take place in institutions (ONS 2000). Frogatt (2002) argues that the regulation of non-registered nurses and carers does not carry a requirement for training and development and that one of the consequences of this is the fragmented and varied approach to staff development in care homes for older people. Certainly the study exploring the training needs of care home staff in end of life care (Sidell et al. 1999) revealed that the focus on mandatory training such as lifting and handling and food hygiene often meant that this was all that staff received. There is a suggestion here that without a specific regulatory requirement for care staff to undergo training and development in end of life care, even though this occupies much of their caring time in care homes, there will not necessarily be a change in this area.

Apart from the gap between rhetoric and practice, there was a tension between the views of death in general as a 'natural and timely' event and the impact of individual deaths on the care staff. By this I mean that care staff had to manage the difficult task of producing death and dying not only as a normal and good event, but also as one which carried individual significance. What I noted was that there were institutional devices which helped staff to manage this dualistic role of treating death as a significant event and also behaving in a professional manner and treating death as natural. It was clear from observations and talking to home staff that from his or her position of power, the head of home directed these scenes of death. Indeed, there was a distinct hierarchy and division of labour in all homes, and junior staff members were not expected to have to make decisions about the care that was given to dying residents around the time of death. Instead, as with the orchestration of dying care, the duty fell to the more senior staff members who had professional expertise of death and dying, if not direct experience, for some senior staff members had not witnessed a death in their career.

My data showed that staff aimed to achieve the features of a good death through the homes' practices and protocols which served to script the end of life care put in place by the head of home. What I observed was that the care was entirely physical and that, mostly, pain was not controlled and instead was tokenistic. For example, no attempts were made to evaluate the efficacy of pain control and it could take several days for GPs to review prescribed analgesics. The routines of care that were established involved regular physical care which centred on turning the residents' body from side to side. Through this action, members of care staff were avoiding continuous pressure which could lead to the development of pressure sores. This was part of the routine of basic nursing care, which was extensively practised in the care of sick and dying residents. On one level, the quality of care given was inscribed on the body, in that the presence of pressure sores would have constituted a mark of poor quality care. Similarly, cleanliness was another visible sign of good care which would be read by the funeral directors, about whose judgement staff told me that they were concerned. The administration of fluids near to the point of death that were not swallowed would fulfil the criteria of good care inasmuch as keeping someone's mouth moist and avoiding thirst served a basic need. However, giving liquids that were not swallowed and which trickled out of someone's mouth, as I witnessed on several occasions, but which were recorded as having been taken, suggested the task fulfilled a more symbolic purpose. I argue that, as with the example of pain relief earlier, the tokenistic quality of giving fluids also reflected the ambiguous nature of a resident's living/dying status. Therefore, despite the routines and protocols which were in place to script a good death, the deaths that I witnessed highlight the extent to which they failed to do so, as much as the extent to which they succeeded.

The ability for care home staff to get to know their residents was one of the major reasons that heads of homes provided for being able to provide good-quality care at the end of a resident's life. This care seemed to be based on the belief that every resident would want to have the same type of death, which would comply with what the staff considered to be a 'good' death.

Implications for end of life care in care homes

Practice Point 6.2

Losing a friend in a care home:

Read the following case study and consider how would you describe the death and its impact upon Bob's attitude to his own death?
How might Bob be supported in his loss?

Fieldnotes

Monday afternoon

One of the care assistants, Melanie, suggested that I might want to talk to Bob because he was 'withdrawn' and she suspected was 'waiting to die'. I made a brief visit to him before I went home and asked him if I could talk to him the next day. I explained that I was looking at the quality of life in the home and I would explain more about it tomorrow. He didn't seem to want to know any detail and agreed to see me at 11 am the next day.

Tuesday morning

I knocked at Bob's bedroom door, which was slightly ajar. Bob told me to come in and I entered his room. He was seated in a wheelchair next to his bed and was doing something with the papers on his dressing table, adjacent to the bed and situated under the small net-curtained window. The room was of average size and contained a bed which was pushed against one wall, a small armchair, a commode and a dressing table covered with photos, papers and Bob's medication, kept in a small plastic ice-cream container.

'Hello Bob, it is good of you to talk to me', I said.

He nodded at me but did not smile. He looked very sad. I asked, 'How long have you lived here, Bob?'

He told me that he had lived in the home for just over 4 years. I asked him if he had any friends in the home and he replied, 'No, I keep myself to myself now – it's better that way.'

I asked him what he meant by 'better'? 'I don't want to make any attachments no more.'

He went on to add, 'I had a very close friend here and we were really good mates, but he died.'

I asked him how his friend's death had affected him and he started to cry (I knew that the death had occurred 2 months previously and had been a sudden death):

'It's completely shaken me, there was no warning, he was gone, just like that (he clicked his fingers) (· · ·) and strangely enough, shortly after his death, I became ill myself! Aye, that was just after Phil's death. We were very close. I didn't go to the funeral 'cos I couldn't manage in the wheelchair, you know? Mind you, they had the funeral tea in the home here, you know, and I was invited. I was pleased about that 'cos I could sort of erm, mark his death some how.'

Commentary:

It seemed clear that Bob was grieving for his lost friend and was afraid to risk another friendship in case he had to endure the pain of loss again. In this way it was possible that his withdrawal was a form of self-protection. Bob told his story very easily without any prompting. He seemed to be preoccupied with his loss, and yet, the care assistant told me that he did not like to talk about his 'lost friend'. Bob also made a connection between the shock of his friend's death and becoming ill, as if the shock made him ill. As he stated, 'It's completely shaken me.'

Bob was pleased that he had been invited to the tea in the home and I would argue that this acknowledgement of his friendship attributed a higher status to his relationship with the deceased resident, Phil, and his place in the bereavement process. It also suggests that making arrangements to get Bob to the funeral would have been too difficult and the funeral tea offered a more convenient alternative. Because Bob was in a wheelchair he would have required special transport *to* and some assistance *at* the funeral, and such an effort might have only been made for a significant person in the life of the deceased. Those residents that I talked to about acknowledging the death of someone close in the home told me that they would attend a home event, but not an outside funeral service. The role of residents at the funeral suggests a more ambiguous role.

Implications for practice

My findings have shown that the focus on residents' bodies and symbolic practices, not as part of responding to their diverse needs but as part of a production of ageing bodies into categories, failed to meet the needs of residents on all levels. This has implications for the personal and professional development of carers. Home managers and inspectors would need to recognise the impossibility and futility of categorising residents into 'states' that bear no relationship to the residents' needs and which only fulfil an institutional purpose. Furthermore, rather than countering the dangers of institutionalisation, 'living' as rehabilitation has produced an institutional form of 'living' that does not bear a direct relationship to the day-to-day experience of residents and their carers. My data also showed how the emotional needs of care staff in homes for older people were not included as legitimate aspects of their caring role. In the delivery of a new type of care, care staff would need to recognise that residents are best placed to dictate their own needs, both as people near to the end of their life, with complex needs, and as people with the capacity to contribute to caring. Many of the residents had been carers for most of their lives and also many had survived multiple losses. My data showed that the caring role of residents through close friendships and their awareness of coping with loss had been largely ignored. Part of this type of recognition would also need to come from the *professional* carers through an awareness of themselves as people with diverse emotional needs and abilities, rather than *producers* of emotional norms.

I argue that such a new culture would need to support a direct engagement with the needs of family carers and dying residents and that such a cultural shift would have the potential to support the provision of more meaningful forms of care. I would also argue that part of a new culture would be one that would recognise and acknowledge residents as people first. However, this is not straightforward. Delivering an appropriate level of care that takes a person-centred approach, as is the rhetoric of good quality care (Hockley and Clark 2002), requires recognition of how that person is produced. Hallam et al. (1999) challenge the notion of the body as a container of an individual self, which ceases to exist after death. Furthermore, Lawton (2000) argues that even in hospice settings that specialise in good-quality care at the end of life, the problematic, disintegrating dying body stands in for individual identity, causing the dying person to withdraw into a marginalised state of isolation and for hospice staff to collude in this sequestration of 'dirty dying'. Without recognition of the self as other than something that resides in a body, and an approach that does not define residents according to their bodily states, the practice of care for residents in care homes cannot easily change.

Finally, therefore, without such an in-depth understanding that such ethnographic studies can bring, rhetoric and practice will remain divided. Forms of care may change, but for practitioners and policy makers to be able to bridge this gap requires more than protocols and resources; although they clearly play a vital role, it requires a new culture underpinned by the findings of the type of research discussed in this chapter that supports a direct engagement with the needs of carers and dying residents and which recognises residents as people first.

Summary of key points

- Death and dying is a regular occurrence in nursing homes.
- Policy changes require that end of life care is available to all who need it.
- There are significant resource constraints that impede the delivery of that type of care.
- The internal constraints include a need for a fundamental shift of emphasis on the need to recognise that dying cannot merely be defined as consisting within a short period of time.
- The recognition that regardless of the formal diagnosis of dying residents' have complex needs would help to raise awareness of the needs for a better quality of end of life care.

References

Bajekal M, Primatesta P and Prior G (Eds) for the Department of Health (2003) *Health Survey for England 2001 – Disability.* London: TSO.

Bajekal M and Purdon S (2003) *Healthy Life Expectancy at Health Authority Level: Comparing Estimates from the General Household Survey and the Health Survey for England.* London: National Centre for Social Research.

Bentham J (1995) Panopticon or the inspection house. In: Bizovic M (Ed), *The Panopticon Writings.* London: Verso, pp. 29–95.

Department of Health (1990) *NHS and Community Care Act.* London: HMSO.

Department of Health (1999) *Community Care Statistics; Home Help: Home Care Services.* London: The Stationary Office.

Department of Health (2000) Health and social services statistics. London: DoH. Available at http://www.dh.gov.uk/en/Publicationsandstatistics/Statistics/index.htm. Accessed on 10 April 2008.

Department of Health (2003) NHS end of life care programme. London: DoH. Available at http://www.dh.gov.uk/en/Healthcare/Longtermconditions/index.htm. Accessed on 02 March 2008.

Frogatt (2002) Changing care practices: beyond education and training to 'practice developments'. In: Hockley J and Clark D (Eds), *Palliative Care for Older People in Care Homes*. Buckingham: Open University Press.

Glaser BG and Strauss AL (1976) Initial definitions of the dying trajectory. In: Schneiden ES (Ed), *Death: Current Perspectives*. Palo Alto, CA: Brown William C & Son.

Goffman E (1961) *Asylums*. London: Penguin Books.

Goffman E (1959/1990) *The Presentation of Self in Everyday Life* (4th reprint). Harmondsworth: Penguin Books.

Hallam E, Hockey J and Howarth G (1999) *Beyond the Body: Death and Social Identity*. London: Routledge.

Hockley J and Clark D (2002) (Eds) *Palliative Care for Older People in Care Homes*. Buckingham: Open University Press.

Komaromy C (2002) The performance of the hour of our death. In: Hockley J and Clark D (Eds), *Palliative Care for Older People in Care Homes*. Buckingham: Open University Press, pp. 138–150.

Lawton J (2000) *The Dying Process: Patients' Experiences of Palliative Care*. London: Routledge.

Mozley C, Sutcliffe C, Eagley H, Cordingley L, Challis D, Huxley P and Burns A (2004) *Towards Quality Care: Outcomes for Older People in Care Homes*. Hampshire: Ashgate.

Office of National Statistics (ONS) (2000) *Social Trends 30*. London: The Stationery Office. Available at www.statistics.gov.uk/. Accessed on 26 November 2008.

Office of National Statistics (ONS) (1999) *Social Trends 30*. London: The Stationery Office.

Office of National Statistics (ONS) (2002) *Social Trends 32*. London: The Stationery Office. Available at www.statistics.gov.uk/. Accessed on 10 April 2008.

Office of National Statistics (ONS) (2005) *Social Trends 32*. London: The Stationery Office. Available at www.statistics.gov.uk/. Accessed on 31 March 2008.

Peace S (2003) The development of residential and nursing home care in the United Kingdom. In: Katz JS and Peace S (Eds), *End of Life in Care Homes*. Oxford: Oxford University Press, pp. 15–42.

Scottish Partnership for Palliative Care (2006) *Making Good Care Better: National Practice Statements for General Palliative Care in Adult Care Homes in Scotland*. Edinburgh: SPPC.

Sidell M, Katz J and Komaromy C (1997) Death and dying in residential and nursing homes for older people: examining the case for palliative care, Commissioned Report. London: Department of Health.

Sidell M, Katz JT and Komaromy C (1999) Investigating the training needs of care. Staff in providing palliative care to older people, Commissioned Report, Department of Health.

Timmermans S (1998) Resuscitation technology in the emergency department: towards a dignified death. *Sociology of Health and Illness*. 20(2):144–167.

Townsend P (1962) *The Last Refuge: A Survey of Residential Institutions and Homes for the Aged in England and Wales*. London: Routledge and Kegan Paul.

Townsend P (1986) Ageism and social policy. In: Phillipson C and Walker A (Eds), *Ageing and Social Policy*. London: Gower.

Tulle-Winton E (2000) Old bodies. In: Hancock P, Hughes B, Jagger E, Paterson K, Russell R, Tulle-Winton E and Tyler M (Eds), *The Body, Culture and Society*. Buckingham: Open University Press, pp. 64–83.

Wilcocks D, Peace S and Kellaher L. (1987) *Private Lives in Public Places*. London: Tavistock Publications.

Wowchunk SM, McClement S and Bond J (2007) The challenge of providing palliative care in the nursing home part 11: internal factors. *International Journal of Palliative Nursing*. 13(7):34.

Chapter 7

Palliative nursing care in hospices

Helen de Renzie-Brett and Denise Heals

Introduction

This chapter examines the development of the hospice movement within the UK and the contribution of hospices to the provision of specialist palliative care. The range and variety of hospice provision is described, identifying the key characteristics of each service. The chapter then discusses the uniqueness of the hospice ethos, the hospice environment and ways of working that enable nurses and other members of the multidisciplinary team to provide holistic care that focuses on individual needs and quality of life. Finally, the importance of providing support for nurses working within this environment is highlighted.

Learning outcomes

Once you have read this chapter and completed the associated practice points, you will be able to:

- Demonstrate a greater understanding of the development of hospices and the associated philosophy of care
- Examine the role of the nurse in the hospice setting
- Explore the function and contribution of the hospice multidisciplinary team
- Appreciate the role of hospices in supporting patients and their families at the end of life
- Recognise the value of appropriate support mechanisms for practitioners

Evolution of hospice care

The nineteenth century saw the emergence of special charitable institutions to care for the dying being developed away from the main general hospitals that were being built at that time (Clark 2004). These institutions were largely founded and run by philanthropists and/or religious orders, with some being called hospices such as St. Joseph's Hospice in Hackney, London. As Clark (2004) describes, the care provided in these places at that time was basic. However, the founders of these institutions provided a basis which others developed in the following century. From the middle of the twentieth century changes began to occur, and Cicely Saunders along with other like-minded practitioners who drew on their personal experiences wrote about how care could be improved for those at the end of life. Consequently, an evidence base for what we now call palliative care gradually developed (Saunders 2006b).

St Christopher's Hospice was opened by Cicely Saunders in 1967 and thus the modern hospice movement emerged, characterised by openness and honesty regarding death and dying and a unique ethos of care. This involved actively engaging with the dying person to ensure they were cared for and their symptoms, whether of a physical, psychological, spiritual and/or social origin, managed effectively. The involvement of, support for and care of families was seen to be an essential part of hospice care (Saunders 2006a), and this care went beyond death so that families continued to be cared for through the grieving process. Evidence from studies exploring end of life care in hospitals around that time showed that such an approach was not always apparent (Bury 1997).

Faull (2005, p. 3) explores the origins of the word hospice and concludes that a hospice

> 'denotes a place where a warm feeling between host and guest is experienced, a place of welcome and care for those in need'.

The environment within a hospice needs to be one that is nurturing, is conducive to listening, and enables patients and their families to feel safe and supported. Thus, a balance is required between an environment that enables practitioners to perform clinical interventions safely, and one that at the same time appears 'homely', being attentive to patient's total needs and enabling them to attend to the priorities in their lives with appropriate support. The philosophy of care outlined above pervades throughout the hospice, being a whole organisational approach, an ethos practiced by all whether senior managers, clinicians or support services staff (Rasmussen et al. 1997). It is reflected in the totality of the hospice environment and approach, and made available by staff for patients and families. Indeed, Clark (1993, p. 129) states that 'hospice is a philosophy and not a place'.

Today, hospice care is often perceived as being provided only in a building (Help the Hospices 2006). Hospice service provision though is not only about inpatient or day patient care, but goes beyond this into the community setting. Care can be provided directly, in the patient's home, by a member of the hospice staff (such as a Community Nurse Specialist or Hospice at Home Carer). Alternatively, it can be given indirectly through the provision of advice and support to other health and social care professionals involved in the patient's care (such as General Practitioners, District Nurses or Community Matrons). This variety of provision enables and supports choice in how and where patients can be cared for, a particular focus of modern health care policy (Department of Health (DoH) 2006). However, the development of hospice services has been haphazard in the UK, with provision lying predominantly outside of the National Health Service (NHS). Consequently, provision across the country is not uniform, resulting in widespread inequity of access to the care that hospices provide. There are currently 223 adult hospices in the UK, of which 63 are run by the NHS, whilst the remaining 160 are independent charitable organisations (Hospice Information 2008). Presently, the majority of patients accessing hospice care have a cancer diagnosis. However, there is evidence that patients with non-malignant diagnoses would benefit from the expertise of hospice services (Skilbeck and Payne 2005) and the *National Service Framework for Long-term Conditions* (DoH 2005) recognises the need for specialist palliative care team involvement at the appropriate time in the many patients' journeys.

Practice Point 7.1

Find out about the services available for patients and their families at your local hospice.

Commentary:

While finding out about your local hospice you should have discovered the type and range of services available for patients at the end of life. These could include inpatient facilities, day care, out-patient care and care for people within their own home. Also, you may have identified how patients are referred to the hospice and any criteria for referral. Finally, is the hospice run by the NHS or is it an independent charitable organisation?

Later in this chapter some of the range of hospice nursing provision is explored, and comparisons can be made with your local hospice.

Nursing in a hospice environment

Currently there are 3226 inpatient hospice beds available in the UK (Hospice Information 2008), with the average length of stay for a patient being 12.9 days (National Council for Palliative Care (NCPC) 2007). There are many reasons for admission to a hospice inpatient unit including assessment and management of physical, psychological, social, and/or spiritual needs, respite care, as well as the provision of a place where the patient may die.

Overall the role of the nurse working within a hospice is essentially one of providing specialist palliative care. This is concerned with quality of care, maximising opportunities and choices whilst enabling patients and families to meet their needs through a comprehensive assessment process. The importance of gathering information to make decisions about the most appropriate approach to use with a specific individual is paramount in the provision of high-quality care.

There appear to be few academic studies examining the role of the nurse working within the hospice environment. However, Rosser and King (2003) examined the experiences of qualified nurses moving into hospice nursing and found that the further development of communication skills was essential in order to facilitate discussions surrounding death and dying. Evans and Hallett (2007), in their study of the work of hospice nurses, offered an insight into the perspectives of the physicality of care balanced with the psychological nature of care, demonstrating the individual and holistic nature of the concept of hospice nursing – being there, giving time for patients and families at the time of dying. It could be argued that there are two key elements in the provision of hospice nursing care which can be categorised as 'hands off', empowering and enabling, and 'hands on' – doing for. Nurses often tend to be task focused, being and feeling more effective when 'doing for' a patient. Within hospice nursing, time is viewed differently. Evans and Hallett (2007) claim this is due to environmental and organisational factors granting nurses 'permission' to spend time with patients. With usually a higher staff–patient ratio than other nursing environments, there is also a change of emphasis. Whilst the 'doing for' role is vital, there is an essential element of 'being with' a patient, something Benner (1984) calls 'presencing'. Along with the essential interpersonal skills of effective communication and listening is the ability to be with a patient and not to do for them, thus recognising the level of intervention and type of approach needed to meet their individual needs and those of their family.

Nursing care may be 'direct care' focused on symptom assessment and management, which could include pain, nausea and vomiting, breathlessness, anxiety and terminal restlessness. It may also be 'indirect care' with the emphasis on advice and support to other caregivers, such as information regarding medication and routes of delivery.

Within hospice nursing, holistic patient-centred care is the central tenet of care provision and is dependent on a partnership/relationship between patients and professionals (Ellis 1997). Those relationships are fundamental to nursing practice, particularly at times of emotional crisis or approaching death (Mok and Chiu 2004). The hospice has been described as a 'safe place to suffer' (Stedeford 1987, p. 73), a place where people who are dying are provided with an environment where they can contemplate life and death. The nurse plays an integral role in that process through the building of relationships, supporting the patient to focus on living whilst acknowledging death (Davies and Oberle 1990) and attending to their needs as they experience them (Jonsdottir et al. 2004). According to Cecily Saunders (1978 cited in Kearney 2000, p. 88), the professional/patient relationship can be viewed as a 'container': the presence of another person being very powerful offering a sense of security, someone who can begin to contain the feelings of another. That other person is often the hospice nurse. The development and maintenance of a good relationship creates a partnership within which nurses can really know their patients and thus attend to their needs, adopting a truly patient-centred approach to care (Whittemore

2000). It is a model of care where the priorities are valuing patients and families, building trust and giving of time and of self.

Practice Point 7.2

As a nurse, the relationship you have with a patient and family is very important particularly when the patient is nearing the end of life.

1. What would you consider to be the key components in establishing and fostering this relationship?
2. How might you establish a relationship with a patient and family in your working environment?
3. How might 'knowing' a patient and family enhance the care you could provide within your working environment?

Commentary:

The key components of the nurse–patient relationship would include the use of sensitive listening and questioning skills, spending time and giving undivided attention, building trust and being as well as doing.

Establishing a relationship could be achieved through respecting the patient and family's uniqueness; attempting to understand their needs and feelings through a sensitive and comprehensive assessment; being caring and compassionate; being responsive and evaluating care interventions; and developing a partnership approach to care by working together with patients and their families in planning and implementing care.

Knowing enables holistic care which is a cornerstone of hospice care. Through careful listening to patient and family 'stories', a greater understanding can be achieved about individual priorities, needs and wishes as death approaches.

As highlighted earlier, hospice care is not just about inpatient provision, and the key aspects of hospice nursing described above extend into other services that enable patients and their families to be supported whilst remaining in their own home. Those services include hospice day care, Community Nurse Specialist roles and 'hospice at home'.

Day care provision within a hospice

Palliative day care aims to provide the principles of palliative care with the emphasis on the multi-professional approach to care, incorporating the physical, psychological and spiritual (Sepulveda et al. 2002), but without the imposition of inpatient admission. A variety of other services are also provided by many day hospices including complementary therapies, along with creative and artistic therapies. The availability of such services is dependent upon resources and the approach and vision of the day care team and organisation (Higginson et al. 2000).

The original philosophy of palliative day care was based on a social model, providing a mechanism by which contact was maintained with patients on discharge from hospital whilst additionally forging and building relationships with other patients during progression of their disease (Herth 1990). However, with the development and availability of a greater range of services, particularly those focusing on meeting physical needs, two models have come to predominate: medical and social. Whereas the medical model focuses on the physical health and care, the social model expresses itself through the building of relationships and social practice points, including creative therapies (Kennett and Payne 2005). In practice, many palliative day care services provide a mixture of the two which is termed the theraputic model of palliative day care (Stevens 2004).

Hospice or palliative day care was first piloted in the UK in 1975, with the establishment of the first purpose-built unit in Sheffield. The number of units has steadily grown since then, with 283 palliative day care services now operating in the UK, offering on average 14.6 places per session, usually from Monday to Friday (Hospice Information Service 2008; NCPC 2006). The majority of these units are attached to a hospice, which may assist in bridging the gap between the community and inpatient care, and also brings benefits through links with the hospice itself. Referral to hospice services can be frightening and confusing for patients and their families. Referral to day care could be perceived as less threatening or less 'final' than admission as an inpatient to the hospice. Also, accessing day care facilities enables patients to access the wider services provided by the hospice (Payne 2006).

Palliative day care is typically a nurse-led service (although some units are led by allied health professionals) with the nurse in charge being responsible for coordinating and managing the service (Stevens 2004). Hospices generally are well supported by volunteers working across a range of departments, adding value to the level and quality of service provided. Day care is no exception, and it is recognised that the use of volunteers is integral to this service provision (Douglas et al. 2003). Volunteers play a variety of roles including that of general helpers, therapists and drivers.

It is important to remember that palliative day care means different things to different people, and patients, families and carers as well as health and social care professionals may all have different perspectives. Professionals may sometimes confuse palliative day care and social day care, and may write off both as 'tea and sympathy' alongside social practice points. The range of interventions potentially undertaken in day care may not always be apparent to those who are unfamiliar with this service. What might look like a 'cosy chat' between a professional and a patient to an inexperienced observer may well involve staff using a considerable depth and breadth of interpersonal and key communication skills (Stevens 2004). Such specialist palliative care skills are essential if people with a life-limiting illness who are living in the community are to be adequately supported (Dosser and Nicol 2006).

Patients may be referred to day care for differing reasons, and their needs may vary according to their particular diagnosis, the stage and progression of their illness, their response to the illness and their social circumstances. Following referral and prior to a first attendance at day care, patients should be visited in the community to assess their suitability for such provision. This is an important part of the assessment process as some may not wish to attend, perhaps feeling threatened by a group approach or feel that day care is not appropriate. These concerns need to be explored so that patients are able to make informed choices about attendance. Also at this time, the aims of attending day care should be clarified. Attendance at day care services may be time limited, with patients being discharged if they have met all their goals previously set during the assessment process or if their condition deteriorates and they are no longer able to travel to the hospice (Hearn and Myers 2001). It will be important for attendance expectations to be explored during the assessment process so that patients are clear about the process.

A variety of benefits of attending palliative day care are reported by patients including opportunities to form supportive friendships with others in similar situations, feeling valued and cared for by the staff and volunteers, being able to explore creative practice points and having access to complementary therapies and medical support (Dawkins and Gallini 2005; Payne 2006; Wilson et al. 2005). Close, supportive relationships can grow between groups of patients and these can present further challenges for staff. For instance, when a fellow patient is unable to continue attending day care or dies, the loss felt by the group can be very acute. Therefore, it is an important function and role for day care staff to ensure that the person is acknowledged and remembered in some way, with feelings explored and support given to other patients.

For the main carer and/or family, the patient's attendance at day care can offer an opportunity for a 'day off' from caring, safe in the knowledge that their loved one is being cared for. However, with the approaching likelihood of death, carers may wish to spend more time with the patient and therefore find it difficult to be parted from him or her when they attend day care. This demonstrates the differing responses and needs experienced by individual patients and their carers, and it is important that when day care attendance is offered, all such perspectives are explored openly, honestly and sensitively (Stevens 2004).

Palliative day care aims to address the needs of the individual patient within a group process. The potential diversity of need can present a challenge for service providers although it is important to remember that no two day care services are exactly the same. Crucially day care provision needs to recognise individuality and deliver flexibility within the principles and philosophy of specialist palliative care balanced with the demands of service provision in the wider community.

The community nurse specialist in palliative care

The provision of specialist palliative care services varies considerably across the UK (National Institute of Clinical Excellence (NICE) 2004). However, what is consistent within any service provision is the multidisciplinary approach to care. The multidisciplinary team typically includes the Community Nurse Specialist (CNS) in palliative care, who is usually an experienced registered practitioner with experience of working in the community setting and having specialist knowledge, skills and expertise in palliative care. The CNS visits people who have been referred to the hospice service in their own homes, in community hospitals and also in nursing and/or residential care homes. They work closely with patients and families and help in their complex needs, helping them to make sense of their situation and experiences and adjust to changes in their lifestyle caused by a life-threatening illness. It has been noted that a significant aspect of the CNS role is the delivery of emotional care and support (Skilbeck and Payne 2003).

The role of the CNS is a multi-faceted one with clinical, consultancy, education and research components (Royal College of Nursing (RCN) 2002). Within their clinical role, CNSs assess the physical, psychological, social and spiritual needs of patients, families and carers and provide specific advice and support as appropriate. Following the principles of palliative care and optimising quality of life for patients living with progressive life-threatening illness in the community setting is a significant element of their work. However, they do not work in isolation. Communication and collaboration with other health and social care professionals in the primary health care teams, relevant agencies and other professionals involved in the patient's care is a fundamental aspect of the CNS role.

Although usually a member of both the CNS team and the wider hospice team, each practitioner will need the ability to work autonomously. Nurse specialists are often assigned to a General Practitioner's (GP) surgery within a defined geographical area. This enables professional relationships to be built with the primary health care team, especially the district nurse who is often the professional most involved with the patient. The provision of specialist, professional advice to such colleagues is an important aspect of the consultancy role, empowering and enabling generalists to provide high-quality end of life care.

Palliative care usually forms a small part of the GP and district nurse caseload, therefore developing and maintaining their own knowledge and skills in relation to contemporary end of life care could present a challenge (Husband and Kennedy 2006). The educational component of the CNS role, encompassing both formal and informal teaching and learning approaches, is therefore crucial in supporting and developing other practitioners. Education of self is equally important, and continuing professional development, including opportunities for research, enables practitioners to keep pace with developments in professional practice and so maintain competence (Nursing and Midwifery Council (NMC) 2002).

The CNS may be the only contact a patient and their family has with the hospice. For other patients, referral to the CNS may be the means by which they access other services provided by the hospice.

Hospice at home

Some hospices in the UK and abroad have gone further than providing a Community Nurse Specialist service and offer, in addition, a range of supportive options for people living with life-threatening conditions at home. Indeed, these so-called 'hospice at home' services may exist even in the absence of a conventional hospice resource (Leach 1999). There are currently 108 hospice at home services in the UK and most exist to provide hospice-type care without the need for hospice admission (Exley and Tyrer 2005; Hospice Information Service 2008). Services vary greatly from the simple provision of untrained carers or volunteers for occasional nursing care to around the clock, multidisciplinary input. Being able to provide rapid response, crisis intervention is particularly important in the prevention of unwanted hospital admission (Travers and Grady 2002).

There are a number of possible criteria for referral to hospice at home. The dying person may be awaiting admission to inpatient care or alternatively, awaiting the setting up of a community care package. In either case, hospice at home provides a 'stop gap', buying time to enable other care arrangements to be made. The person may be experiencing acute exacerbation of symptoms, or the family may have particularly pressing psychosocial or general support needs. Here, hospice at home can provide crisis intervention and/or respite care. Finally, the person living at home who is reaching the end of life may require short-term, intensive support to enable dying at home (Sullivan et al. 2005). Clearly, across a range of patient experiences, hospice at home provides a useful addition to the armoury of hospice services.

Bereavement care

As has been seen throughout this chapter, care within the hospice environment extends beyond the patient to family and friends. Providing adequate support through the grieving process is an important aspect of this provision, as without it health and well-being can be affected (Egan and Arnold 2003). Given the uniqueness of people, their circumstances and life experiences, reactions to loss are likely to be highly individual. In light of this, the bereavement support available needs to be flexible and individualised, and hospices may choose to offer a range of services. The results of a recent survey amongst hospices (Field et al. 2004) identified the following as potentially being available: one-to-one support, provision of informational literature, memorial, remembrance or anniversary services and group support. The survey noted that one-to-one support was the most common type of provision. This service is again one in which volunteers provide invaluable support with Field et al.'s (2004) study demonstrating that two thirds of bereavement services used volunteers.

Nurses are in a particularly good position to provide support due to their often close involvement with families and the likelihood that they will have been present at the moment of death (Greenstreet 2004; Lyttle 2005). Indeed, nurses have been identified as key providers of bereavement support (Field et al. 2004). Crucial in the process of bereavement support is recognising those at greatest risk of grief that is complicated or does not appear to be resolving.

Practice Point 7.3

Within your work environment what information and/or support is available for patient's families and friends who are experiencing or have experienced a loss?

Commentary:

As a nurse you have the opportunity to listen and talk with patients' families and friends, and this is an important aspect of support, particularly if relationships have been built up over time. Potential sources of information and/or support might include booklets/leaflets providing specific advice and guidance, and other members of the multidisciplinary team such as the chaplain or social worker.

The hospice multidisciplinary team

As a hospice nurse it is important to recognise and accept one's individual professional limitations and know who else might have the skills to help and support the patient from within the multidisciplinary team. Cicely Saunders qualified as a nurse, medical social worker and doctor, seeing that each of these professions brought specific knowledge and skills to the complex scenario of caring for the dying. Undertaking a detailed assessment and developing an associated individualised care plan to meet physical, psychological, spiritual and social care needs that can then be comprehensively evaluated necessitates a comprehensive team approach.

The use of a team approach to address patient symptoms and concerns has been recognised as good practice (Fisher 2006) and successive government initiatives have endorsed this multidisciplinary approach through the identification of quality measures in specialist palliative care provision. Firstly, the NICE Guidance on Cancer Services (2004) states that assessment of holistic care needs must be undertaken using a team approach, and secondly, the Manual of Cancer Services (DoH 2004) states that specialist palliative care teams must work together to ensure a multidisciplinary approach to care delivery and decision-making.

Practice Point 7.4

Identify a patient whose care you were involved in who was nearing the end of life. What difference might the involvement of a hospice have made to their care and that of their family and carers?

Commentary:

The specialist knowledge and expertise of the multidisciplinary team may have been able to provide advice and guidance on symptom control (e.g. pain, nausea and vomiting, breathlessness or terminal restlessness) through pharmacological and/or non-pharmacological means. They may have been able to assist in helping the patient and their family explore difficult issues relating to loss, transition, death and dying as well as providing bereavement support. Assistance in advance care planning and a greater awareness and understanding of the choices available at the end of life may have been helpful.

The hospice team may also have been able to provide support to you and others in the care team where difficulties were being experienced.

It is well recognised that nursing patients at the end of life is associated with significant stress for the professionals involved (Newton and Waters 2001). Hospice nursing is a balance between caring for the living whilst acknowledging dying and death, and this naturally has an impact upon the nurse. Through acknowledging the deaths of others, ones own mortality is recognised. A hospice nurse cannot escape or shy away from the fragility of life and the finality of death, therefore attending to one's own needs is very important. Three particular stress factors have been noted for the palliative CNS. These are the building of relationships with patients and families in their own homes and the constant exposure to sadness, pressures of workload and relationships with other health care professionals (Newton and Waters 2001). Support mechanisms and strategies, both formal and informal, have a significant role to play in maintaining the physical and psychological health of these workers.

For nurses new to hospice work, a mentor enables an easier transition at a time of uncertainty of role, skills and abilities in caring for the dying person (Rosser and King 2003). For experienced hospice nurses, support strategies are also very important, and these may include formal support structures such as clinical supervision, critical incident analysis, education, reflective practice and de-briefing at the end of each shift. The NMC (2002) supports the establishment of clinical supervision as a part of clinical governance and in the interests of improving patient care. Sensitive and supportive line management should also be an element of the organisational structure of the hospice.

Practice Point 7.5

Explore what support mechanisms are available to you in your current work environment. Which of these might help you as you cope with the demands of caring for the dying? Consider both the formal and organisational support structures as well as where you find support on a more informal or personal basis.

Commentary:

You may have identified formal/organisational mechanisms such as ward/unit/department staff meetings, appraisal/personal development review meetings, clinical supervision, employee assistance programmes and/or regular one-to-one meetings with your manager or senior staff member. Informal mechanisms may include peer/colleague support, family, friends, social networks and the ability to take 'time-out'.

Key aspects within any of these mechanisms are the importance of confidentiality and someone who will listen in a supportive and constructive manner.

Conclusion

Hospices have contributed significantly to improving care for the dying person and their family through direct care provision, education and research activity. Recent government supported developments in end of life care provision, such as the Liverpool Care Pathway (Ellershaw and Wilkinson 2003), have their basis in the hospice model of care.

This chapter has outlined the development of hospices within the UK and discussed the uniqueness of the hospice ethos, environment and ways of working with patients and their families. The nursing contribution in a variety of different settings and/or roles within the hospice environment and the significance of the nurse–patient relationship and multidisciplinary working in providing holistic care have been explored.

References

Benner P (1984) *From Novice to Expert: Excellence and Power in Clinical Nursing Practice.* CA: Addison-Wesley.

Bury M (1997) *Health and Illness in a Changing Society.* London: Routledge.

Clark D (1993) *Partners in Care? Hospices and Health Authorities* (Occasional Papers in Social Administration). Aldershot: Avebury.

Clark D (2004) History, gender and culture in the rise of palliative care, Chapter 2. In: Payne S, Seymour J and Ingleton C (Eds), *Palliative Care Nursing: Principles and Evidence for Practice.* Maidenhead: Open University Press, pp. 39–54.

Davies B and Oberle K (1990) Dimensions of the supportive role of the nurse in palliative care. *Oncology Nursing Forum.* 17(1):87–94.

Dawkins L and Gallini A (2005) Gaining the views of service users in a specialist palliative day care setting. Cancer Nursing Practice. 4(10):35–39.

Department of Health (2004) *Manual for Cancer Services*. London: Department of Health.

Department of Health (2005) *National Service Framework for Long-Term Conditions*. London: Department of Health.

Department of Health (2006) *Our Health, Our Care, Our Say: A New Direction for Community Services*. London: Department of Health.

Dosser I and Nicol JS (2006) What does palliative day care mean to you? *European Journal of Palliative Care*. 13(4):152–155.

Douglas H-R, Normand CE, Higginson IJ, Goodwin DM and Myers K (2003) Palliative day care: what does it cost to run a centre and does attendance affect use of other services? *Palliative Medicine*. 17(7):628–637.

Egan K and Arnold R (2003) Grief and bereavement care: with sufficient support, grief and bereavement can be transformative. *American Journal of Nursing*. 103(9):42–52.

Ellershaw JE and Wilkinson S (Eds) (2003) *Care of the Dying: A Pathway to Excellence*. Oxford: Oxford University Press.

Ellis S (1997) Patient and professional centred care in the hospice. *International Journal of Palliative Nursing*. 3(4):197–202.

Evans M J and Hallett CE (2007) Living with dying: a hermeneutic phenomenological study of the work of hospice nurses. *Journal of Clinical Nursing*. 16(4):742–751.

Exley C and Tyrer F (2005) Bereaved carers' views of a hospice at home service. *International Journal of Palliative Nursing*. 11(5):242–246.

Faull C (2005) Chapter 1: the context and principles of palliative care. In: Faull C, Carter Y and Daniels L (Eds), *Handbook of Palliative Care* (2nd edition). London: Blackwell Publishing, pp. 1–21.

Field D, Reid D, Payne S and Relf M (2004) Survey of UK hospice and specialist palliative care adult bereavement services. *International Journal of Palliative Nursing*. 10(12):569–576.

Fisher K (2006) Specialist palliative care for patients with non-cancer diagnosis. *Nursing Standard*. 21(4):44–47.

Greenstreet W (2004) Why nurses need to understand the principles of bereavement theory. *British Journal of Nursing*. 13(10):590–593.

Hearn J and Myers K (Eds) (2001) *Palliative Day Care in Practice*. Oxford: Oxford University Press.

Help the Hospices (2006) *Public Perceptions of Hospice Care*. London: Help the Hospices.

Herth K (1990) Fostering hope in terminally ill people. Journal of Advanced Nursing. 15(11):1250–1259.

Higginson IJ, Hearn J, Myers K and Naysmith A (2000) Palliative day care: what do services do? *Palliative Medicine*. 14(4):277–286.

Hospice Information (2008) *Hospice and Palliative Care Directory, United Kingdom and Ireland 2008*. London: Help the Hospices.

Husband J and Kennedy C (2006) Exploring the role of community palliative care nurse specialists as educators. *International Journal of Palliative Nursing*. 12(6):277–284.

Jonsdottir H, Litchfield M and Pharris MD (2004) The relational core of nursing practice as partnership. *Journal of Advanced Nursing*. 47(3):241–250.

Kearney M (2000) A place of healing: working with suffering in living and dying. Oxford: Oxford University Press.

Kennett C and Payne M (2005) Understanding why palliative care patients 'like day care' and 'getting out'. *Journal of Palliative Care*. 21(4):292–298.

Leach E (1999) Community nursing. Where the heart is. *Nursing Times.* 95(28):30–31.

Lyttle CP (2005) Bereavement visiting in the community. *European Journal of Palliative Care.* 12(2):74–77.

Mok E and Chiu PC (2004) Nurse–patient relationships in palliative care. *Journal of Advanced Nursing.* 48(5):475–483.

National Council for Palliative Care (NCPC) (2006) National survey of patient activity data for specialist palliative care services. MDS full report for the year 2005–2006. London, NCPC.

National Council for Palliative Care (NCPC) (2007) National survey of patient activity data for specialist palliative care services. MDS full report for the year 2006–2007. London, NCPC.

National Institute for Clinical Excellence (2004) Guidance on Cancer Services: *Improving Supportive and Palliative Care for Adults with Cancer – The Manual.* London: NICE.

Newton J and Waters V (2001) Community palliative care clinical nurse specialists' descriptions of stress in their work. *International Journal of Palliative Nursing.* 7(11):531–540.

Nursing and Midwifery Council (2002) *Supporting Nurses and Midwives Through Lifelong Learning.* London: NMC.

Payne M (2006) Social objectives in cancer care: the example of palliative day care. *European Journal of Cancer Care.* 15(5):440–447.

Rasmussen B, Sandman PO and Norberg A (1997) Stories of being a hospice nurse: a journey towards finding one's footing. *Cancer Nursing.* 20(5):330–341.

Rosser M and King L (2003) Transition experiences of qualified nurses moving into hospice nursing. *Journal of Advanced Nursing.* 43(2):206–215.

Royal College of Nursing (2002) A framework for nurses in specialist palliative care. Competencies Project. London, RCN.

Saunders C (2006a) St. Christopher's Hospice, Chapter 17. In: Saunders C (Ed), *Cicely Saunders: Selected Writings 1958–2004.* Oxford: Oxford University Press, pp. 115–118.

Saunders C (2006b) *Cicely Saunders: Selected Writings 1958–2004.* Oxford: Oxford University Press.

Sepulveda C, Marlin A, Yoshida T and Ullrich A (2002) Palliative care: the World Health Organization's global perspective. *Journal of Pain and Symptom Management.* 24(2):91–96.

Skilbeck J and Payne S (2003) Emotional support and the role of Clinical Nurse Specialists in palliative care. *Journal of Advanced Nursing.* 43(5):521–530.

Skilbeck JK and Payne S (2005) End of life care: a discursive analysis of specialist palliative care nursing. *Journal of Advanced Nursing.* 51(4):325–334.

Stedeford A (1987) Hospice: a safe place to suffer? *Palliative Medicine.* 1(1):73–74.

Stevens E (2004) Palliative day care – more than tea and sympathy. Abstract of presentation at 14th Congress on the Care of the Terminally III, Montreal. *Journal of Palliative Care.* 20(3):231.

Sullivan KA, McLaughlin D and Hasson F (2005) Exploring district nurses' experiences of a hospice at home service. *British Journal of Community Nursing.* 10(11):496–502.

Travers E and Grady A (2002) Hospice at home 1: the development of a crisis intervention service. *International Journal of Palliative Nursing.* 8(4):162–168.

Whittemore R (2000) Consequences of not 'knowing the patient'. *Clinical Nurse Specialist.* 14(2):75–81.

Wilson DM, Kinch J, Justice C, Thomas R, Shepherd D and Froggatt K (2005) A review of the literature on hospice or palliative day care. *European Journal of Palliative Care.* 12(5):198–202.

Section Three

Palliative Nursing Care for People with Specific Illnesses

Chapter 8

Palliative nursing care in heart failure

Margaret Kendall

Introduction

Over the last 25 years an upsurge of interest and research into the care of dying people has resulted in improved symptom control and support. Yet even with these welcome developments not all dying patients benefit from the expert services of palliative care teams (Gibbs et al. 2006).

The World Health Organization, in its definition of palliative care, articulates an approach associated with life-limiting illness. However, access to these services outside the field of cancer is limited. The National Service Framework for Coronary Heart Disease (DoH 2000) included the recommendation that a palliative care intervention should be included in end stage disease.

There is evidence to indicate that requests to provide a palliative intervention for patients with non-malignant disease are becoming more frequent. Discussion with some palliative care practitioners reveals that there may be a reluctance to accept referrals for patients who do not have a malignancy. Some practitioners believe that they do not have the skills and knowledge base required to care for diseases other than cancer. Others appear fearful that a precedent may be set and there is much discussion of the metaphorical 'floodgates' opening, and creating such demand that the current service providers would be unable to cope. However, there appears to be a dearth of evidence on this subject, although studies from Scott (2001) and Pettingell (1999) both produce some evidence that purports to refute this claim.

Discussion with the cardiology teams to ascertain the perceived complexity of need of the end stage heart failure patients, and approximate numbers for referral to palliative care, may lead to surprises on both counts. It appears that the needs of patients as they are dying are not that different from the needs of cancer patients (Lewis and Stephens 2005). Many patients do not wish to have an ongoing intervention from palliative care. Rather they prefer a collaborative approach with joint support from both cardiology and palliative care as and when they need it.

Having provided interventions for patients with heart failure it is apparent that there is a steep learning curve required for both specialities: to learn the intricacies of care pertinent to the individual fields of practice. Patients and carers derive substantial benefit from a palliative care intervention, but ongoing liaison with cardiology teams remains of paramount importance.

Learning outcomes

Once you have read this chapter and completed the associated practice points you will be able to:

- Describe the needs of the patients and their families
- Discuss the opportunity to 'hear', through narrative, how the patients actually feel about their disease
- Describe specific symptom management for end of life care
- Explain how to apply the principles of palliative care to diseases other than malignancy

Prevalence

Heart failure has become a major cause of morbidity and mortality in Britain (Gibbs et al. 2001) with a prevalence of 3–20 per 1000 population, increasing rapidly in those people who are aged 65 years and above (Davis et al. 2001). Gibbs (2001) suggests the mortality rate is 31–48% at 1 year from diagnosis of heart failure and 76% at 3 years. Murray and Lopez (1997) speculate that this incidence is likely to rise by 70% over the next decade. These mortality figures are higher than some cancers and yet there is little research about the palliative care needs of this patient population. Only 6.9% of the total numbers of referrals to specialist palliative care services in Britain in 2002–2003 were for non-cancer related disease. Approximately 16% of this total percentage of referrals was for cardiovascular disease (Eve 2004).

Physical problems

A portion of the SUPPORT study by Lynn et al. (1997) examines the case of 92 patients who died during hospitalisation. Of these 35% had severe pain and 43% had dyspnoea of increasing severity. Of those who remained alive 1 year after the commencement of the study, 18% had pain and 32% dyspnoea, indicating this was an ongoing problem. The incidence of pain in this group of patients is lower than the corresponding patients who have cancer, but in the last three days of life these symptoms escalated. Data is comparable to the last three days of life of cancer patients who were placed on the Liverpool Care of the Dying Pathway (Ellershaw et al. 2001).

Studies have indicated that patients with heart failure are often symptomatic, disabled and their symptoms have a significant impact on their lifestyle and quality of life (Anderson et al. 2001; McCarthy et al. 1996). One of the major difficulties in caring for patients is the recognition when a patient is dying as opposed to an exacerbation of their disease which is correctable (Zambroski 2006). Physical symptoms are frequently influenced by psychological, spiritual and social issues, hence the appropriateness of a holistic approach to care and the importance of the involvement of different members of the multidisciplinary team. Communication issues have also been highlighted to be of vital importance (Rogers et al. 2000).

> 'Sometimes it's just too much. You know, the constant struggle. Everything I do is an effort; getting up in the morning; struggling to get washed and dressed; then there's the tablets. Oh so, so many. Everyday it's the same.' (Kendall 2004)

Symptom management

Management of symptoms should continue alongside active cardiac management. This is where a collaborative approach is of paramount importance (Daley et al. 2006). Where is it appropriate for active management of cardiac symptoms to continue, the palliative needs of the patient should be sympathetic to this active management. A holistic approach should be applied which will take into account the physical, psychological, spiritual and social aspects of the disease for both the patient and the family (Stuart 2007). Because of the longevity of the disease process, with some patients having heart failure for 3–4 years, patients often feel the need to protect their family and friends from the burden of the disease process. Patients may speak of the need to keep going, in spite of increasing burden of symptoms, particularly if they have an awareness that their life may be drawing to a close:

> 'It makes me feel terrible. I'm not that sort of person you know. It's hard to ask for help. Have always been the one who did the things. I hate to ask anyone to do anything. I struggle on rather than ask. I mean it's not the man thing is it? I'm the head of the family. She shouldn't be doing things like that for me. It's my job to look after her. So you see I don't ask... won't ask. I think that having this (heart failure) has had a big impact on her as well. It's changed her, life-wise for a start. She won't say. Like I won't say. I think she's heard more today that I have ever said but if you share things it puts more burden on them.' (Kendall 2004)

It is important to consider whether there are particular things worrying or frightening the patients and also to explore the meaning of a symptom with the patients: for example if there is an exacerbation of pain or dyspnoea or do they make the assumption that their condition is worsening.

Practice Point 8.1

Plan the referral processes you may make for a patient who has heart failure with an expected prognosis of less than 1 year.

Commentary:

It may be of help to consider the following:

Is the patient known to the district nursing team? How often do they visit?
Is the patient known to specialist palliative care? Would it be appropriate to link the patient into an outpatient clinic run by that service or would a domiciliary visit be more appropriate?
Has the patient expressed any particular preferences for place of care?
Does the local hospice accept referrals for patients with non-malignant disease?
What is the age of the main carer?
Are any aids and adaptations required at home?

There are particular symptoms which are associated with end stage heart failure for which a specialist palliative care intervention may be appropriate. However, within the confines of this chapter it is not possible to go into the specific management in depth. The working party at Merseyside and Cheshire have devised advice on pharmacological and non-pharmacological management of the following symptoms:

- Breathlessness
- Cough
- Pain
- Nausea and vomiting
- Cachexia and anorexia
- Constipation
- Psychological issues
- Peripheral oedema
- Dry mouth
- Withdrawal of medication
- Financial benefits
- Terminal heart failure – the last few days of life

Advice on all these topics is available from the network website www.mccn.nhs.uk.

A palliative intervention for symptom management should be used in conjunction with national and local guidelines for the management of heart failure, including NICE guidance (2003).

Who to refer?

It is important to realise that not every patient with heart failure would benefit from, or needs to have, a specialist palliative care assessment. However, it is equally important to have some indication for the patients that should be referred. In April 2005 a working party of palliative care specialists and cardiology specialists was developed within the Merseyside and Cheshire region. This group aimed to formulate guidelines for health care professionals who were caring for patients with end stage heart failure. Also it was recognised that the development of referral criteria would facilitate the identification of those patients for whom referral to specialist services would be appropriate.

Referral criteria

Any referral to another service should be at the discretion of the referrer and in conjunction with clinical assessment. It is often helpful if the initial visit (either at home or in a clinical environment) has both the referrer and the specialist practitioner present. This joint approach often reassures the patient that they are not being passed to another service. Also it reinforces the concept that the professionals are working in collaboration for the benefit of the patient and the family.

Merseyside and Cheshire guidelines

Patient and medical team (Consultant and/or GP) should be aware that the referral has been made and they agree with the referral. Plus two or more of the following:

1. Patient is aware that they have a confirmed diagnosis of heart failure
2. Patient has advanced heart failure (New York Heart Association Grade 3 or 4 at the discretion of the referring team)
3. It is anticipated that the patient is within the last 12 months of life
4. The patient has had three admissions to hospital within the last 12 months with symptoms of heart failure.
5. Physical or psychological symptoms despite optimal therapy (+/− deterioration in renal function)

(www.mccn.nhs.uk)

Symptom specifics

Pain

The use of opiates for patients with heart failure is usually permissible. However, unlike the incidence of cancer related pain, pain in heart failure is often caused by a specific incident and thus is unpredictable. Many patients do not wish to take regular analgesics, often because of the amount of other medications they are already taking. It is often more appropriate therefore to use immediate release preparations of opiates rather than sustained release because of their speed of action. It should also be remembered that a high proportion of patients with heart failure may have a non-specific generalised pain, for example musculoskeletal. Not all these pains may be opioid responsive, so alternative medications should be considered as well as opioids.

Pain does not necessarily only have physical components. Psychological, spiritual and emotional issues can exacerbate pain. Because the disease trajectory for heart failure if often much longer than that of a malignant disease, the impact of this may have a significant bearing on the amount of psychological distress a patient experiences. A full needs assessment of the pain should be undertaken. This will include:

- What the pain feels like
- How often it occurs?
- Are there any mitigating factors?
- Is there any other pathology that needs to be taken into account?
- Does the pain require a pharmacological intervention or would a non-pharmacological approach, for example occupational therapist or physio-therapist, be more appropriate?

Following the assessment if it is appropriate to consider treatment with medication the principles of the World Health Organization (WHO 1996) analgesic ladder should be applied (Fig. 8.1).

If starting immediate release morphine use a low dose, for example 2.5 mg, and repeat dose 4 hourly as required. Low-dose morphine is also beneficial for management of dyspnoea. Renal function should be checked prior to commencing opioids; if there is diminished renal function, advice regarding medication should be sought from the palliative care team.

Constipation

Practitioners should be aware that the use of any regular analgesic will give rise to constipation. In heart failure the problem may be triggered by reduced intake of food and fluids, general immobility, and the use of diuretics. The problem is preventable if laxatives are prescribed as a prophylactic measure. Most patients will need to have both a stool softener and a stimulant. These are available in combined medications. Note that *the use of co-danthramer is contraindicated*

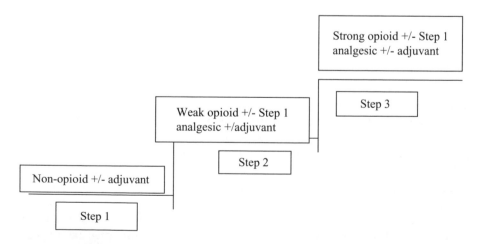

Fig. 8.1 The World Health Organisation Analgesic Ladder (WHO 1996)

in patients who do not have a malignant disease. A good combination is Senna 2 tablets nocte, with liquid paraffin plus magnesium hydroxide (milk of magnesia) 10 mL BD. This is especially useful as it may help to relieve coexisting gastric symptoms.

Nausea and vomiting

Patients with heart failure may have multiple reasons why they experience these symptoms. The actual cause of the symptom should be ascertained on an individual basis. The use of antiemetics is advisable, especially if the problem is related to the commencement of opiates. Regular administration usually 30 minutes before meals is advisable, although the use of *cyclizine is contraindicated in patients with heart failure.* If patients are unable to swallow oral antiemetics alternative modes of administration, such as continuous subcutaneous infusions (CSCI), should be considered.

Practice Point 8.2

Reflect on the care of a patient with heart failure you have known. With reference to symptom management what medications would you consider for a similar patient?

Commentary:

It may be helpful to consider:

What is the patients' dietary intake?
How mobile is the patient?
Do they have difficulty swallowing?
Does the patient have pain? If so is it constant or caused by activity?
Is the patient wakeful at night? What might be the cause of this?
Does the patient have any other medical condition?

End of life care

In 2006 the English government recognised the need to have extra investment for services to patients at the end of life. Additional monies were also set aside to provide further training for those staff looking after patients who were dying. The End of Life Care (EoLC) Programme was set up to improve the care at the end of life, irrespective of the place of care or diagnosis. The three tools which underpin this process are the Gold Standards Framework (GSF), Preferred Place of Care (PPC, recently renamed Preferred Priorities of Care) and the Liverpool Care of the Dying Pathway (LCP). All these documents are available via the internet via the Department of Health website (www.dh.gov.uk) or by direct link to www.endoflifecare.nhs.uk. The application of all these tools to patients with heart failure will ensure a cohesive approach to care through the final stages of life. It is perceived that patients will have a greater choice as in where they wish to be cared for, and where they may die. Also they provide the opportunity to forward plan and thus reduce the number of emergency admissions to hospital for patients who wish to die at home. However, in spite of these initiatives recent research indicates that patients and relatives are still unaware that they have choice in care modalities and communication with health care professionals still failed to address these issues (Selman et al. 2007).

Key points

- Heart failure and the conditions managed by palliative care specialists share many features: inexorably progressive debilitation, a deteriorating quality of life, and unless conscientiously addressed, distressing symptoms, especially at the end of life
- In end stage heart failure a strategy is needed to ensure a timely progressive move away from invasive treatment towards supportive terminal care
- The specific views of the patients in question, regarding how and when they would like to be treated are often not sought or go unheeded
- Palliative care specialists have developed treatment strategies which effectively control many of the distressing symptoms which patients report, and for which conventional cardiological treatments are ineffective or inappropriate
- There is no practical reason why the regular use of opiates should not be considered as a routine medication for the management of dyspnoea of chronic heart failure
- The basic principles of palliative care – good communication and close attention to symptom control – should be adapted to improve the quality of life for heart failure patients (Johnson 2007)

Practice Point 8.3

What considerations would you make for end of life care for a patient with heart failure?

Commentary:

It may be useful to think about the following:

How would you approach the subject of end of life care?
Has a preferred place of care document been written?
What medications may be required at the end of life?
What plans would you need to put into place, for example proactive prescribing?

Conclusion

Addressing the needs of patients without a diagnosis of malignancy highlights important issues for palliative care services. By enhancing the provision of care for this group of patients we will address another of the inequalities within health care.

The breadth of the palliative care needs in heart failure patients requires better recognition. It is the responsibility of all health care practitioners to acknowledge this need, and use their skills and expertise to improve patients' quality of life. Good care at the end of life is a universal right and should not be reserved solely for those patients with cancer. Now is the time to collaborate and accelerate the changes for the benefit of all patients.

'When I feel ok, life is good. Sometimes I try to forget that I'm dying, try to make everything ok. But at my age you keep meeting it. Like Pat, saw him about 10 days ago and he was fine. Then got a call to say he'd gone. That makes you think. Next time it could be me. That scares me, not death itself, but having to leave everything. Fear, leaving my wife, all this. I'm frightened of leaving it all. But on bad days it would be so easy to roll over and just go... But at my age I try to accept it. I know I can't go on forever. No, I don't want to live forever, but die? But some days I don't call it living.' (Kendall 2004).

References

Anderson H, Ward C, Eardley A, Gomm S, Connolly M, Coppinger T, Corgie D, Williams J and Makin W (2001) The concerns of patients under palliative care and a heart failure clinic are not being met. *Palliative Medicine.* 15(4):279–286.

Daley A, Matthews C and Williams A (2006) Heart failure and palliative services working in partnership: report of a new model of care. *Palliative Medicine.* 20(6):593–601.

Davis R, Hobbs F and Lip G (2006) History and epidemiology. In: Davies MK, Gibbs C and Lip G (Eds), *ABC of Heart Failure* (2nd edition). London: BMJ Books, p. 1–5.

Department of Health (2000) *National Service Framework for Coronary Heart Disease: Modern Standards and Service Models.* London: HMSO.

Ellershaw J, Smith C, Oversill S, Walker S and Aldridge J (2001) Care of the dying: setting standards for symptom control in the last 48 hours of life. *Journal of Pain and Symptom Management.* 21(1):12–17.

Eve A (2004) Minimum data set (MDS) statistics. National Council for Hospice and Specialist Palliative Care Services, unpublished.

Gibbs C, Davies M and Lip G (2001) *ABC of Heart Failure* (2nd edition). London: BMJ Books.

Gibbs J (2001) Heart disease. In: Addington-Hall J and Higginson I (Eds), *Palliative Care for Non-Cancer Patients.* Oxford: Oxford University Press, Chapter 3, pp. 30–37.

Gibbs L, Khatri A, and Gibbs J (2006) Survey of specialist palliative care and heart failure: September 2004. *Palliative Medicine.* 20(6):603–609.

Johnson M (2007) Management of end stage cardiac failure. *Postgraduate Medical Journal.* 83:395–401.

Kendall M (2004) Does the lived experience of patients with end stage heart failure indicate the need for a specialist palliative care intervention? A phenomenological study. Unpublished dissertation.

Lewis C and Stephens B (2005) Improving palliative care provision for patients with heart failure. *British Journal of Nursing.* 14(10):563–567.

Lynn J, Teno J, Phillips R, Albert W, Desbians N, Harrold J, Claessens M, Wenger N, Kreling B and Connor A (1997) SUPPORT: perceptions by family members of the dying experience of older and seriously ill patients. *Annals of Internal Medicine.* 126:97–106.

McCarthy M, Addington Hall J and Lay M (1996) Dying from heart disease. *Journal of the Royal College of Physicians of London.* 30(4):325–328.

Murray C and Lopez A (1997) Global mortality, disability, and the contribution of risk factors: Global Burden of Disease Study. *Lancet.* 349(9063):1436–1442.

NICE (2003). *Chronic Heart Failure: Management of Chronic Heart Failure in Adults in Primary and Secondary Care.* London: NICE.

Pettingell Y (1999) Palliative care for all. Nursing Management (Harrow). 6(4):8–9. In: Scott J (Ed) (2001), *Palliative Care Approaches for Heart Failure Patients: An Unmet Need? Coronary Health Care.* 5(: 3): 115–117.

Rogers A, Addington-Hall J, Abery A, McCoy A, Bulpitt C, Coats, A, and Gibbs J (2000). Knowledge and communication difficulties for patients with chronic heart failure: qualitative study. *British Medical Journal.* 32(7261):605–607.

Scott J (2001) Palliative care approaches for heart failure patients: an unmet need? *Coronary Health Care.* 5(3):115–117.

Selman L, Harding R, Beynon T, Hodson F, Coady E, Hazeldine C, Walton M, Gibbs L and Higginson I (2007) Improving end-of-life care for patients with chronic heart failure: 'Let's hope it'll get better, when I know in my heart of hearts it won't'. *Heart.* 93(8):963–967.

Stuart, B (2007) Palliative care and hospice in advanced heart failure. *Journal of Palliative Medicine.* 10(1):210–228.

World Health Organization (1996) *Cancer Pain Relief* (2nd edition). Geneva: World Health Organization.

Zambroski C (2006) Managing beyond an uncertain disease trajectory: palliative care in advanced heart failure. *International Journal of Palliative Nursing.* 12(12):566–573.

Chapter 9

Palliative care in chronic obstructive pulmonary disease

Sarah Russell and Vikki Knowles

Introduction

This chapter is concerned with the end of life care of patients with chronic obstructive pulmonary disease (COPD). It begins by reviewing the burden that a diagnosis of COPD brings before looking at specific nursing issues. The first issue that is considered is communication. Following this, the ethical considerations required when caring for a person with COPD are examined. Symptom management issues are then explored before the chapter finishes by discussing end of life care practices and care pathways.

Learning outcomes

Once you have read this chapter and completed the associated practie points you will be able to:

- Examine the physical, emotional, social, psychological and spiritual burden of COPD
- Describe the communication needs at the end of life in COPD
- Discuss symptom control at the end of life in COPD
- Explain the use of care pathways at the end of life

Burden of disease

Chronic obstructive pulmonary disease is an incurable illness and the fourth leading cause of death worldwide (Pauwels et al. 2001). The palliative care approach has much to offer these patients including commitment to a multi-professional approach, attention to physical, psychological, emotional, spiritual and social aspects of care as well as a familiarity with death and dying issues. Individuals with COPD live with the diagnosis and experience of the illness over years, often in a continuous state of poor health with intermittent exacerbations and subsequent hospital admissions (Goodridge 2006). Prognosis is poor, and the 5-year mortality rate for individuals with COPD ranges from 40 to

70% depending upon disease severity (Nishimura and Tsukino 2000). Overall the survival rate for individuals with severe COPD is worse than that of cancer (Gore et al. 2000). Symptoms in the last year of COPD include poor quality of life, social isolation, loneliness, anxiety, depression, panic, fear, frustration, fatigue, sleep disturbances, breathlessness, respiratory secretions, cough, wheezing, fear of suffocation, great impairments of activities of daily living and poor social, economic and physical function (Elkington et al. 2005; Gore et al. 2000). There is evidence that individuals with COPD do not receive palliative care to the same extent as cancer patients, despite a similar disease burden (Claessens et al. 2000). COPD patients have limited contact with health services, rare involvement with specialist respiratory or palliative care nurses and poor coordination of care (Skilbeck and Payne 2005). The American College of Chest Physicians (Selacky et al. 2005) position statement on end of life care for patients with cardiopulmonary disease affirms that the prevention, relief, reduction and soothing of symptoms 'without affecting a cure' should be an integral part of cardiopulmonary medicine.

Communication

Communication is a key part of the interaction between the patient and the health care professional in terms of psychological support, information giving in connection with treatments, medications and rehabilitation strategies and for having and dealing with the consequences of difficult conversations during and at the end of life (See Table 9.1). The challenge of prognostication in COPD (discussing the uncertainty of how long the patient has left to live and identifying the final days or weeks of life) is widely reported (Goodridge 2006; Yohannes 2007). It has been said to lead to 'prognosistic paralysis where clinicians prevaricate when considering end of life issues' (Murray et al. 2005). End of life issues are infrequently discussed with people with COPD, despite the fact that patients often desire to have such conversations (Curtis et al. 2002; Curtis et al. 2005). Discussions are often late in the disease trajectory and take place in less than ideal settings such as intensive care (McNeely et al. 1997). Conversations exploring and allowing expression of the meaning of the illness and value of self are important not only during the terminal phase of the illness but also throughout the course of it. Bereavement follow-up is also a key part of good palliative care.

There are a variety of communication and breaking bad news skills models used in health care today, and applicable to the care of people with COPD. These include facilitative behaviours (e.g. open questions, use of silences, reflection and acknowledgement), preparation (e.g. checking facts, appropriate venue and participants), breaking of the bad news (e.g. warning shot, the bad news, expression of feelings and emotions, and clarifying patients concerns) and follow-up (e.g. summarising, agreeing an action plan, offering follow up conversations and communicating with the multidisciplinary team; see

Table 9.1 Studies of communication challenges in COPD.

Author	Comment
Wenger et al. (2000), Golin et al. (2000)	Studies of resuscitation discussions with COPD patients identified a mismatch in that patients were able to make decisions about resuscitation but unable to communicate them to physicians.
Edmonds et al. (2001)	Lung cancer patients were more likely to have known they were dying and for a longer period of time than chronic lung disease patients.
Wenrich et al. (2001)	Study of 137 cancer and chronic illness terminally ill patients; views on patient–physician communication; identified key areas of talking honestly and straightforwardly, being willing to talk about dying, giving bad news in a sensitive way, listening to patients, encouraging questions, and being sensitive to timing of such discussions.
Morgan (2003)	Discussion of the patient–doctor relationship highlighted the significant difference between the content and process of communication. Points out that patients' perceptions of doctors' inadequacies in communication arise from what the doctors communicate (content) as well as how they communicate (process).
Gaber et al. (2004)	Review of 100 COPD outpatients; views on discussion of resuscitation; concluded that resuscitation could be discussed with patients without causing distress.
Curtis et al. (2004)	Review of the differences between COPD, cancer and HIV patients' perspectives on end of life care provision; identified specific need for COPD patients to know more about the disease processes, treatments, prognosis and what dying might be like.
Evans and Hallett (2007)	Highlighted the importance of the role of comfort to those who are dying, 'helping persons to deal with the heavy burden of death awareness by entering their world in a compassionate and a connected interpersonal relationship'.
Knauft et al. (2005)	Discussion of communication with oxygen-dependent COPD individuals; report that only 32% of patients had an end of life discussion and describe barriers such as patients wanting to concentrate on staying alive, not being sure which doctor would continue their care and not knowing what type of care they wanted.
Shah et al. (2006)	Described the difficulty in predicting when non-cancer patients will die and fear of causing distress when raising such issues – but in discussion with 40 patients from a teaching hospital and hospice (20 with cancer, 20 with COPD, heart failure or renal disease) revealed patients did not object to questions about end of life care.
Yohannes (2007)	Suggests that patients and general practitioners may be unwilling to discuss end of life care because of a lack of confidence and time to have such discussions, uncertainty about prognosis and lack of knowledge about available care.
White et al. (2007)	Identified that although in the ITU setting withdrawing life support may be discussed, long-term survival (prognosis) often was not.
Clayton et al. (2007)	Systematic review of adults with advanced progressive life-limiting illness with less than 2 years to live, including but not restricted to cancer, end stage pulmonary disease, end stage cardiac failure, and motor neurone disease; and/or the caregivers (including bereaved relatives) of such patients; and qualified health care professionals. Concluded that avoidance can lead to poorer patient satisfaction and psychological morbidity. If information provision is not honest and detailed, patients may perceive that health care professionals are withholding potentially frightening information. Although many health care professionals believe introducing the topic will unnecessarily upset the patient and dispel any hope, evidence suggests that patients can engage in such discussions with minimal stress and maintain a sense of hope even when the prognosis is poor. In addition, awareness of prognosis is associated with greater satisfaction with care and lower depression levels in patients.

www.breakingbadnews.co.uk). Discussions about important issues affecting COPD patients should ideally occur at an earlier stage and utilise strategies such as those described above. Advance care planning, which highlights wishes and preferences around place and management of death can be challenging for patient, carer and health care professional. However, facilitating the asking of 'What if?' questions in the event of their disease continuing to worsen, will aid and guide management at the end of life. There are a variety of communication training programmes available for health care professionals and staff should access them in order to be both confident and competent in communicating with patients at the end of life.

Ethical considerations

Good ethical practice is implicit within good end of life care using the principles of:

1. Respect for autonomy: respecting the decision-making capacities of autonomous persons; enabling individuals to make reasoned informed choices
2. Beneficence: balancing of benefits of treatment against the risks and costs; the health care professional should act in a way that benefits the patient
3. Non-maleficence: the health care professional should not harm the patient. All treatment involves some harm, even if minimal, but the harm should not be disproportionate to the benefits of treatment
4. Justice: distributing benefits, risks and costs fairly; the notion that patients in similar positions should be treated in a similar manner

(Beauchamp and Childress 2001)

As patients deteriorate and clinical decisions become more difficult, ethical principles help health care professionals to make appropriate clinical choices.

Practice Point 9.1

Consider the last person with COPD that you were involved in the care of. How would you assess the burden of their disease, and how would you facilitate a discussion about end of life decisions and issues?

Commentary:

You should be able to describe the assessment tools and communication skills that you will need to assess, manage and communicate with a COPD patient at the end of life. Clinical areas use many different assessment tools to ensure that patients receive the highest quality of care. However, one of the problems of advocating a solitary method of assessment is that it runs the risk of ignoring the complexities that surround gathering information and making sense of the variations in individual patients' holistic needs (Vernon (2001). Therefore, your clinical area should have assessment tools that are valid and reliable to assess the issues that affect your patient group. Assessment tools should not be onerous for patients to complete, as this will reduce the level of completion and thus the accuracy of the assessment. Finally, all staff who use assessment tools should have the knowledge and skills to do so. For further information on the many tools that are available to assess physiological, psychological, spiritual and social needs, McDowell and Newell's (1996) book on *Measuring Health* is a good place to start. The level of communication skills that are required to assess patients' needs will depend on the complexity of their issues. The *Knowledge and Skills Framework* (NHS Employers 2006) considers the ability of NHS employees to communicate effectively in their role as a key competency. The level of skill that is required for each post is determined by the job description. These issues will be discussed in more detail in Chapter 18 'Palliative Nursing Education and Continuing Professional Development'.

Symptom control

Symptoms in a patient with COPD are influenced by the degree of airway obstruction as well as co-morbidities and complications that are often present. These include muscular wasting and weakness, relative malnutrition and cor pulmonale. Determining when the terminal phase in COPD has been reached is extremely challenging. However predictors of impending death for COPD patients have been defined and may help facilitate discussion between patients and their clinician at an appropriate time. It is suggested that patients who have severe irreversible air flow obstruction, severely impaired and declining exercise capacity and performance status, older age, the presence of co-morbidities and a history of recent hospitalisation for exacerbation are more likely to die within 6–12 months (Hansen et al. 2007). Tools such as the **B**ody mass index, airflow **O**bstruction, **D**yspnoea, **E**xercise capacity index (BODE) may be useful in predicting mortality (Celli et al. 2004) because there is evidence that prognosis and severity are closely related. Other measurements such as decline in lung function of COPD may not always predict prognosis as the disease is punctuated by acute exacerbations with stepwise changes in activity and lung function (Mannino et al. 2003). Assessment of severity of lung function impairment, frequency of exacerbations and requirement for long-term oxygen therapy (LTOT) may help identify patients entering the final 12 months of life (Seamark et al. 2007). Other variables influencing prognosis may be nutritional status and associated co-morbidities (Melbostad et al. 1997). Typically patients may experience:

- Consistent respiratory symptoms such as breathlessness, cough and chest wall pain
- Increased frequency of hospital admissions or acute care with acute exacerbations particularly in the last year of life

- Anxiety, depression, fear, panic attacks, fatigue, anorexia, thirst, poor mobility, communication issues and poor quality of life
- Breathlessness is the most common presenting symptom in COPD (Bellamy and Brooker 2004). Patients who experience chronic breathlessness also experience acute episodes of severe breathlessness during infective exacerbations

The difficulty in determining the most appropriate time to address end of life issues may impact on agreement of a suitable plan of care. Consequently care may be aimed at active management even towards the terminal phase of the disease process, which may be inappropriate and have a detrimental effect on the dying process.

The palliative care approach with its emphasis on the physical, emotional, psychological, social and spiritual impact of the disease has much to offer the COPD patient and carer during and at the end of their illness. Careful attention to symptom assessment, management and review is the priority. Attention to detail will maximise the quality of life potential for both the patient and carer (see Table 9.2). In the UK, the National Institute of Clinical Excellence (NICE) (2004) guidelines emphasise a stepwise management of COPD based on symptom control rather than severity of lung function. However, disease-specific treatments may still occur alongside symptom control measures.

Table 9.2 Pharmacological management of symptoms in COPD.

Medication	Rationale
Beta$_2$ agonists: salbutamol, terbutaline Long-acting beta$_2$ agonists: salmeterol, formoterol Anticholinergics: ipratropium bromide Long-acting anticholinergic: tiotropium	Impact on the sensation of breathlessness by reducing air trapping in the smaller airways leading to reduction in the residual volume of the lungs; may not improve lung function measurements.
Oral theophyllines:	Relieve breathlessness, impact on lung deflation and reduction in residual lung volume.
Opioids: morphine and diamorphine	Decrease ventilatory demand by altering the processing of central motor signals, altering central perception of breathlessness.
Anxiolytics: lorazepam and diazepam	Reduce apprehension and provide mild sedation.
Antidepressants:	Reduce impact of depression on the ability to cope with symptoms
Combination treatment: Seretide, Symbicort	Reduce the frequency of exacerbations. Patients who present with two or more exacerbations have been shown to benefit from the addition of combination therapy.

Adapted from Chadwick and Russell (2008), Merseyside and Cheshire Cancer Network (2006) and Watson (2006).

Breathlessness, pain and cough

The use of opioids

Opioids such as morphine and diamorphine have been used to treat breathlessness, pain and cough for a number of years in the cancer respiratory patient. In the treatment of the COPD patient they have their place with careful assessment, monitoring and review.

Breathlessness

Morphine reduces inappropriate and excessive respiratory drive and substantially reduces the ventilatory response to hypoxia and hypercapnia. By slowing respiration it makes breathing more effective (Watson 2006). Concerns for its use in COPD patients predominately revolve around questions of respiratory depression. In a systematic review of the use of opioids, Jennings et al. (2001) concluded that there was a highly statistically significant benefit of using opioids on the sensation of breathlessness. A stepwise, low-dose increment is always recommended, for example an initial dose of 2.5 mg immediate-release oral morphine, carefully monitored and repeated every 4 hours, and titrated upwards every 24 hours. In some circumstances, the initial starting dose may be lower than 2.5 mg immediate release oral morphine and frequency may be 12 hourly rather than 4 hourly. Slow release (e.g. 12 hourly) preparations can also be used rather than the immediate release ones, but in some circumstances patients may prefer the immediate release preparations. Nebulised opioids have also been trialled in some areas but this approach is not routinely used or recommended.

Pain management

Careful assessment of pain to identify cause will be necessary (e.g. for intercostal blockage and neuropathic pain). For immediate-release morphine, initial starting doses and management approach will be similar to those used for breathlessness above. A note of caution is that a patient who may be on high doses of morphine for pain may benefit from starting on lower doses as described above for breathlessness rather than the usual calculated PRN pain-relieving doses. Parenteral opioids can be used at the end of life for those patients no longer able to take oral medications. Subcutaneous infusions with drug combinations of opioids, benzodiazepines, anticholinergics and antiemetics may benefit a patient in terms of consistent symptom control when no longer able to swallow (Dickman et al. 2005). Careful conversion of oral to parenteral doses is necessary as well as explanation to the patient and carers about the aim which is to maximise symptom relief and not to hasten death. Palliative care teams and hospices are very familiar with the use of opioids and subcutaneous infusions at the end of life and advice should be sought from them. When using opioids in any regimen, careful monitoring and review as well as the co-prescribing of a laxative and antiemetic to proactively reduce the side effects of constipation and nausea are recommended (Twycross et al. 2002).

Oxygen therapy

Evidence of the benefit of oxygen therapy at the end of life is inconclusive. Clear guidelines support the use of long term oxygen therapy (LTOT) in the management of COPD with chronic hypoxaemia (NICE 2004), but the evidence for the use of short-burst oxygen for palliation of symptoms without hypoxia is less clear. Studies have demonstrated a survival benefit for patients with chronic hypoxia using LTOT for a minimum of 15 h/day, although there may be no improvement in symptoms (Lacasse 2001). The prescribing of palliative oxygen at the end of life is not unusual. Patients may not meet the requirements for LTOT, but it probably does have a place in symptom control at the end of life. It should be introduced on a trial basis, accompanied by subjective and objective measures of the patient's response (where possible by the use of dyspnoea scales and pulse oximetry), before being introduced on a long-term basis. Useful questions to consider may be:

- How many hours a day is the oxygen to be used (as required or on a constant basis)?
- What should the flow rate be? (blood gas analysis is essential prior to the provision of LTOT)

Non-invasive ventilation (NIV)

Many patients with end stage COPD will present with hypercapnic respiratory failure, both as part of the disease progression and also during infective exacerbations. It is recommended that NIV should be considered early when patients present with respiratory failure during exacerbation of COPD as NIV has been shown to reduce mortality, avoid the need for endotracheal intubation and reduce the possibility of treatment failure (Picot et al. 2004). Patients with end stage disease may also present with chronic hypercapnic respiratory failure; however, there is little evidence supporting the role of domiciliary NIV although trials are now ongoing into its efficacy. Patients meeting criteria for LTOT who develop hypercapnic respiratory failure but cannot tolerate low flow oxygen may benefit from long-term NIV, However, these patients should be referred to specialist centres for individual consideration of treatment (NICE 2004). Decisions regarding initiation of domiciliary NIV should be made following a consideration of the wishes of patients and carers, quality of life and support available within the community.

Bronchodilators

Bronchodilator therapy to open the airways is the first line of treatment in COPD where the goal is to achieve maximal bronchodilator effect. COPD is classified as irreversible airways disease, but bronchodilator therapy can have significant impact on the sensation of breathlessness by the effect achieved on the smaller airways. Air trapping is reduced which reduces the functional reserve capacity of the lungs reducing the sensation of breathlessness, although this may not show as an improvement in lung function as measured using spirometry. This effect can be achieved by the use of high-dose short-acting beta$_2$ agonists such as salbutamol four times daily via a spacer device, or alternatively via a nebuliser compressor four times daily. The use of the combination bronchodilator Combivent™ as a nebulised solution is also effective. Long-acting bronchodilation can be achieved using either long-acting beta agonists (salmeterol or formoterol) or long-acting anticholinergics (tiotropium). Patients who continue to experience significant distress from breathlessness may also benefit from the addition of oral theophyllines; these can also lead to an improvement in symptoms without improvement in spirometry by relaxing the smooth muscle, thus enhancing the effects of the beta agonists (BTS/NICE 2004). Response to treatment should be assessed by tools which assess the impact that breathlessness has on the individual such as the Breathlessness Assessment Guide (Corner and Driscoll 1999). Drug therapies used to help suppress cough may include cough linctuses, codeine linctuses, low-dose oral morphine solutions and methadone solution (advice from a specialist palliative care team should be sought with morphine and methadone solutions). Non-pharmacological measures such as acupuncture, fans to circulate the air around a patients face, relaxation and breathing control techniques, aromatherapy and visualization have also anecdotally been found to be useful. The support of the physiotherapist and occupational therapist to maximize independence is also essential.

Infective exacerbations

Infective exacerbations can impact significantly on the symptoms of breathlessness and disease progression. They should be treated promptly with the appropriate antibiotic (therapy if the sputum is purulent) and an oral corticosteroid (prednisolone, usually 30 mg daily for 7–14 days) to reduce airway inflammation. The use of combination therapy consisting of an inhaled corticosteroid, fluticasone and long-acting beta$_2$ agonist, salmeterol (Seretide) or the combination of budesonide with the long-acting beta$_2$ agonist formoterol (Symbicort) has been shown to reduce exacerbation rates in moderate to severe COPD. Reductions in exacerbation rates have also been seen with the use of tiotropium and mucolytics. It is recommended that a multi-drug approach be taken in order to take advantage of the effects of each class of bronchodilator.

Sputum and Secretions

Antimuscarinic bronchodilator treatment should be considered to enhance the bronchodilator effect. This can be given as either ipratropium bromide four times daily via a spacer device or via a nebuliser compressor, or alternatively in the long-acting formulation of tiotropium once a day. Mucus hypersecretion can be a problem for COPD patients. The combination of anticholinergics to reduce mucus secretion and beta agonists may improve mucus clearance. Patients who produce large volumes of sputum and experience frequent infective exacerbations may benefit from mucolytic therapy. Mucolytic therapy can reduce sputum viscosity and thus enhance clearance. Parenteral anticholinergics such as hyoscine hydrobromide and glycopyrronium may also be of use, particularly in the terminal care setting.

Anxiety, fear and depression

Depression is common in patients with COPD (Gore et al. 2000). It is suggested that it may influence discussions about end of life care, either by leading patients to rate the quality of these conversations poorly or influencing their treatment choices (Curtis et al. 2005). Depression may also influence patients to want more or less treatments (SUPPORT Investigators 1995). Accurate assessment and appropriate pharmacological and psychological antidepressant treatment should be considered (especially to understand the underlying causes and difference between depression and anxiety). Selective serotonin reuptake inhibitors (SSRIs) such as sertraline, citalopram or mirtazepine may be used (Twycross et al. 2002). Tricyclic antidepressants should be avoided in patients with concurrent heart failure because of possible cardiotoxic side effects. The onset of the antidepressant effect of these drugs may take several weeks; caution should also be taken with the concurrent use of non-steroidal anti-inflammatory drugs due to an increased possibility of gastrointestinal bleeding. Night sedation may also be necessary. Psychological support may range from cognitive behaviour techniques to counselling and complementary therapies. Benzodiazepines such as lorazepam, midazolam and diazepam can help with panic, associatede with hyperventilation and fear of suffocation. Short-acting benzodiazepines such as lorazepam and midazolam are helpful in crisis situations.

Practice Point 9.2

Consider the last COPD patient that you nursed and review the following document: 'Chronic obstructive pulmonary disease: national clinical guideline for management of chronic obstructive pulmonary disease in adults in primary and secondary care' (NICE 2004). It can be accessed at http://www.nice.org.uk/guidance/index.jsp?action =byID&r=true&o=10938.

Commentary:

Are you able to identify a symptom control management plan for your patient and describe the rationale for your plan of care that is in keeping with best practice as suggested by the NICE (2004) guidance? Quality assurance is a phrase used to classify the policies and procedures developed within health care to assess and evaluate the quality of service provision. It should be an integral part of all clinical practice, although assessing health care requires a versatile approach to ensure that all aspects of quality such as effectiveness, acceptability, efficiency, access, equity and relevance are appraised (Hughes and Higginson 2006). This inevitably means that all nursing practices and patient interventions should be continually reviewed to ensure they meet accepted best practice and as a result, the nursing team should be continually updating policies and procedures.

The last days or hours of life

Prognostication in COPD is challenging. However, the palliative care approach already described is just as appropriate in the last year as the last days of life. The principles of careful assessment, monitoring, review and evaluation remain paramount. In the last few days of life it becomes necessary to shift gear to the terminal phase where the focus moves away from cure. The multidisciplinary team will need to be in agreement about goals and management plan. Discussions with the patient and carers are essential in order to support them through this time. If there is uncertainty about length of time to live, this should be shared where possible with the patient and carers. The literature to date reviewed in Table 9.1 reveals that although these conversations may be difficult to have, patients and carers value empathetic, honest conversations. Inappropriate medications and interventions such as venapuncture and vital signs checking may also no longer be appropriate. As well as emotional, practical and psychological support at the end of life, physical symptom control may well involve medications to relieve breathlessness, pain, secretions, agitation and nausea and vomiting. Local policy will dictate symptom control guidelines and dose ranges, but they

Table 9.3 Common parenteral drugs used at the end of life in COPD.

Symptom	Parenteral/subcutaneous drugs	Comment
Pain	Diamorphine or morphine	Take into account whether already on oral opioids for pain
Breathlessness	Diamorphine or morphine Midazolam	Take into account whether already on oral opioids for pain
Secretions	Glycopyrronium or hyoscine hydrobromide	Consider positioning as well as drug therapy
Agitation	Midazolam or levomeprazine	Exclude contributing factors such as psychological distress, urinary retention, constipation, infection or nicotine withdrawal
Nausea and vomiting	Haloperidol or cyclizine or levomeprazine	Take into account other prescribed medications and anxiety

Adapted from Chadwick and Russell (2008), Merseyside and Cheshire Cancer Network (2006) and Watson (2006).

may include drug combinations as shown in Table 9.3. Advice should be sought from specialist palliative care teams regarding dose ranges and combinations.

End of life tools

American studies identify that the majority of patients with COPD wish to die in their own home yet relatively few patients achieve this (Weitzen et al. 2003). Elkington et al. (2005) in the UK revealed that 67% of patients with COPD died in hospital. In the UK, the End of Life Initiative and the NICE (2004) Supportive Care Guidance recommend the use of the Gold Standards Framework (GSF), Liverpool Care Pathway (LCP) and Preferred Place of Care (PPC) and/or Advanced Care Planning. Similar tools can also be found in the United States with the 'Go Wish Card Game' developed by the CODA alliance (Menkin 2007). The underlying principles to these tools are the concept of planning ahead and open communication between patient, family, health care professionals and lay carers in order to be able to plan and discuss end of life preferences. These toolkits help stimulate practical discussions about care as well as expression of feelings and emotions. It may also be postulated that they provide a vocabulary to discuss end of life preferences.

The GSF (www.goldstandardsframework.nhs.uk) is a systematic approach to optimising multiprofessional care through identifying, assessing and planning the care of any patient nearing the end of life. There are seven key tasks of Communication, Coordination, Control of Symptoms, Continuity including out of hours, Continued learning, Carer support and Care in the dying stage (known as the 7 Cs). This framework has also developed a Prognostic Indicator Guidance which includes patients with COPD. Further discussion of this tool can be found in Chapter 5.

A similar prognostic indicator has also been developed by community hospices in Maryland USA, by similar organisations in Canada and by the End of Life/Palliative Resource Centre in America (www.eperc.mcw.educ).

The LCP was developed to transfer the hospice model of care into other care settings. It has proved helpful for health care practitioners working in secondary care in providing a holistic evidence-based framework of care for the dying patient. The LCP has eleven goals, which are broken down into the areas of symptom control, psychological and spiritual support and communication. The pathway is commenced when certain criteria are present. Once the patient has reached this stage of their illness the pathway provides a clear holistic guide to the appropriate management which is suitable for all patients with end stage lung disease (www.lcp-mariecurie.org.uk). A further in-depth discussion of the LCP can be found in Chapter 4.

Advance directives can be used to set out who will represent the patient in the event of their inability to express their wishes, treatment preferences and preferred place of care. This gives clinicians a clear picture of the patient's wishes avoiding the potential for unwanted heroic measures to be instigated (www.goldstandardsframework.nhs.uk).

Practice Point 9.3

In your area of clinical practice are end of life tools in use? Review the use of both the tools mentioned above. Information on them can be found in Chapters 4 and 5 of Section 1 of this book.

Commentary:

You should be able to identify the key principles within end of life tools and describe how to incorporate them into your clinical practice. The End of Life Programme in England (http://www.endoflifecare.nhs.uk/eolc) has identified the use of these two tools as being effective in ensuring that optimal end of life care is provided to all those who require it regardless of diagnosis or place of care. In Scotland representations have been made to the government and it is hoped that these tools will also be formally recognised as part of a national end of life care strategy. In preparation for this an End of Life Care lead has recently been appointed. Similarly Wales and Northern Ireland are developing strategies to ensure good end of life care is available to all.

Summary

This chapter has discussed the issues surrounding the provision of palliative care for patients with COPD covering:

- Burden of disease including physical, psychological, emotional, spiritual and social needs including communication issues
- Ethical issues
- Symptom control at the end of life, including the use of the relevant tools

Having read this chapter and having completed the reflective activities you should have a greater understanding of the needs of patients with COPD at the end of life. This should allow you to identify and manage the issues that affect the COPD patients in your care more effectively. However, it is known that competent and confident practice only comes once a nurse has had time to integrate new knowledge and skills fully into their practice and as such it may take some time to fully change the way you care for this group of patients

References

Beauchamp TL and Childress JF (2001) *Principles Biomedical Ethics* (5th edition). Oxford: Oxford University Press.

Bellamy D and Booker R (2004) *Chronic Obstructive Pulmonary Disease in Primary Care. All You Need to Know to Manage COPD in Your Practice* (3rd edition). London: Class Health.

BTS/NICE (2004) Chronic obstructive pulmonary disease: full guideline. *Thorax.* 59(Suppl 1):42–51.

Celli BR, Cote CG, Marin JM, Casanova C, Montes de Oca M, Mendez RA, Pinto Plata V and Cabral HJ (2004) The body-mass index, airflow obstruction, dyspnea, and exercise capacity index in chronic obstructive pulmonary disease. *New England Journal of Medicine.* 350(10):1005–1012.

Chadwick S and Russell S (2008) *End Stage Respiratory Guidelines.* Berkhamsted, Hertfordshire: Hospice of St Francis, unpublished.

Claessens MT, Lynn J and Zhong Z (2000) Dying with lung cancer or chronic obstructive pulmonary disease: insights from SUPPORT. *Journal of the American Geriatric Society.* 48(Suppl 5):S146–S153.

Clayton JM, Hancock KM, Butow PN, Tattersall MH, Currow DC, Adler J, Aranda S, Auret K, Boyle F, Britton A, Chye R, Clark K, Davidson P, Davis JM, Girgis A, Graham S, Hardy J, Introna K, Kearsley J, Kerridge I, Kristjanson L, Martin P, McBride A, Meller A, Mitchell G, Moore A, Noble B, Olver I, Parker S, Peters M, Saul P, Stewart C, Swinburne L, Tobin B, Tuckwell K and Yates P (2007) Clinical practice guidelines for communicating prognosis and end-of-life issues with adults in the advanced stages of a life-limiting illness, and their caregivers. *Medical Journal of Australia.* 186(Suppl 12):S77, S79, S83–S108.

Corner J and Driscoll M (1999) Development of a breathlessness assessment guide for use in palliative care. *Palliative Medicine.* 13(5):375–384.

Curtis JR, Engelberg RA, Nielsen EL, Au DH and Patrick DL (2004) Patient–physician communication about end-of-life care for patients with severe COPD. *European Respiratory Journal.* 24(2):200–205.

Curtis JR, Engelberg RA, Wenrich MD and Au DH (2005) Communication about palliative care for patients with chronic obstructive airways disease. *Journal of Palliative Care.* 21:157–164.

Curtis JR, Wenrich MD and Carline JD (2002) Patients' perspectives on physician skill in end-of-life care: differences between patients with COPD, cancer, and AIDS. *Chest.* 122:356–362.

Dickman A, Schneider J and Varga J (2005) *The Syringe Driver: Continuous Subcutaneous Infusions in Palliative Care* (2nd edition). Oxford: Oxford University Press.

Edmonds P, Karlsen S, Khan S and Addington-Hall J (2001) A comparison of the palliative care needs of patients dying from chronic respiratory diseases and lung cancer. *Palliative Medicine.* 15(4):287–295.

Elkington H, White P, Addington-Hall J, Higgs R and Edmonds P (2005) The healthcare needs of chronic obstructive pulmonary disease patients in the last year of life. *Palliative Medicine.* 19(6):485–491.

Evans MJ and Hallett CE (2007) Living with dying: a hermeneutic phenomenological study of the work of hospice nurses. *Journal of Clinical Nursing.* 16(4):742–751.

Gaber KA, Barnett M, Planchant Y and McGavin CR (2004) Attitudes of 100 patients with chronic obstructive pulmonary disease to artificial ventilation and cardiopulmonary resuscitation. *Palliative Medicine.* 18(7):626–629.

Golin C, Wenger NS, Liu H, Dawson NV, Teno JM and Desbien NA (2000) A prospective study of patient–physician communication about resuscitation. *Journal of American Geriatrics Society.* 48(5):S52–S60.

Goodridge DM (2006) COPD as a life limiting illness: implications for advanced practice nurses. Topics in Advanced Practice Nursing eJournal. 6(4). Accessed on 23 February 2008.

Gore JM, Brophy CJ and Greenstone MA (2000) How well do we care for patients with end stage chronic obstructive pulmonary disease (COPD)? A comparison of palliative care and quality of life in COPD and lung cancer. *Thorax.* 55:1000–1006.

Hansen EC, Waller J and Woodbaker R (2007) Explaining chronic obstructive pulmonary disease (COPD): perceptions of the role played by smoking. *Sociology of Health and Illness.* 29(5):730–749.

Hughes R and Higginson IJ (2006) Discussion of quality and audit in health. *Journal of Health and Social Policy.* 22(1):29–38.

Jennings AL, Davies AN, Higgins JPT and Broadley K (2001) Opioids for the palliation of breathlessness in terminal illness. Cochrane Database of Systematic Reviews, Issue 3.

Knauft E, Nielsen EL, Engelberg RA, Patrick DL and Curtis JR (2005) Barriers and facilitators to end-of-life care communication for patients with COPD. *Chest.* 127(6):2188–2196.

Lacasse Y, Rousseau L and Maltais F (2001) Prevalence of depressive symptoms and depression in patients with severe oxygen dependent chronic obstructive pulmonary disease. *Journal of Cardiopulmonary Rehabilitation.* 21(2):80–86.

Mannino DM, Buist AS, Petty TL and Enright PL (2003) Lung function and mortality in the United States: data from the First National and Nutrition Examination Survey follow up study. *Thorax.* 58:388–393.

McDowell I and Newell C (1996) *Measuring Health* (2nd edition). Oxford: Oxford University Press.

McNeely PD, Hebert PC, Dales RE, O'Connor M, Wells AG, McKin D, and Sullivan KE (1997) Deciding about mechanical ventilation in end-stage chronic obstructive pulmonary disease: how respirologists perceive their role. *Canadian Medical Association Journal.* 156(2):177–183.

Melbostad E, Wijnand E and Magnus P (1997) Chronic bronchitis in farmers. *Scandinavian Journal of Work Environment and Health.* 23(4):271–280.

Menkin ES (2007) Go wish: a tool for end of life care conversations. *Journal of Palliative Medicine.* 10(2):297–303.

Merseyside and Cheshire Cancer Network (2006) Specialist palliative care referral guidelines and symptom control for patients with end stage chronic respiratory disease. Available at www.mccn.nhs.uk. Accessed on 20 November 2008.

Morgan M (2003) Doctor patient relationship. In: Scrambler G (Ed), *Sociology as Applied to Medicine* (5th edition). Oxford: Saunders.

Murray SA, Boyd KA and Sheikh A (2005) Palliative care in chronic illness. *British Medical Journal.* 330(7492):611–612.

National Institute Clinical Excellence (NICE) (2004) Chronic obstructive pulmonary disease: national clinical guideline for management of chronic obstructive pulmonary disease in adults in primary and secondary care, NICE Guideline Number 12. London: NICE.

NHS Employers (2006) *The NHS Knowledge and Skills Framework: A Short Guide to KSF Dimensions.* London: NHS Employers.

Nishimura K and Tsukino M (2000) Clinical course and prognosis of patients with chronic obstructive pulmonary disease. Current Opinions in Pulmonary Medicine. 6:127–132.

Pauwels RA, Buist AS, Calverley PMA, Jenkins CR and Hurd SS (2001) Global strategy for the diagnosis, management and prevention of chronic obstructive pulmonary disease. *American Journal Respiratory and Critical Care Medicine.* 163(5):1256–1276.

Picot J, Lightowler J and Wedzicha JA (2007) Non-invasive positive pressure ventilation for treatment of respiratory failure due to exacerbations of chronic obstructive pulmonary disease. *Cochrane Database of Systematic Reviews.* Issue 4.

Seamark DA, Seamark CJ and Halpin DM (2007) Palliative care in chronic obstructive pulmonary disease: a review for clinicians. *Journal of the Royal Society of Medicine.* 100(5):225–233.

Selecky PA, Eliasson AH, Hall RI, Roslyn F, Schneider RF, Varkey B and McCaffree R (2005) Palliative and end-of-life care for patients with cardiopulmonary diseases – American College of Chest Physicians position statement. *Chest.* 128(5):3599–3610.

Shah S, Blanchard M, Tookman A, Jones L, Blizard R and King M (2006) Estimating needs in life threatening illness: a feasibility study to assess the views of patients and doctors. *Palliative Medicine.* 20(3):205–210.

Skilbeck JK and Payne S (2005) End of life care: a discursive analysis of specialist palliative care nursing. *Journal of Advanced Nursing.* 51(4):325–334.

SUPPORT Principal Investigators (1995) A controlled trial to improve care for seriously ill hospitalised patients: the study to understand prognoses and preferences for outcomes and risks of treatments. *Journal of the American Medical Association.* 274(20):1591–1598.

Twycross R, Wilcock A, Charlesworth S and Dickman A (2002) *Palliative Care Formulary* (2nd edition). Oxon: Radcliffe.

Vernon S (2001) Use of standardised scales in community nursing assessment. Journal of Community Nursing Online. 15(9). Available at http://www.jcn.co.uk/journal.asp?MonthNum=09&YearNum=2001&Type=backissue&ArticleID=392. Accessed on 11 April 2008.

Watson M (2006) *Adult Palliative Care Guidance* (2nd edition). West Sussex/Northern Ireland: Sussex Cancer Networks/Palliative Medicine Group.

Weitzen S, Teno JM, Fennell M and Mor V (2003) Factors associated with the site of death: a national study of where people die. *Medical Care.* 41(2):323–335.

Wenger NS, Phillips RS, Teno JM, Oye RK, Dawson NV, Liu H, Califf R, Layde P, Hakim R, and Lynn J (2000) Physician understanding of patient resuscitation preferences: insights and clinical implications. *Journal of the American Geriatric Society.* 48(Suppl 5):S44–S51.

Wenrich MD, Curtis JR, Shannon SE, Carline JD, Ambrozy DM and Ramsey PG (2001) Communicating with dying patients within the spectrum of medical care from terminal diagnosis to death. *Archives Internal Medicine.* 161(6):868–874.

White DB, Engelberg RA, Wenrich MD, Lo B and Curtis JR (2007) Prognostication during physician–family discussions about limiting life support in intensive care units. *Critical Care Medicine.* 35(2):442–448.

Yohannes AM (2007) Palliative care provision for patients with chronic obstructive pulmonary disease. Health and Quality of Life Outcomes Online. 5:17. Available at http://www.hqlo.com/content/5/1/17. Accessed on 20 November 2008.

Further reading

http://www.thoracic.org/sections/publications/statements/pages/respiratory-disease- adults/palliative-care.html.

American Thoracic Society (ATS) founded in 1905 specialises in pulmonology, critical care, sleep medicine, infectious disease, pediatrics, allergy/immunology, thoracic surgery, behavioural science, environmental and occupational medicine. The ATS publishes statements, workshop reports and clinical guidelines, and establishes the latest standards of care for a variety of adult and paediatric respiratory, critical care and sleep disorders. Publication in 2008 of position statement on palliative care in respiratory disease and critical illness.

www.communityhospices.org.

This is an American hospice organisation that provides information on palliative care for patients, families and care professionals. Their website says:

'At Community Hospices we believe that terminally ill individuals deserve to live their remaining days pain and symptom free in the company of friends and family. We are dedicated to providing the highest quality inpatient and homecare hospice services for our patients and their families.'

www.palliativedrugs.com.

This site provides essential, comprehensive and independent information for health professionals about the use of drugs in palliative care. It highlights drugs given for unlicensed indications or by unlicensed routes and the administration of multiple drugs by continuous subcutaneous infusion.

Websites

www.breakingbadnews.co.uk. Accessed on 15 January 2009.

www.endoflifecare.nhs.uk/eolc. Accessed on 15 January 2009.

www.goldstandardsframework.nhs.uk. Accessed on 15 January 2009.

www.lcp-mariecurie.org.uk. Accessed on 15 January 2009.

Chapter 10

Palliative care for people who have dementia

Stephen D. M. Smith

Introduction

This chapter explores key issues relevant to the provision of palliative care for people who have dementia and their carers. The focus relates to nursing; however, there is a need for nurses to have a broad understanding of this subject; in terms of the way multiple services are involved in the provision of care for the person with dementia and their carers.

In order to provide a context for this chapter, epidemiological issues and definitions of dementia will be identified. The author will then describe a needs assessment process undertaken as part of the West Lothian Dementia Palliative Care Project. This needs assessment, although local to West Lothian in Scotland, highlights and mirrors key palliative dementia care issues identified throughout the UK.

The key nursing issues identified by the needs assessment were:

- Provision of person-centred care
- Management of pain and other symptoms
- Supporting carers of people with dementia

Learning outcomes

Once you have read this chapter and completed the associated practice points, you will be able to:

- Discuss the magnitude of the problem of dementia and the impact of this for nurses who work in a variety of care settings
- Identify key nursing issues relevant to the provision of person-centred care, pain and symptom control, support for family carers and end of life care
- Describe approaches to caring for people with dementia that will have the following positive outcomes: for the person with dementia to be treated as an individual, to maximise individual and effective management of pain and distress and for the carer to experience support appropriate to their needs and wishes

Background information

Dementia is defined as:

'A generic term indicating a loss of intellectual functions including memory, significant deterioration in the ability to carry out day-to-day activities, and often, changes in social behaviour' (Scottish Intercollegiate Guidelines Network 2006, p. 1). Alzheimer's disease is the most common form of a dementia. Vascular dementia and Lewy Body disease are other examples of dementia related diseases'

(Alzheimer Scotland – Action on Dementia 2006).

Epidemiology

It is acknowledged that the number of people affected by dementia in the UK is steadily rising on an annual basis. This is because dementia, as a syndrome, predominantly affects older people and the number of older people is rising in proportion to the rest of the population. There are significant concerns that in the next two decades, there will not be enough people of working age to provide care for the large numbers of people who will be affected by dementia.

Recent estimates suggest that there are currently 700 000 people in the UK affected by dementia. This is expected to rise to 940 110 by 2021 (Alzheimers Society 2007). NHS Health Scotland (2003, p. 11) states, 'The baby boomers of the 1970s and 1980s will be in their 70s and 80s in the 2030s, and with lower fertility from the 1970s, the overall population structure in Scotland is changing dramatically. Whilst greater longevity is also relevant, these broader demographic factors are the main reason why the projection for 2031 shows significant mass ageing.'

These population changes are significant and will have a major impact on the delivery of health and social services in the future. As such dementia, as part of older people's care, can be viewed as a highly political issue where there is a sense of urgency to plan and develop responsive services. It is evident that nurses will encounter people who have dementia in all care settings, hospital, care homes, in primary care and (potentially to a far lesser extent) in hospices. In 2007, the Alzheimer's Society commissioned research on the social and economic impact of dementia in the UK. The report identified that dementia care costs the UK government £17 billion a year and that the care provided by family carers saves £6 billion annually.

An important factor in regard to palliative care for people who have dementia is the period of time people live with these diseases. Prognosis is variable, with some people living up to 10 years or more following diagnosis (Morgan 2005). This prognosis is an important factor when considering palliative care for people who have dementia.

Palliative dementia care in practice

It is interesting to note how in the British healthcare system, people with different but equally debilitating diseases can be treated quite differently in terms of the care they receive. Services available to people with dementia are generally less well developed and coordinated, compared to those available to people with advanced cancer. This is in spite of the fact that people with dementia and their families have been identified as having very similar needs to those living with a cancer diagnosis (McCarthy et al. 1997).

It could be argued that from a theoretical perspective dementia care has much in common with the palliative care approach (Scottish Partnership for Palliative Care 2006). In the clinical context, however, the two approaches are only commonly integrated during end of life care. This limited connection results in people with dementia receiving inconsistent and sub-optimal support during the early stages of their disease, leading to a negative impact on their quality of life. Issues such as identifying and documenting individual future wishes and care preferences, organising finances and making legal decisions, such as determining power of attorney arrangements, may not be addressed (Scottish Intercollegiate Guidelines Network 2006). These are important activities that require the person to have the mental capacity which may be lost later in the disease. Addressing these issues early on could have a positive impact on both existing and future quality of life. There are examples of such an approach being attempted early on in dementia care, but it is not applied consistently and is dependent upon individual mental health, primary and social care services. A positive example of recent service development that addresses these issues is the development of memory clinics, where people have access to a structured programme of support early on in their illness. These supportive interventions do not require to be provided by palliative care professionals or specialists, but may be more appropriately provided by those already involved including psychiatrists, social workers and mental health nurses. In 2007 a national initiative in Scotland led to the development of a care pathway for people with dementia that specified who, how and when these care interventions should be provided (NHS Quality Improvement Scotland 2007).

Palliative care for people who have dementia is identified in dementia care literature and has developed from a social care perspective as opposed to the traditional medical holistic model of palliative care as apparent in models of palliative cancer care. Issues such as communication, making connections with the person who has dementia, the care environment, working with people who have behaviour that is challenging, provision of physical care and managing common symptoms and supporting carers are key issues within the dementia care literature.

Needs assessment aims and process

Conducting a needs assessment was the initial activity of the West Lothian Dementia Palliative Care Project: a three and a half year action research project, completed in August 2007, managed by NHS Lothian and funded by the Big Lottery Fund. The needs assessment was conducted in 2004. The project coordinator conducted a combination of semi-structured interviews and focus groups with people who have dementia, their carers and service providers. Reports compiled, following the completion of interviews and focus groups, were reviewed with participants and the final content agreed. All reports were independently analysed by the project coordinator and a member of the project steering group.

Identified needs and evidence – person-centred care

The notion of providing holistic care as part of a palliative care approach is now familiar to anyone involved in palliative care. Definitions of palliative care classify holistic care in terms of physical, psychosocial and spiritual elements.

In his 1997 book, *Dementia Reconsidered*, Tom Kitwood attributed many of the difficulties surrounding dementia care at the time to the adoption of a medical model of dementia. He was highly critical of the biomedical approach and how it was reflected in the care and services people with dementia received. Kitwood was shocked when he witnessed the treatment of people with dementia. He observed people being demeaned and disregarded and their personhood undermined. A particular focus of his work related to authentic contact and communication with people who have dementia. Kitwood (1997) described his approach as person-centred care; he defined personhood as 'a standing or status that is bestowed on one human being to another in the context of relationship and social being' (p. 8). To maintain personhood involved the following: 'enabling the exercise of choice, the use of abilities, the expression of feelings and living in the context of a relationship' (Kitwood 1997, p. 60).

It is feasible that a palliative care approach, incorporating physical, social, psychological and spiritual aspects, whilst caring for people as individuals, using good communication and respecting autonomy and dignity, could provide a care and support system for people with dementia and their carers (Scottish Partnership for Palliative Care 2006). As an approach it is holistic and in keeping with Kitwood's (1997) person-centred approaches. Hughes et al. (2005) support this argument, stating that the palliative care approach equates to person-centred care in dementia. A potential advantage of the palliative care approach, in comparison to Kitwood's (1997) person-centred and personhood theories, is its applicability in practice. Palliative care professionals have developed practical assessment and intervention methods that provide a clinical and importantly a practical application of this approach, for example the Liverpool Care Pathway for the Dying and the SIGN guidelines for the control of cancer pain (Ellershaw et al. 2003; King et al. 2005; Scottish Intercollegiate Guidelines Network 2008-guidelines revised November 2008).

As part of the dementia palliative care needs assessment process, participants identified key challenges in providing person-centred care. Packer (2000) questions whether person-centred care does actually occur in daily practice. A particular challenge exists in care settings where a large number of people are cared for together. 'The key to providing useful support is knowing the individual and his/her needs. Every individual has a unique personality, all are different as is the response and impact of dementia.' (Comments from a service provider, NHS Lothian 2004.)

The challenge for nurses working with people who have dementia is how to understand the person, their likes and dislikes, their interests, occupation, their relationships with family and friends and identifying what things are important to them. Engaging people who know the person with dementia is a useful way of developing this type of knowledge. The challenge for nurses is to provide care that takes all of these person-centred issues into consideration. Particularly in care settings where a group of people are cared for, there is a need to look at routines and how care is given. There may be a need for nurses to adapt the way care is provided if individual needs are to be met.

Practice Point 10.1

What assessment activities could nurses undertake to get to know and understand the person with dementia and then adapt care to meet their individual needs?

Commentary:

There are particular communication approaches which can help in the assessment of the person with dementia. The person himself or herself should be involved in the assessment. Even if their dementia is advanced and there is limited verbal communication, a person can convey their reaction to situations by their behaviour and the sounds they make. From this, an understanding of preferences and choice can be developed which can then act as a guide for nurses/carers. A key aspect of this type of observational assessment requires nurses to observe over time and discuss their observations as a team, particularly documenting observations carefully and in detail. During the activities of the West Lothian Dementia Palliative Care Project (2007), a repeated experience occurred when staff came together and shared their observations and different perspectives of the behaviour and actions of people with dementia. This collective understanding initiated prompts for carers to try different approaches to providing care based on their observations and evidence. This sounds logical and straightforward; however, it requires a team that has a commitment to meet together regularly, and during these meetings manages to focus on questions such as, How do they behave and why do they behave in this way? What is the perception of the person with dementia? What are they thinking? These discussions are typical of nurses/carers who are interested in the person, their past and their wishes and understanding what is important to them. Importantly these discussions are not an end in themselves, but rather form the basis of rationales for trying different ways of providing individualised care.

Other communication strategies have been identified by a range of authors. These are not exclusively related to identifying individual, person-centred needs, but recognised as good practice when communicating with people who have dementia and who have some difficulty with communication (Buijssen 2005; Health Education Board for Scotland 2003; Regnard et al. 2007; Ward et al. 2005). This is a very important if not vital area of dementia care and one that has been written about in depth. Some of these communication strategies are as follows:

Use simple language.
Ask one question at a time and specifically use closed questions.
Adopt a patient and understanding demeanour and if possible, stop the assessment if the person becomes agitated. An agitated person who feels a degree of pressure will be less able to participate in any discussion.
It could be worth repeating the question at a different time when the person's ability to concentrate is better.
Is there a better time of day to hold a discussion?
Does the person respond well to a particular nurse? Perhaps they should engage the person in assessments.

There are also fundamental questions which might aid communication such as:

Does the person wear spectacles?
Is a hearing aid required and is it working?

The environment may impact upon successful communication; noise, lighting and the activity of those around are factors that could inhibit effective communication.

Other assessment approaches that assist in getting to know the person as an individual are speaking with their family and finding out about their past and what is important to them. These can be discussions held jointly with family and friends and the person with dementia. Possibly family members, in conjunction with the person with dementia, may have made a life storybook and this could give vital information about the person. Specifically this would include information about their family, work, places of importance, hobbies, activities and daily routines. If not, would the activity of completing a life storybook be useful? The value of this type of work is that the information gained can enable a greater understanding of the individual, so that their care can be made more person centred. A key organisational issue is how this information is shared amongst the care team and how it is acted upon to support person-centred care.

Management of pain and distress

'She had a really bad time in the ward; she had pneumonia and suffered a bit of pain with her arthritis. It took a long time to get on top of the arthritis pain.' (Comments from a carer, NHS Lothian 2004)

The carer in this excerpt describes a situation where nursing staff began to associate how a patient's behaviour was related to her pain; then by working alongside other members of the multidisciplinary team, pain relief was achieved.

Pain assessment

In the statement quoted above, the key challenges of pain assessment and management for someone who has severe dementia and communication challenges are evident. There was a need to observe and consider this lady's behaviour, as she was unable to communicate verbally. In keeping with many older people, she suffered from arthritis and experienced pain as a result of this. She appeared to be in significant distress, crying and screaming, biting and ripping her bed sheets. When staff considered that her distressed behaviour might be related to pain, a process of ongoing assessment and a trial of analgesia took place. In time her distressed behaviour reduced and evidence pointed to her distress being a result of untreated pain. This course of action appears straightforward; however, there is a real challenge for nurses is to be constantly vigilant as to the potential problem of pain for people who have dementia and who have difficulty with verbal communication (Weiner et al. 1999).

A substantial body of literature now exists which highlights undetected and untreated pain for people who have dementia and recognises pain assessment as a significant clinical challenge (Kovach et al. 2002; Krulewitch et al. 2000; Lefebvre-Chapiro 2001; Morrison and Sui 2000; Weiner 1999). A number of pain assessment tools are available for people with dementia which have been validated to varying degrees. Those which seem to be most commonly used, at least in the UK, are the Abbey Pain Scale (Abbey et al. 2002) and the Doloplus II (Lefebvre-Chapiro 2001).

Key issues for nurses assessing pain for people who have dementia are getting to know the person, discovering whether they have had problems with pain in the past and using a validated assessment tool, relevant to the person's situation. This is preferable to nurses using their own criteria to assess pain, based on individual knowledge and experience. The work of the West Lothian Dementia Palliative Care Project (2007) highlighted the positive impact of staff working together to complete assessments, particularly where a person's behaviour was being considered. Many perspectives are better than one and a sense of confidence ensues when a collective decision is reached. It is also important to use the person with dementia's existing abilities and not to assume they will be unable to participate in an assessment.

Assessing and managing distress

What is distress? People with dementia can experience distress for a multitude of reasons. Examples include frustration at diminishing abilities, finding they are unable to do things they used to and experiencing an altered perception of other peoples' behaviour or their surroundings. Regnard et al. (2006) argued that for people who have little or no verbal communication it is necessary to identify distress first, and then consider possible causes. This research focused originally on people who had intellectual disability, but during the work of the West Lothian Dementia Palliative Care Project (2007) the principle was adopted for people with dementia who had difficulty in communicating. A core part of the principle is identified in the statement, 'distress may be hidden but it is never silent, changes in behaviour, posture and expression are evident' (Regnard et al. 2006). These authors developed an assessment tool called the Disability Distress Assessment Tool (DisDAT). The principle of the tool is getting to know the person and understanding how they behave when they are distressed and when they are content. Once this assessment has been completed, behaviours that are associated with distress can be further investigated by identifying possible causes and initiating appropriate responses.

Many of the principles applied to the assessment of pain, as identified above, can also be applied to the assessment of distress. It is an individual experience and expressed in a unique way. Some people will become quiet and subdued, whilst others will be agitated and restless. A key question for those caring for people who appear distressed is asking what they are experiencing, thinking or perceiving. Is there a physical problem such as infection or pain? Is their something about the environment, for example stimulation from increased noise or light, which is distressing them? In providing care, are we doing something which causes irritation or do they not understand what is happening? Trying to find a cause for distress can be difficult and time-consuming, but ongoing team discussion and debate, clear documentation of behaviours and involvement of those who know the person best are all important. The principle for nurses should be one of adapting and testing different care practices. Pharmacological interventions to reduce distress can be tried. However, in a similar way to the use of analgesia, a cautious approach is required and continuous assessment necessary (Scottish Intercollegiate Guidelines Network 2006).

Managing pain

In terms of managing pain it is advisable to follow a local pain guideline and undertake trials of analgesia if pain is considered to be a potential problem. The best evidence available is the same for people with dementia as for those who have other conditions and experience pain, namely following the World Health Organization analgesic ladder (SIGN 2008-guidelines revised November 2008). It is important to remember that older people can be very sensitive to analgesia; therefore, a cautious approach is necessary and ongoing assessment essential. Starting with low doses of analgesia and increasing doses slowly is important. For older people, the additional problems of polypharmacy and inadequate fluid intake cannot be ignored when considering using analgesia, further highlighting the need for caution.

A significant advance in clinical practice for people who have dementia are transdermal analgesic patches. These are available in different preparations and strengths and provide additional options for pain relief. Patch administration is less invasive and less frequent and therefore provides a solution for those people who struggle to cooperate taking medication, or for whom there are other reasons, such as swallowing difficulties, which makes the administration of medicines difficult. Although there are many positive reasons for using analgesia in the form of a patch, care needs to be taken to avoid toxicity. Symptoms of toxicity include tremor, drowsiness, hallucinations and appearing frightened or anxious. This can be a very distressing experience but can be avoided with careful assessment and management. Fortunately the trend in analgesic patch development is to make a greater range of strengths available; therefore, options now exist to use lower doses.

Practice Point 10.2

What actions can nurses take to identify when a person with dementia who has communication difficulties may be experiencing pain?

Commentary:

Some key activities include finding out what pain problems the person has currently or has had in the past. Do they take any form of pain relief medication or engage in activities that are aimed at reducing pain, for example exercise programmes, use of special cushions or chairs? How do they behave when they are content and what behaviours do they display when experiencing some form of distress? A key factor, worthy of consideration by nurses and carers, is when a change of behaviour becomes evident. It is important to give active consideration to a potential problem of pain and investigate this thoroughly, avoiding making assumptions about the likely cause of changed behaviour. There are many other reasons why a person's behaviour may change, for example the presence of infection. Discussions between members of the multidisciplinary team and checking out concerns and questions with the person with dementia and their family/friends are important activities that will reduce the possibility of undetected and untreated pain and distress.

Carer support

There is a definite need for nurses to be aware of and act upon the immensely difficult situations experienced by family carers of people who have dementia. Literature identifies multiple challenges for family carers. The Health Education Board for Scotland (NHS Health Education 2003) provided guidance for carers covering a wide range of issues. These include developing a knowledge and understanding of dementia itself, learning to cope with the caring role, dealing with financial and legal issues, the practical issues of providing daily care, identifying where help can be sought and in the latter stages, issues related to admission to a care home.

> 'It's important to acknowledge feelings of grief, guilt and anger and the variation of coping strategies carers adopt,' ... 'A three-pronged approach of support is useful for carers; (1) education and information from professionals, (2) ongoing professional support, (3) mutual support from other carers.'
>
> (Service provider, NHS Lothian 2007)

It is important to recognise that families can care for their relative for prolonged periods of time, in some instances up to 10 years (Lishman 1998). For those families who take on a caring role, the difficulties and stresses are well documented. 'The manifestations of dementia often cause great physical, emotional and social strain on the lives of family caregivers' (Maas et al. 2004). Furthermore, Brodaty et al. (2003) have described how family carers experience higher levels of depression and poorer physical health compared to control groups of people who do not provide care.

One strong emotion often experienced by carers of people with dementia is guilt. Buijssen (2005) states that family carers can experience guilt at the point of diagnosis, when they begin to understand the reasons for recent behavioural changes. Carers might feel that they should have been more understanding, that they should have identified problems sooner and that they should have been more active in seeking help and securing a diagnosis. As Buijssen (2005) has described, 'there can be remorse regarding lost time, when more could have been done together, when questions remained unsaid and issues unresolved'. During periods when family carers are doing all they can for the person with dementia, guilt can still be experienced. Carers can place impossible demands upon themselves, namely that their family member must be happy and all their physical needs met. This is frequently not possible and failure is almost inevitable. Issues of guilt when the person with dementia is admitted to a care home or hospital can also be very significant.

Annerstedt et al. (2000) stressed the importance of identifying breaking points, when family carers can no longer cope with their caring role. These often happen when the person with dementia has an impaired sense of identity of the caregiver or indeed misidentifies them, when the time spent caring is substantial, when the person has clinical fluctuations and when there are problems at night and the carer's sleep is disturbed. It is evident that over time, as the dementia process progresses, a carer is likely to experience a combination of the above situations. It is almost impossible to accurately conceive the impact of caring. Consider for example an elderly wife whose husband has dementia. How does an older person cope with disturbed sleep, the ongoing daily work of caring and the sadness, loss and frustration of her husband no longer recognising her as his wife? In terms of the impact on carers, there can be few more demanding situations.

Practice Point 10.3

What can the nurse do to support family carers caring for someone with dementia?

Commentary:

A number of interventions have been identified and used to help family carers look after people with dementia at home. These include education and training programmes, support groups, counselling and breaks from caring (Brodaty et al. 2003). For nurses who have regular contact with carers, demonstrating an empathic, knowledgeable understanding of their situation, combined with a proactive approach to continuing supportive interventions, is a useful strategy. Carers, such as those people who have dementia they care for, are individuals. Their support needs will be individual and unique to them. Having continuity in support, namely a professional who gets to know them as an individual and can identify with them and their individual challenges and frustrations, but who can also negotiate and initiate appropriate support, is invaluable.

End of life care for people with a dementia

There are a number of key issues identified in the literature regarding end of life care for people who have dementia. One is concerned with how professional carers think about people with dementia and whether they link this type of care to a palliative care approach or to another model of care, such as care for someone with a neuropsychiatric condition (Downs et al. 2006). The theory identified here states that the links made will affect the care provided. Dementia and palliative care professionals would argue this is preferential to fitting people into a specific model that may limit care practices (Hughes et al. 2004).

An issue related to this is that people with dementia, at the end of their lives, are likely to be cared for in care homes or other continuing care settings. Care homes have been identified as 'de facto hospices' for people with dementia (Phillips et al. 2006). It has also been identified that providers of care within these care settings require support to adopt person-centred palliative care approaches. Pain and symptom management, and advance care planning are two particular areas in which training may have to be provided (Bosek et al. 2003). These authors also highlight the benefits of multidisciplinary team working and engagement with social workers and spiritual advisers in care homes to develop understanding of team values and beliefs about death, which could have a direct impact on care.

Another important end of life issue is the appropriateness of interventions such as antibiotics and feeding tubes. At the end of life, the use of such treatments could be contrary to good clinical practice if they result in distress with little benefit to the patient (Evers et al. 2002). A further example of this is inappropriate hospital admission, where a person is taken from their care environment, such as a care home, to have acute treatment in hospital. With advanced planning, such a situation and the consequent distress it may cause could be avoided.

The ethical issues raised by the use of such interventions require debate, but decisions are often determined by the collective approach adopted by the practitioners involved. This situation has a further implication. There is a need for family and nurses to act as advocates for the person with dementia, identifying and agreeing to an overall plan of care that determines the type of interventions that are appropriate for the individual (Mitchell et al. 2004; Phillips et al. 2006). Consistent with a number of issues in this chapter, this is best achieved when the members of the multidisciplinary team work together in a proactive way following an agreed overall approach.

Conclusion

This chapter has highlighted key palliative care needs for people who have dementia and their carers. Approaches that nurses can adopt to address issues regarding the provision of person-centred care, pain and distress management, support for carers and end of life care have been identified. Literature relating to person-centred dementia care is entirely consistent with and identifiable as following a palliative care approach.

References

Abbey J, De Bellis A, Piller N, Esterman A, Giles L, Parker D and Lowcay B (2002) Abbey pain scale. Dementia Care Australia. Available at www.dementiacareaustralia.com.

Alzheimer Scotland – Action on Dementia (2006) *About Dementia: Some Facts and Figures*. Edinburgh: Alzheimer Scotland – Action on dementia.

Alzheimer's Society (2007) *Dementia UK*. London: Alzheimer's Society.

Annerstedt L, Elmstahl S, Ingvad B and Samuelsson S (2000) Family caregiving in dementia: an analysis of the caregiver's burden and the breaking point when home care becomes inadequate. *Scandinavian Journal of Public Health*. 28(1):23–31.

Bosek MSD, Lowry E, Lindeman DA, Burck JR and Gwyther LP (2003) Promoting a good death for persons with dementia in nursing facilities: family caregivers' perspectives. *JONA'S Healthcare, Law, Ethics and Regulation*. 5(2):34–41.

Brodaty H, Green A and Koschera A (2003) Meta-analysis of psychosocial interventions for caregivers of people with dementia. *Journal of American Geriatric Society.* 51:657–664.

Buijssen H (2005) *The Simplicity of Dementia: A Guide for Family and Carers.* London: Jessica Kingsley Publishers.

Downs M, Small N and Froggatt K (2006) Explanatory models of dementia: links to end-of-life care. *International Journal of Palliative Nursing.* 12(5):209–213.

Ellershaw J and Wilkinson S (Eds) (2003) *Care of the Dying: A Pathway to Excellence.* Oxford: Oxford University Press.

Evers MM, Purohit D, Perl D, Khan K and Marin DB (2002) Palliative and aggressive end of life care for patients with dementia. *Psychiatric Services.* 53(5):609–613.

Health Education Board for Scotland (2003) *Coping with Dementia: A Handbook for Carers.* Edinburgh: NHS Health Scotland.

Hughes JC, Hedley K and Harris D (2004) The practice and philosophy of palliative care in dementia. *Nursing and Residential Care.* 6(1):27–30.

Hughes JC, Robinson L and Volicer L (2005) Specialist palliative care in dementia. *British Medical Journal.* 330(7482):57–58.

King N, Thomas K, Martin N, Bell D and Farrell S (2005) 'Now nobody falls through the net': practitioners' perspectives on the Gold Standards Framework for community palliative care. *Palliative Medicine.* 19(8):619–627.

Kitwood T (1997) *Dementia Reconsidered: The Person Comes First.* Buckinghamshire: Open University Press.

Kovach CR, Noonan PE, Griffie J, Muchka S and Weissman DE (2002) The assessment of discomfort in dementia protocol. *Pain Management Nursing.* 3(1):16–27.

Krulewitch H, London MR, Skakel VJ, Lundstedt GJ, Thomasen H and Brummel-Smith K (2000) Assessment of pain in cognitively impaired older adults: a comparison of pain assessment tools and their use by non-professional caregivers. *Journal of the American Geriatric Society.* 48(12):1607–1611.

Lefebvre-Chapiro S (2001) The DOLOPLUS ® 2 scale – evaluating pain in the elderly. *European Journal of Palliative Care.* 8(5):191–194.

Lishman WA (1998) *Organic Psychiatry: The Psychological Consequences of Cerebral Disorder* (3rd edition). Oxford: Blackwell Science.

Maas ML, Reed D, Park M, Specht JP Schutte D, Kelley LS, Swanson EA, Tripp-Reimer T and Buckwalter KC (2004) Outcomes of family involvement in care intervention for caregivers of individuals with dementia. *Nursing Research.* 53(2):76–86.

McCarthy M Addington Hall J and Altmann D (1997) The experience of dying with dementia. *International Journal of Geriatric Psychiatry.* 12:404–409.

Mitchell SL, Kiely DK and Hamel MB (2004) Dying with advanced dementia in the nursing home. *Archives of Internal Medicine.* 164(3):321–327.

Morgan K (2005) Living with dementia: then and now. *Generations Review.* 15(1):2–3.

Morrison RS and Sui AL (2000) A comparison of pain and its treatment in advanced dementia and cognitively intact patients with hip fracture. *Journal of Pain and Symptom Management.* 19(4):240–248.

NHS Health Scotland (2003) *Coping with Dementia: A Handbook for Carers.* Edinburgh: NHS Health Scotland.

NHS Lothian (2007) *West Lothian Dementia Palliative Care Project.* Edinburgh: NHS Lothian.

NHS Quality Improvement Scotland (2007) *Draft Standards for Integrated Care Pathways for Mental Health*. Edinburgh: NHS QIS.

Packer T (2000) Does person centred care exist? *Journal of Dementia Care*. 8(3):19–21.

Phillips J, Davidson PM, Jackson D, Kristjanson L, Daly J and Curran J (2006) Residential aged care: the last frontier for palliative care. *Journal of Advanced Nursing*. 55(4):416–424.

Regnard C, Reynolds J, Watson B, Matthews D, Gibson L and Clarke C (2006) Understanding distress in people with severe communication difficulties: developing and assessing the Disability Distress Assessment Tool (DisDAT). *Journal of Intellectual Disability Research*. 51:277–292.

Regnard C, Reynolds J, Watson B, Matthews D, Gibson L and Clarke C (2007) Understanding distress in people with severe communication difficulties: developing and assessing the Disability Distress Assessment Tool (DisDAT). *Journal of Intellectual Disability Research*. 51(4):277–292.

Scottish Intercollegiate Guidelines Network (2008) *SIGN Control of Pain in Patients with Cancer*. Edinburgh: Scottish Intercollegiate Guidelines Network.

Scottish Intercollegiate Guidelines Network (2006) *SIGN 86 Management of Patients with Dementia*. Edinburgh: Scottish Intercollegiate Guidelines Network.

Scottish Partnership for Palliative Care (2006) *Making Good Care Better: National Practice Statements for General Palliative Care in Adult Care Homes in Scotland*. Edinburgh: Scottish Partnership for Palliative Care.

Ward R, Vass AA, Aggarwal N, Garfield C and Cybyk B (2005) What is dementia care? 1. Dementia is communication. *Journal of Dementia Care*. 13(6):16–19.

Weiner DK, Peterson B and Keefe F (1999) Chronic pain associated behaviours in the nursing home: residents versus caregiver perceptions. *Pain*. 80(3):577–588.

Weiner D, Peterson B, Ladd K, McConnell E and Keefe F (1999) Pain in nursing home residents: an exploration of prevalence, staff perspectives and practical aspects of measurement. *Clinical Journal of Pain*. 15(2):92–101.

Chapter 11

Palliative nursing care in other neurological conditions

This chapter is concerned with the provision of palliative nursing care for people who are diagnosed with other neurological conditions. The four specific illnesses that are discussed within this chapter have been selected as there is growing evidence to show that the palliative care approach can improve both the quality of life and death for those diagnosed with these conditions. Each sub-section will provide an overview of the illness before discussing the challenges and benefits of providing palliative nursing care to the group being discussed. It has to be noted that as the incidence of these conditions varies widely nurses providing general palliative care may come into contact with people diagnosed with some of these illnesses more than others.

Huntington's disease

Anne Thomson

Introduction

This section provides the reader with an overview of Huntington's disease (HD) including the clinical features of the disorder and the role played by genetic testing. It explores the experience of living with a hereditary illness like HD and examines the effects on family members. It also discusses the physical, psychosocial and spiritual symptoms encountered in HD and palliative care issues affecting HD sufferers and their families.

Learning outcomes

Once you have read this section and completed the associated practice points, you will be able to:

- Demonstrate a knowledge of HD and its progression
- Reflect on the impact that living with a hereditary disease has on patients and families
- Explain why a palliative care approach can help in the management of HD
- Discuss when to make a referral to Specialist Palliative Care Teams

Background

Huntington's disease is a progressive, neurodegenerative disease caused by a single faulty gene. It is an autosomal dominant disorder affecting males and females equally. The prevalence of the disorder is estimated at 1 in every 10 000. However, there do appear to be areas with higher incidence and in Scotland, for example, prevalence is 1 in every 7000–8000 (MacGill 2003). Given the genetic nature of this disease, it is estimated that for each affected person there may be another 6–9 individuals living at risk of the disease.

HD symptoms usually present between the ages of 35 and 45 although juvenile and late onset variants of the disease exist. Juvenile HD and late onset account for 10% of patients presenting with symptoms. Death occurs 15–20 years from the onset of symptoms; however, with improvements in diagnosis and care management some patients are living longer. There is currently no known cure for HD and therefore management for diagnosis is palliative.

The role of genetic testing

The HD gene was discovered in 1993 and subsequently a single blood test was developed to determine whether or not a person had the gene. Testing is only available for people who are 18 years old or above, and should be carried out at regional genetics clinics. Genetic counsellors will provide information and counselling over a period of months to allow each individual to make an informed choice about being tested. In practice, only 15–20% of individuals actually proceed to testing (Quarrell 1999). The majority of people seem to prefer to live with the hope that they do not have the gene, rather than the knowledge that they do.

Regardless of the result of the test, post-test counselling takes place. The risk of suicide is greater in the HD population and even higher in those who have recently been tested positive (Robins et al. 2000). Even a negative test result can cause psychological problems, as those who test negative can experience feelings of guilt that they do not have the disease whilst their siblings are affected. They may also have feelings of regret over the long period of time they might have spent worrying about developing the illness.

For couples considering a having children, genetic counselling is available to enable them to discuss their options and the likelihood that they will have a baby who is positive for the gene.

Clinical features of Huntington's disease

Huntington's disease manifests itself through its effects on three domains: motor, cognitive and psychiatric (Fig. 11.1). However, the pattern of disease varies in each individual and in its early stages HD can be difficult to recognise. Signs and symptoms at this stage may include restlessness, mild uncontrolled or uncoordinated movements, irritability, poor concentration, memory problems

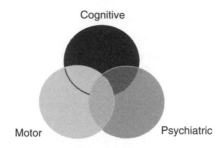

Fig. 11.1 Domains affected by Huntington's disease.

and depression. Unless there is a known family history it is possible for people to be misdiagnosed, especially as symptoms can be vague and their onset insidious.

As HD progresses, symptoms become much more problematic. Among the motor effects is moderate to severe chorea, which can affect ability to walk, speak and carry out basic functions. Impaired vision, balance and gait lead to concerns about safety, and particular challenges are encountered when the person's ability to swallow becomes compromised. Cognitive effects include slowed thinking, impaired judgement and difficulties with planning, organising, prioritising and decision-making. Carers may also be faced with challenging behaviours. Psychiatric effects include depression, mood swings, changes in personality, psychosis and increased risk of suicide.

Care at this stage is often fragmented because of the wide variety of symptoms and the number of medical specialities and different care agencies involved (Aubeeluck and Moscowitz 2008; Simpson 2006). As a result it is common to find poorly coordinated and often inadequate care management.

The end stages of the illness are usually characterised by complete loss of physical function and severely impaired or absent communication. Individuals are fully dependent on others for all aspects of care. Cause of death is often bronchial pneumonia secondary to HD caused by repeated aspiration.

The effect of Huntington's disease on families

Sulaiman (2007) has graphically described the impact of HD on family life:

> 'This illness can seem like a juggernaut ploughing through the family, so massively, awesomely unstoppable that each family member ends up almost paralysed by it.'

Every family's experience of HD is unique, but significant disruption of family life and changes to individuals' roles are commonplace.

Keenan et al. (2007) studied children brought up in an HD family and found that while some children are relatively unaffected, others experience very significant changes of role. Many young people take on household responsibilities including cleaning, cooking and care of younger siblings. Many also carry out personal care tasks for the affected parent and some assume the role of principal carer.

> *'People should know what I live through. I'm not just an ordinary girl ... I used to care for my mum all the time until we got 24-hour care.'*

> (13-year-old)

Even as children reach adulthood, the effects of watching and caring for a parent continue.

> *'I love my mum to bits, I always want to help her as much as I can, but it gets so much at times. I cry a lot and I've had time off work. And every time I go in and open her door I'm always dreading in case I see her lying there with a cracked skull.'*

> (21-year-old)

The 50% risk that each child has of developing the disease creates huge stresses and can result in a range of physical, emotional and psychological symptoms:

> *'Ever since I found out I have really bad nightmares ... it makes me as tired in the morning as when I went to bed, if not more ... I watch myself too as I know it can start early in life.'*

> (24-year-old)

Palliative care issues for people with Huntington's disease

Practice Point 11.1

Think about the effects that HD can have on the quality of life (ideally reflect on someone you have been involved in caring for) and consider how a palliative care approach might be beneficial.

Commentary:

A number of authors have suggested that palliative care is the most appropriate model of care to address the issues raised by a hereditary illness such as HD (Dawson et al. 2004; Mallet and Chekroud 2001). Priorities include control of distressing symptoms, provision of psychological support and attention to practical needs.

Control of motor symptoms

The person with HD typically develops involuntary movements, which initially may just seem like fidgetiness or a nervous restlessness, but which usually develop into obviously abnormal movements that are difficult to control. This movement is referred to as chorea.

Chorea can often be managed with the use of antipsychotic or neuroleptic medication. However, unwanted side effects such as sedation need to be considered and may be more distressing than chorea itself (Kent 2004). Many patients are untroubled by their chorea or dystonia, and unless it is affecting functional capability it is often in the patient's best interests not to treat.

Chorea management should touch on wider issues such as the creation of a safe environment, the choice of suitable seating and the achievement of adequate nutrition. Altered gait and balance problems can cause anxiety for all concerned. Falls are common and can be a source of significant morbidity (Rosenblatt et al. 2004). Walking and other safety aids (such as handrails) may be impossible to use because of chorea or may be rejected by the patient who has no insight into his or her individual needs. However, if occupational therapy assessment is introduced early, there is more time for the patient to adapt to any aids supplied.

Rigidity can be helped with antispasmodic medication in conjunction with passive movements and exercise (Kent 2004). Early referral to a physiotherapist and admission to an exercise programme that concentrates on balance, muscle strength and flexibility can be useful. Family members need to be involved to support and encourage the patient to comply.

Dysarthria can be a real source of frustration for the patient and attempts to communicate can result in outbursts of anger or distress. Speech can become slurred, dysrhythmic, variable in volume and increasingly difficult to under-stand (Rosenblatt et al. 2004). There are many techniques that families and staff need to introduce to try to maintain speech for as long as possible. Allowing longer time to answer questions, asking closed questions, using short simple sentences, using visual clues and keeping background distraction to a mini-mum can all help (Kent 2004). Regular assessment by a speech and language therapist is essential.

Dysphagia varies from patient to patient, but inevitability causes a number of practical and ethical problems. Early and ongoing involvement of a dietician and speech and language therapist is essential to provide advice and support on management of associated problems. Advice from a physiotherapist on chest-clearing exercise and positioning during eating can be helpful, because as the disease progresses, the risk of choking increases. Cognitive impairment may cause the person to eat inappropriate food, overfill their mouth or eat too quickly. Swallowing is a complex process and motor problems can affect the coordination of the muscles involved. This can lead to aspiration and chest infection, and as the condition deteriorates the patient is at risk of pneumonia.

Choking is another highly distressing symptom for patients and families. Simple measures can be instigated to try to prevent choking including modifying the diet, gentle prompting to chew food, and encouragement to slow down and take drinks between mouthfuls (Kent 2004). Invariably however, as the disease progresses swallowing becomes worse, and families and staff will require advice on first aid measures should choking occur.

The continued feeding of a patient with a swallowing disorder presents both practical and ethical challenges, but if a patient continues to want food and drink despite the risks then strategies should be put in place to overcome the problems. Families and care staff will require support and advice about the risks involved and how to manage them. At some stage the issue of artificial feeding should be discussed. Patients need information to help them exercise informed choice, and all relevant professionals should be involved in the discussion. van Broekhoven-Gutters et al. (2000) have shown that artificial feeding may add to quality of life but can also prolong life and suffering. It is important therefore that the patient and those closest to them are given adequate information about the pros and cons of artificial feeding.

Practice Point 11.2

Consider the ethical issues that arise when a patient with HD whose swallowing has become compromised is unable to communicate his or her choice about artificial feeding.

Commentary:

If a patient becomes too unwell to communicate or is deemed not to have capacity, then decisions over artificial feeding may have to be taken by his or her family in consultation with the multidisciplinary team. Ideally, sensitive issues such as artificial feeding would have been discussed with the patient at an earlier stage in the disease process (and/or an advance directive may have been written). In the absence of such information, the guidelines produced by Rabeneck et al. (1997) and the General Medical Council (2002) may aid decision-making.

Other symptoms and their control

The prevalence and characteristics of pain in HD are poorly understood, but there is anecdotal evidence that at least some patients experience little or no pain. Nevertheless careful assessment is required and the use of an appropriate pain assessment tool may be useful. There are several pain tools that could be tried but referral for specialist pain assessment may also be appropriate.

Oral problems are common in HD and can result from changes in mood and function caused by the disease. For instance, there may be a disinclination to maintain personal hygiene routines such as regular teeth cleaning, and the situation may be exacerbated by loss of dexterity associated with chorea. Because patients with HD are often encouraged to eat high-calorie foods, rates of severe dental caries are increased. This in turn can worsen dysphagia and dysarthria (Nance and Westphal 2002). Dental treatment in patients with chorea can be difficult, but regular check-ups and good oral hygiene advice early in the disease are vital to prevent major problems later on.

Weight loss is common in HD for a variety of reasons. Nance and Westphal (2002) have suggested that some patients require 4000–5000 calories per day. However, dietary intake may be poor due to the inability to obtain and prepare food, reluctance to eat in front of others, difficulty eating due to chorea or a reliance on others to be fed. Low mood and depression affect appetite and fear of choking may also be an issue. Dietary assessment is required to determine calorie requirements and the dietician may recommend dietary changes and/or supplements. An occupational therapist may be able to provide aids and adaptations to make eating easier.

Psychiatric issues including depression, psychosis, mania, challenging behaviour and increased risk of suicide are all encountered in people with HD. Of these, depression is the most common, affecting more than 50% of patients as well as carers and those living at risk of developing the disease. Depression should be treated and should lead to improvement in quality of life. If unrecognised and untreated, it can lead to serious morbidity. Robins Whalin (2007) has shown that the incidence of suicide is significantly higher than in the general population and professionals caring for the patient with HD should be aware of the risk.

The management of challenging behaviours such as irritability and aggression should begin with careful assessment and identification of possible causes such as environment, individuals, pain, fear and frustration (Paulsen 1999). Useful techniques include establishing routines, improving communication skills, simplifying the environment and reducing distractions. Referral to psychiatric services for specialist advice may be required.

Many of the symptoms of HD are exacerbated by stress. A number of non-pharmacological interventions have proven useful in reducing stress for both patient and carers (Kent 2004). These include physiotherapy, relaxation and complementary therapies.

The wider issues of Huntington's disease

Spiritual issues

People with HD often struggle with existential issues and questions such as 'Why me?' and 'Why us?' There may be guilt about passing on the gene to children, and the sufferer, aware of the progressive nature of the disease, may wonder how they will let people know their feelings when they are unable to speak. For some families the stigma and secrecy that often surrounds HD can stop them talking about the range of emotions and feelings they are experiencing. Communication problems may make it difficult to reflect on past experiences and losses and to express any feelings about the future. Also, families affected by HD can find their religious or personal belief systems challenged by the diagnosis.

End of life care

The majority of people with HD die of complications which are secondary to their disability. The most common cause of death is bronchopneumonia, but other causes are related to immobility, general debility and malnutrition (Moskowitz and Marder 2001; Rosenblatt et al. 2004). The inability to communicate symptoms can lead to patients developing and even dying from undiagnosed co-morbidities. A previous lifestyle characterised by non-compliance with medication, or a reluctance or inability to attend for routine screening procedures also place HD sufferers at increased risk of co-morbid, potentially life-threatening conditions.

There is a real paucity of research regarding end of life care in patients with HD. There are also no recognised prognostic indicators for HD, and predicting the end of life can be extremely challenging. However, the use of recognised care pathways such as the Gold Standards Framework (Thomas 2003) and the Liverpool Care Pathway (Ellershaw and Wilkinson 2003) may help in the transition to the end of life phase.

Loss, grief and bereavement

In HD families, loss is not confined to one family member, and some families suffer multiple bereavements. There are also losses related to other aspects of life including losses of role, employment, financial security, status, independence and home. Individuals may suffer complicated grief and may require the intensive bereavement support that some specialist palliative care teams offer.

Carers

The responsibility for caring for someone with HD often falls to family members (Pickett et al. 2007). The genetic dimension of the disease and its long-term care implications may mean that HD family members experience more intense problems than carers of people with other illnesses. Fifteen years ago Shakespeare and Anderson (1993) found that service provision for HD families was often inadequate and unsuitable, and that families felt burdened by the demands placed upon them. There is little evidence to suggest that this has changed. Aubeeluck and Buchanan (2006) have found that quality of life for carers is poor and family breakdown caused by violence, aggression and challenging or anti-social behaviours is common. As the onset of symptoms tends to occur at a relatively young age, employment is often compromised and this can bring the added burden of financial hardship. Nurses and other professionals have to be aware of the demands on carers and the need to refer to regional and local agencies for support and respite services (Kristjanson et al. 2006b).

The role of specialist palliative care units

Specialist palliative care units and hospices may not always be the most appropriate care setting for patients with specific neurodegenerative conditions, especially those with a related behaviour or personality disorder (Travers et al. 2007). However, some patients may benefit from inpatient, day care or respite services and individual specialist assessment should be accessed. All staff can benefit from the practical advice, education and support of the specialist palliative care team. Such support may prove invaluable in the management of some of the more complex issues which arise when caring for patients and families affected by HD.

Care planning

A key element in palliative care is care planning, and this is central to the management of any family affected by HD. The plan should encompass all the holistic aspects of management: physical, social, psychological and spiritual. Travers et al. (2007) have shown that a recognised care management pathway is an invaluable tool for key workers, improving continuity of care and decision-making. The Scottish Huntington's Association also recognises the need for a clear framework of guidelines and is developing an integrated care pathway to assist in care management (Scottish Huntington's Association 2006).

Care planning must also address the more sensitive issues of future care including artificial nutrition, resuscitation and organ donation. The fact that HD causes cognitive impairment must be recognised, and advanced directives should be completed while the patient is still deemed capable. Simpson (2006) suggests that to alleviate any concerns about the validity of advanced directives they should be discussed with those closest to the patient and a lasting power of attorney put in place to represent the patient when they are no longer able to communicate.

Conclusion

Huntington's disease is a profoundly debilitating and distressing disorder. Patients and families affected by HD not only have the greatest need for support among of any of the neurodegenerative diseases, but are also among those most likely to benefit from a palliative approach (Kristjanson et al. 2006a). Complex symptom control and spiritual needs are often difficult to assess, and combined with the inability of a patient to communicate, can be particularly challenging to manage. Nurses are in an ideal position to play a key role in coordinating a multidisciplinary, proactive plan of care for families affected by this disease. They can also identify and highlight problem areas for families and refer on to appropriate agencies. As there is no known cure for Huntington's disease, palliative care is essential to ensure that the care provided focuses on optimising quality of life.

Motor neurone disease

Carole Ferguson

Introduction

This section provides the reader with an overview of the main problems that motor neurone disease (MND) presents to the patient, family, friends and professionals who are all involved in the palliative care of people diagnosed with this condition. It begins by reviewing the epidemiology and incidence of motor neurone disease and showing how a diagnosis is made. It then proceeds to discuss the only drug treatment available for MND before examining the common problems associated with the illness. The final section examines the benefits of providing specialist palliative care to these people before looking at bereavement issues for family members left behind.

Learning outcomes

Once you have read this sub-section and completed the associated practice points you will be able to:

- Consider the current issues surrounding the care of the MND patient
- Describe the current interventions available to help alleviate symptoms.
- Discuss the benefits of providing palliative care to people with MND

What is motor neurone disease?

MND is a progressive illness involving the degeneration of upper and lower motor neurones. Currently there is no known cause or cure and because of this the main focus of clinical care is to provide the highest possible quality of life through managing symptoms and physical or emotional suffering. It is a disease that can be extremely rapid, with diagnosis and death being within months of each other. Thus the care of patients with MND is different from some other life-limiting illnesses.

Epidemiology

Where ascertainment is complete the incidence of sporadic MND is geographically relatively constant ranging from 0.86 to 2.5 per 100 000 per year. The average duration of the disease is 3 years, while the mortality is 80% at five years (Hocking et al. 2006). Prevalence rates may be estimated at three times the incidence rate of about 6 per 100 000 on any given date (McGuire and Nelson 2006).

In population-based studies mean and median ages at onset are approximately 65 years and mean and median disease duration from clinical onset to death are approximately 3 years. Familial cases make up 5–10% of patients diagnosed with MND. As noted MND occurs over a wide age range but is predominantly in the middle aged and elderly, the age-specific incidence rising to 1:10 000 when aged 65–68 years. The male to female ratio of incidence is 1.4:1.0 (British Brain and Spine Foundation (BBSF) 2000).

In Scotland a register of all definite cases of MND is in existence and from this there was a prospective study of adult onset MND in Scotland conducted which laid out the demography and clinical features of incident cases. Data from this epidemiological study shows that there are approximately 122 new cases per year in Scotland, while in the UK there are around 5000 people living with

MND any one time (BBSF 2000). In the Scottish study, the average age onset of symptoms was 65.2 years for males and 67.2 for females, while the mean for onset of symptoms to diagnosis was 1.3 years, median survival from onset 2.1 years and the male to female ratio of incidence was 5:4. (Scottish Motor Neurone Disease Register 1992). So although conducted nearly 20 years ago, newer studies report the same information in relation to incidence and age of onset (Hocking et al. 2006), showing that there has been little achieved in the ability to prevent or cure this illness.

Diagnosis

Making a diagnosis of MND as early as possible is important for the patient for psychological, economical, ethical and neurological reasons (Vucic et al. 2007). However, it remains the norm that from onset of symptoms to diagnosis the path is complex and there is no one specific test that will give a definite diagnosis (BBSF 2000). Often the symptoms are vague and intermittent at the start and there is a time delay before the patient seeks medical advice.

Most general practitioners will only see one case of MND in a lifetime of practice (average 25 years). Often referral is made to other specialists such as ear, nose and throat, rheumatology, orthopaedics before the patient sees a neurologist due to the vagueness of symptoms. Motor neurone degeneration causes the muscle wasting which is seen in MND. Most patients have a mix of upper and lower motor neurone degeneration which causes the muscle wasting (Oliver et al. 2007).

Lower motor neurones are located in the spinal cord and brain stem; they extend out to the peripheral nerves and make direct contact with and activate the muscle fibres. Lower motor neurone degeneration causes muscle weakness, wasting and fasciculation, a twitching sensation for the patient which can usually be seen as a rippling under the skin in the arms, legs and chest.

Upper motor neurones lie within the cortex in the frontal lobe of the brain and project downward to join with and activate the lower motor neurones. Deterioration of upper motor neurones causes muscle spasticity and deep tendon reflexes are exaggerated. Most patients diagnosed with MND have a mixture of both upper and lower signs. Where only lower motor signs are present it is called progressive muscular atrophy. Where only upper signs are present it is called primary lateral sclerosis. Both these types of MND progress more slowly and survival time is longer.

The muscles of the eye, bowel and bladder have neurones from the sensory and autonomic nervous systems and are therefore unaffected (Hocking et al. 2006). However, there are issues which can lead to problems with toileting, which will be discussed further.

The four main forms of the disease are summarised in Table 11.1; however, it should be noted that as the disease progresses there may be significant overlap resulting in more comprehensive muscle wasting and weakness.

Table 11.1 Four main forms of motor neurone disease.

Type	Key facts	Symptoms
Amyotrophic lateral sclerosis (ALS)	Occurrence: 65–75% Involves upper and lower motor neurones. Average survival 2–5 years	Muscle weakness, spasticity, emotional lability, fasciculation, weight loss and hyperactive reflexes.
Progressive bulbar palsy (PBL) (a form of ALS)	Occurrence: 25% Both upper and lower motor neurones may be affected. Predominantly affects women. Average survival 6 months to 3 years.	Dysarthria, dysphagia, pharyngeal weakness, regurgitation of fluid via nose, tongue atrophy and fasciculation, emotional lability
Progressive Muscular Atrophy (PMA)	Occurrence: <10% Mainly affects lower motor neurones. Predominantly affects men. Younger age of onset. Average survival 5 plus years	Muscle weakness and wasting, weight loss and fasciculation.
	Occurrence: approximately 2% Only upper motor neurones affected. Men are affected twice as often as women. Onset usually after 50 years Survival similar to normal life span	Muscle weakness, limb stiffness and increased reflex response

Adapted from Motor Neurone Disease Association (2001).

The revised El Escorial criteria for diagnosis of MND/ALS (Mitsumoto et al. 2006) were recently updated. These were originally established at a conference in the Spanish Castle El Escorial and are used for inclusion criteria for trials, and underline the importance of establishing a definite diagnosis of MND.

The El Escorial criteria suggest that the diagnosis of amyotrophic lateral sclerosis (ALS) requires:

(a) the presence of:
1. evidence of lower motor neuron (LMN) degeneration by clinical, electrophysiological or neuropathological examination,
2. evidence of upper motor neuron (UMN) degeneration by clinical examination, and
3. progressive spread of symptoms or signs within a region or to other regions, as determined by history or examination.

together with

(b) the absence of:
1. electrophysiological and pathological evidence of other disease processes that might explain the signs of LMN and/or UMN degeneration, and

2. neuro-imaging evidence of other disease processes that might explain the observed clinical and electrophysiological signs. (http://www.wfnals.org/guidelines/1998elescorial/elescorial1998 criteria.htm)

It is extremely important that the diagnosis is given well spending time with the patient and their family ensuring that questions are answered and that they understand the information being offered (Oliver 2006).

Drug therapy

Currently there is only one drug, Riluzole, which has been clinically tested and proven to be of some benefit to this group of patients and as such is offered to most patients. This drug is a glutamate release antagonist and was found to prolong survival by about 3 months after 18 months' treatment (Miller et al. 2007). There is also evidence that survival benefit might be even greater, 4–19 months (Traynor et al. 2003).

The clinical nurse specialist role

As an expert in the field of MND the clinical nurse specialist (CNS) is the person to whom all newly diagnosed patients should be referred. All CNS are based in neurological centres and work closely with the neurologists. Referral is normally made once a definite diagnosis of MND has been established. This may be some time after the initial consultation with the neurologist, following tests and a number of follow-up appointments. The diagnosis may not come as a major shock as the patients and their relatives may well have been told that the nature of the problems may not be treatable.

Following referral an early home visit may be offered to the patients; this is often within a few days of diagnosis. Most families are receptive to this offer. This visit enables the patients and their families to begin to establish a relationship with the CNS who remains one of the constants throughout their disease progression. It allows patients and families to ask questions in the privacy of their own home and to receive information at a pace that is suitable to them. It helps the CNS to gain knowledge of the family and to gather information about their home and personal circumstances that have a direct bearing on the type and amount of care and support that the patient and family will require not only at the present but also in the future. It has to be noted that support has to be tailored to each individual and their family/caregivers, as some people prefer to have minimal contact whilst others are anxious to have the maximum input available. The level of input will vary depending on the stage of the illness. A study in West Berkshire found that the input of the CNS improves care and patient and family satisfaction by reducing time spent in hospital, facilitating rapid referral to other agencies and providing a patient-centred service that supported both the patient and family (Quinn 2006).

Case management

As the muscle wasting progresses the symptoms experienced by people with MND become more wide ranging and challenge the caregivers. A multidisciplinary approach with good case management is essential to help ensure that the quality of life of the patient is maximised (McDermott and Shaw 2008).

Management of symptoms experienced by patients with MND is a truly multidisciplinary task (BBSF 2000). The expertise of the neurologist at diagnosis followed by the care from the general practitioner and the community staff with the expertise of the palliative care specialists should ensure that the patient's journey through a disease that is one of multiple losses and changing needs is well managed.

Patient care is managed in a variety of settings. Some centres have a multidisciplinary clinic where the patient sees all the relevant professionals in one location. An example of this is the clinic held at King's College Hospital in London. The team consists of a neurologist, nurse specialist, care coordinator, speech and language therapist, dietician, occupational therapist and physiotherapist. Access to respiratory consultant and palliative care consultant is also available. Patients come prepared to spend a considerable length of time at the clinic as they feel this is beneficial to their care. Their care is then continued at a more local level with return to the clinic at approximately three-monthly intervals. This is considered the gold standard. More clinics across the country are now able to offer a service that is more comprehensive. Contact details for centres across the UK can be found at www.mndassociation.org.uk.

Predominantly people with MND wish to remain in their own home with caregivers attending to their physical needs along with the support from relatives and friends. This can be complex to organise and the care is often managed by a designated person from the multidisciplinary team, such as the district nurse. The holding of case discussions/case conferences involving all the team is a valuable exercise, ensuring all team members are aware of the plan for the patient. The physical, hands-on nursing care given to patients with MND is given by carers, community nurses and family and friends. The use of the Gold Standards Framework (Thomas 2003) as discussed in Chapter 5 would ensure good community-based palliative care.

Common problems

Ongoing muscle deterioration leads to problems with speech, swallowing and breathing. These are the most common issues for patients with MND and their families. This section discusses these further.

Speech and swallowing

As MND progresses speech deteriorates, with slurring of words, loss of volume and loss of useful speech being the main problems. Alternatives to speech such as writing, using a communication aid (Scott and Foulsom 2000), should be introduced at the earliest appropriate opportunity, enabling the patient to be familiar with them before being totally reliant on them. Computer programmes are available to help with communication especially where hand function is deteriorating, and this enables the person to be in control of the computer through a single switch. Although there is a wide choice of 'high-tech' gadgets many people will choose to manage with simple alphabet boards using eye movements to indicate words. Most family members and carers who are in regular contact with the patient will be able to understand speech that is poor.

Practice Point 11.3

Consider the best way to approach communication with a patient in these circumstances?
  What difficulties could this pose for you?

Commentary:

Honesty is the best policy with these patients as they will realise when you have not understood what they are saying. It becomes easier the better you know the person. Expert advice can be obtained from speech and language therapists and they in turn may well look for advice and guidance from agencies such as the Scottish Centre of Technology for Communication Impaired (SCTCI). SCTCI is a specialised resource available for the West of Scotland. It employs a manager who is a speech and language therapist, and another therapist and a technician run this service. Information on this service can be found at http://callcentre.education.ed.ac.uk/Useful_Links/ICTSLS_ULB/ictsls_ulb. html. You could also contact the MND Association (MNDA; www. mndassociation.org) that would let you know about all the services in your area although there are not services like this in all areas of the UK, confirming the patchiness of care availability.

Swallowing becomes a problem as the bulbar muscles deteriorate and affects around 90% of MND patients as the disease progresses (Oliver et al. 2007). The speech and language therapist has a major role in assessing the function of these muscles and the patients' ability to swallow safely (Wagner-Sonntag and Prosiegel 2006). The major problem with a poor swallow is of aspiration. With a poor cough reflex chest infection is a major hazard for patients with MND, and pneumonia is not uncommon in this group of patients. Many people with MND are reluctant to have input from speech and language therapists as they are under the impression that all they can do is help with speech. Once it is explained that monitoring of swallow is important most people are willing to have their advice and expertise.

Eating for most of us is a social and enjoyable activity which people do not want to lose. Augmented feeding has to be considered for many patients; however, they often do not wish to think of gastrostomy assuming that they will no longer be able to have an oral intake. Nonetheless if swallowing is considered safe with adaptation of diet to exclude food that is difficult to swallow many people are able to continue with both oral and gastrostomy intake, at least for a short while after gastrostomy has been placed.

Early discussion of the alternative to oral intake, that is gastrostomy, enables the patient and their family to make an informed choice about the procedure. Early insertion of gastrostomy is preferred (Miller et al. 1999) and oral intake and use of gastrostomy is well managed by patients. This requires time and discussion which is usually repeated prior to a decision.

The first step is to have the patient assessed with respiratory function being of major importance. Evidence suggests that a predicted force vital capacity of less than 50% is indicative of respiratory insufficiency and could put the patient at risk of respiratory problems if insertion with endoscopy was chosen (Gregory et al. 2002). Endoscopic placement of gastrostomy, percutaneous endoscopic gastrostomy, is referred to as PEG. Alternative placement under radiological guidance is considered a lesser risk for the respiratory system due to the smaller amount of sedation used. This entails radiological guidance to place the tube referred to as a RIG. A naso-gastric tube is placed prior to the procedure and placement is carried out in the X-ray department.

A unit caring for MND patients in England recently identified that the organisation and planning process for insertion and follow-up care of gastrostomies for patients under their care was often disorganised and poorly planned. After a lengthy multidisciplinary consultation on a local and regional basis, a pathway was developed to facilitate gastrostomy insertion and although it has had limited use, to date it has demonstrated an improvement in the care with both patients and health care professionals reaping the benefit (Oliver et al. 2007).

Respiratory symptoms

As the diaphragm weakens the respiratory system of the patient is under increased strain and the patient may complain of breathlessness, frequent wakening at night, not feeling refreshed after a night's sleep and daytime solomnence.

The use of non-invasive ventilation with bi-level positive pressure at the onset of respiratory insufficiency increases survival in comparison with those who cannot use non-invasive ventilation (Aboussouan et al. 1997). Tolerance is reduced in patients with bulbar onset and compliance of treatment is therefore poor (Bourke and Gibson 2004).

Sialorrhoea, the result of poor lip seal and/or impaired ability to swallow saliva can be a major problem which does not always respond to treatment. Treatment would be with anticholinergic agents. The reverse can also be found where thick tenacious secretions can cause distress – this can be due to dehydration and mouth breathing. The use of chest physiotherapy and nebulised saline can help with this.

Further useful advice regarding specific drugs and dosages can be found in a publication named *Motor Neurone Disease – A Problem-Solving Approach for General Practitioners and Health Care Professionals* which is produced by the Scottish Motor Neurone Disease Association (SMNDA). It can be sourced at www.smnda.org

Bowel and bladder issues

Constipation is another problem that is seen in people with MND. This can be due to poor abdominal muscles and the lack of power to expel faeces; it can also be affected by altered diet, inadequate fluid intake and also by drugs that the patient may be taking. Immobility also plays its part. Advice on diet, fluid intake and the use of laxatives can usually alleviate the situation. Immobility and the difficulties of physically getting to the bathroom are also large contributory factors for both bowel and bladder.

Some patients will after discussion with district nurses and other health care professionals opt to have a urinary catheter which will reduce the number of transfers between seats and bed, etc. they have to make in order to visit the toilet.

Cognitive dysfunction

Until relatively recently it was the widely held view that MND did not cause cognitive change and that only a small percentage had dementia due to temporal lobe problems. It is now acknowledged that in about 3% of sporadic cases and 15% of familial cases a temporal lobe dementia might be present (Neary et al. 2000). It is also recognised that people with MND may have some cognitive impairment that is subtle and only seen on neuropsychological testing (Goldstein 2006). Emotional lability with uncontrollable laughter and crying is also seen in patients with MND.

Psychological, social and spiritual impact

MND is a progressive illness with no spells of remission, no known cure and a drug that is of limited use. The diagnosis is often devastating for patients and their families. It is a disease of loss. The patient relentlessly loses the ability to carry out tasks that were previously done without thought. It is often rapid and loss can sometimes be identified on a day-to-day basis.

MND weakens muscles and with this comes a fatigue that becomes more marked as the disease progresses. There is no treatment for this but advice on management of lifestyle is often helpful (Ream 2008).

Time factors in relation to planning ahead for future needs have to be taken into consideration. Assessment of need is required sooner rather than later and this can be difficult to achieve as the person is often still numbed by the diagnosis. The need to plan ahead is often very difficult for the patient and their family to cope with. They see the situation as it is in the here and now and are unable to look ahead and plan accordingly.

The input from occupational therapy at the Social Work Department at this stage is vital. Adaptations to property take time given that plans have to be drawn up and approved and grant applications have to be made. Tradesmen then have to be appointed to carry out the works; during this time the patients' condition will be deteriorating and their needs changing. Sadly adaptations are often unsuitable once they have been completed.

Practice Point 11.4

Consider what at this stage you can offer to the patient and their family or carers to help them?
How can you help them to accept intervention from professionals?

Commentary:

Encouraging people to talk can hopefully bring anxieties and fears to the fore and these can then be addressed. Whilst focusing on the anxieties and fears of the patient and their family, it is also worth considering the fears of the professionals many of whom will feel inadequate as they do not have the answers to many of the questions. The patients and their families who are angry may direct this anger to the very people who are trying to help them through their frustration and feelings of powerlessness over the disease and the loss of control. This can cause hurt to all and it is sometimes worth considering the input from psychological services to help patients and families to live with the loss and change that are occurring in their lives.

It is extremely important to remember the carers and the strain that is put on them. They are adapting to change often becoming exhausted by the physical role they are fulfilling, feeling socially isolated, hating the intrusion of carers, feeling resentful of their loved one and becoming angry and frustrated as the caring role becomes more difficult (McIntyre and Lugton 2005).

Respite care at home or in a day care setting can help the carer to have a few hours when they should be encouraged to do something for themselves. Respite care on an inpatient basis is extremely difficult but if there is a need for symptoms to be assessed then admission to a palliative care unit may well be beneficial to all concerned.

Specialist palliative care

The use of the expertise of specialist palliative care is extremely helpful. In a disease that has no cure and an unpredictable path it is useful to involve palliative care earlier rather than later (Oliver 2002). Input from palliative care when discussing gastrostomy and non-invasive ventilation is desirable. Whilst taking the opportunity to explore anxieties and fears it is useful to introduce the hospice and the role that palliative medicine can play. The help and advice that is available should be made known to the patient and their family. Explaining the role that the hospice fulfils is essential in dispelling pre-conceived ideas that exist about hospice care. Planning ahead, looking at the options of making advanced directives and living wills, leaving memories for younger children or grandchildren, making a will and leaving precise plans for funerals are all very difficult to do but are often the things that given the opportunity the patient wants to discuss. The unpredictable nature of MND may lead to rapid deterioration and death can occur more quickly than expected. It therefore makes it desirable to have discussed these important issues.

End of life care

In earlier discussion patients may well have expressed a preference as to where they wish to die or where possible this should be honoured. In some cases death can be sudden and before a recognisable end of life stage is reached. Some families have expressed concern that this has happened and they were not prepared for it. For others the end of life can last for a number of weeks with symptoms gradually worsening. Upper respiratory tract infection in conjunction with a rapid deterioration over a period of a few days is the most common end stage of life.

Managing symptoms is different for every patient. For some increasing respiratory weakness means that they are drowsy and are neither distressed nor in pain. For others there are signs of terminal restlessness. At the end of life most patients will have their medication reviewed and medication that is not essential withdrawn. The use of opioid analgesia which reduces the cough reflex relieves dyspnoea and controls pain along with an anti-cholinergic to reduce secretions plus a sedative to reduce anxiety is the medication that is most often used. The delivery of this via a syringe driver at relatively low dose is the preferred choice for symptom relief (Scottish Motor Neurone Disease Association 2004). Regardless of the place of death good nursing care and the involvement of family at this stage is vital, as the way a person dies stays with family long after the death has occurred.

The *Preferred Place of Care* (PPC) document is one of three national tools in the NHS End of Life Programme and follows the patient through their illness experience across health and social settings with the aim of improving palliative care for patients (Storey and Pemberton 2002). To date this has been used predominantly for patients with cancer; however, it has been implemented in a region of England for patients with MND and has helped health care professionals facilitate difficult conversations surrounding end of life care and identifying patients' needs. As a result and success of this project, it has since been shared with other MND services throughout the country (Storey et al. 2006).

Bereavement

Where death has been sudden and relatively unexpected it can leave the bereaved with mixed emotions: relief that their loved one is no longer suffering and that they have been relieved of the burden of care; or a feeling of having been cheated out of time with the person to say the things that they wanted to and loss of the time that they had planned to take to devote to them.

Where death has been more expected many are still left with the finality of the event and the feeling that they were not prepared to let go. The loss of the person with MND leaves their partner bereft of the support that has been in place for the months or years of illness, and their home is also empty of equipment that has been an essential part of their loved one's life.

Support over the coming months from a variety of people will help the carer to come to terms with their loss and move into a different phase of their life. Counselling is available from the Scottish Motor Neurone Disease Association which has a network of counsellors who have knowledge of MND and training from Cruse Bereavement Care. It is available for those who have cared for or have been involved with a person with MND. Counselling is also available for those with MND family and carers at any time. The Motor Neurone Disease Association also has a list of helpful organisations on its website http://www. mndassociation.org/life_with_mnd/getting_more_information/ useful.html.

The website also includes a list of the national MND care centres who provide much of the professional advice and support for MND patients and their families during and after the patient's death.

Summary

Working with people with MND and their families is both challenging and rewarding. As it is a fairly rare disease many professionals do not have the experience to manage these patients and their families well. There are numerous common issues that arise with MND patients and their carers, but by using a multi-agency approach many of these can be addressed. The use of the MND clinical nurse specialist as a key to the provision of timeous care should be considered as should making use of the national care centres and the SMNDA and the MNDA. By utilising all these resources, good palliative care can help those with MND to live as active a life as possible, within the constraints of their illness and also help them to have a peaceful death.

Multiple sclerosis

Richard Warner

Introduction

The purpose of this sub-section is to introduce the reader to the application of the principles of palliative care for people living with multiple sclerosis (MS).

Learning outcomes

Through reading this sub-section and engaging in the associated practice points the reader will achieve three key learning outcomes associated with this patient group. The reader will:

- Identify key features of living with MS that may predispose the individual to risk of premature death

- Develop an appreciation of symptom management
- Appreciate the meaning of quality of life for people with MS

Understanding physical aspects of multiple sclerosis

Multiple sclerosis is a chronic disease of the central nervous system. The process of the disease is characterised by demyelination and axonal degeneration. These processes result in patients experiencing acute attacks of symptoms (relapses), transient worsening of symptoms and a progressive accumulation of neurological impairment. There is currently no cure for MS. Typically patients who initially follow a relapsing form of disease receive a diagnosis in early adulthood. This relapsing form often changes to a progressive pattern. Patients who primarily follow a progressive form of disease are often diagnosed later in adulthood (Cottrell et al. 1999). A younger age at diagnosis is thought to predict a longer period of survival (Brønnum-Hansen et al. 2004).

MS can cause a range of symptoms, including bladder and bowel dysfunction, sexual dysfunction, spasticity and weakness, impairment of balance and coordination, fatigue, cognitive impairment, speech, swallowing and visual problems. In addition a person with MS can experience neuropathic pain or musculoskeletal pain secondary to abnormalities of movement. Depression is common. There are other less common neuropsychiatric disorders that could be broadly classified under the label of emotionalism (National Collaborating Centre for Chronic Conditions 2003). Emotional liability, pathological laughing and crying and forms of euphoria have been described in association with MS (Feinstein 1999).

Survival and Prognosis

Death as a direct result of MS is exceptionally rare (Burgess 2002). One study examined the causation of death for 50 cases of unexpected death in patients with MS, whose death required autopsy (Riudavets et al. 2005). This study only revealed nine cases where cause of death was believed to be directly related to MS. This was assumed as no other cause of death could be established. The authors of the study speculate that MS may have affected the hypothalamus and medulla, which in turn might impact on the control of cardiovascular, respiratory or thermoregulatory functions. Despite these data it is considerably more likely that people with MS will die from either other diseases (i.e. atherosclerotic cardiovascular disease) or from complications secondary to MS. The risk of death due to complication is directly related to levels of neurological impairment. With increasing levels of motor impairment and dysphagia people with MS are at risk of pneumonia and aspiration. In this sense MS in itself should not be considered to be a terminal disease. Life expectancy for the population of people with MS is only marginally reduced compared to the general population (Midgard et al. 1995). Closer examination of published data reveals that the group of people with MS who experience profound and complex disability are at greater risk of premature death as a consequence of complications. In other words just because a person has MS does not predispose them to premature death. There is a reasonable likelihood that the person with MS will live for decades from diagnosis and actually die from other illness. Clinical practitioners should look to identify specific features of the disease and profound neurological impairment and then ensure that management strategies are in place to mediate risk.

The personal experience of living with multiple sclerosis

Given the natural history of the disease it is important to develop an idea of palliation that is concerned with the personal experience of living with MS. This approach will be applicable to a greater number of people living with MS rather than just those who face complex neurological impairment.

Using mixed method case study Warner (2006) was able to demonstrate that despite similarities between objective levels of functional activity, people with MS would construct very different experiences of perceived impairment and social disability which were dependent on their sense of personal identity. Identity was driven by experience of interaction with their immediate communities and their sense of loss associated with expectation of life. This sense of loss was also found by Wollin et al. (2006) during a survey of people with MS who had complex impairment. Although people had lived with MS for many years and were now facing profound impairment and disability they still expressed a sense of loss. They believed that MS had denied and limited the opportunity to fulfil expectation in their lives with regard to work, relationships and leisure. So although people were in employment, long-term relationships and had family, they still believed that they would have had a more fulfilling experience of these if MS had not been present. Equally they still believed that they had to continually fight for services to attend to their needs. It is important to recognise that a person's sense of emotional well-being probably has a greater influence over their perceived quality of life than physical impairment alone (O'Connor et al. 2001). In summary, people with MS find that living with the condition has a pervasive and negative effect on all aspects of life and this is compounded by social disability (Khan et al. 2006). The consequence of this can be a deep and profound sadness: a sense of loss. Depression is common for people with MS. Features of depression such as irritability, frustration and discouragement seem to be more prevalent than feeling of guilt and low self-esteem often found in other patient groups who experience depression (Minden et al. 1987). The population of people with MS are thought to be under treatment for depression. It is important that all health care professionals are sensitive to depressive changes in their patients. For people with MS this is particularly so for two reasons. Firstly, severity of depression in MS, particular in men, is a strong predictor of suicidal ideation and intent (Turner et al. 2006 and Feinstein 2002). Secondly, depression and mental health, in some studies, appears to exceed physical and cognitive impairments as a predictor of poor quality of life (Ghaffer and Feinstein 2007).

Studies reveal that issues such as health distress and limitations on emotional role play as much a part in determining the person's perception of quality of life as physical impairment (O'Connor et al. 2001). Atkin (2000) found in a large-scale qualitative study that people with disability from a range of patient groups felt more satisfied in life when they achieved a balance between 'body, mind and spirit'. Through interviews the study found that people valued being able to perform expected roles. For the people with disability this meant being able to construct and live in a 'reciprocal social world' (Atkin 2000, p. 31). The patients did not diminish or deny any impairments or the consequential social disability that might arise. However, they did expect to be able to establish the normative social dynamics of adult relationships. Numerous studies have reported that symptoms such as fatigue, cognitive impairment, depression, limited mobility, bladder dysfunction and pain can lead to social disability. In a recent study of 204 patients who had a mean duration of 9 years of disease, only 35% remained in full-time employment with 63% still driving a car (Khan et al. 2006).

The nursing response to multiple sclerosis

As I have implied the role of palliative care should include developing interventions to mediate the risk of premature death as well as aiming to improve aspects of quality of life. Please consider the following scenario:

Mr X has lived with MS for 33 years. He has minimal function in all limbs. He requires a suprapubic catheter to aid bladder function. He is unable to defaecate without the use of enemas. He has increased tone in both lower limbs that he finds painful particularly during hoisting and after sitting for long periods. His speech is slurred and he has recently started to cough when drinking fluid. He requires assistance to eat and drink. His family, who he lives with, recognise that he has difficulty with memory and concentration. He has not lost any weight recently or had any chest infections. The family believe that Mr X has always been reluctant to look to formal health care for assistance with living with his MS. The family receive no formal care package. District nurses attend to administer enemas and to change catheters at appropriate intervals.

Practice Point 11.5

Spasticity
Please attempt to identify one pharmacological and one non-pharmacological intervention to address increased tone. What other issues should be considered that might cause an increase in tone?

Commentary:

Tone is said to be increased when resistance is felt as a limb travels through normal range of movement. This is thought to be because of damage to the upper motor neurones of the corticospinal tract. Patients often complain of stiffness and difficulty in extending or moving an affected limb. For the person with advanced disease it is highly likely that they will already be experiencing extensive spasticity. This can not only render purposive movement limited but can affect the safety and comfort of seated, prone and hoisted posture. It is important to involve both occupational therapists and physiotherapists in the assessment of positioning to mediate the risk of contracture at joints as well as the development of pressure sores.

National clinical guidelines suggest that first-line pharmacological treatment should be with baclofen or gabapentin (NICE 2003). Interestingly credible systematic review of antispastic treatments for MS concluded that the evidence base was too limited to recommend specific treatments (Shakespeare et al. 2000). This is in part a reflection of the inconsistent use of outcome measures for trials and debate surrounding the reliability and validity of available measurement techniques.

It is important to recognise that any change in the patient's presentation of spasticity or spasm could be a reflection of the presence of other problems. For example, urinary tract infection, tight clothing, pain, anxiety and positioning discomfort can all exacerbate the symptom. For the person with advanced disease it is likely that they will already have experience of antispastic agents, so goals for treatment should be centred on very specific activities or the promotion of comfort (Currie 2001). Passive stretching regimes can be incorporated in other care activities such as washing and dressing. It is often possible for physiotherapists to teach carers how to implement such exercises.

Practice Point 11.6

Dysphagia
What are the ethical issues associated with the decision to use nutritional support?
    Would it be necessary to establish whether Mr X has the capacity to make decisions regarding nutritional support?

Commentary:

Multiple sclerosis lesions affect nerve conduction originating from the brainstem. This can affect coordination of both laryngeal and pharyngeal motility (Abraham and Yun 2002). A proportion of such patients will experience liquid bolus penetration of the airways due to impairment of epiglottic positioning or movement. This, in turn, will predispose these people with MS to develop pneumonia. Speech and language therapists are often involved in assessing swallowing ability and devising interventions (Squires 2006). Interventions will range from employing an altered textured diet through to receiving all nutrition and fluid via a percutaneous endoscopic gastrostomy. Despite such interventions mortality at one year for people with MS has been reported at 14.2% of a study of 911 patients (Jones 2007).

The concept and practice of gaining consent has been well described by the Department of Health in guidance to NHS professionals (Department of Health 2001a). The documents' opening statement recognises that patients have a 'fundamental legal and ethical right to determine what happens to their own bodies' (Department of Health 2001a, p. 9). In addition, nursing can look to its own professional standards for conduct (Nursing and Midwifery Council 2004). Registered nurses must respect a patient's right to decide whether health care interventions are appropriate for themselves even if such decisions would lead to harm or even death. In this sense the formulation of plans of care should be seen as a dynamic process centred around the patients wishes that are developed over time in consultation with the patients' family and health and social care workers. It is also important to recognise the concept of capacity (Mental Capacity Act 2005).

The Mental Capacity Act (2005), which came into force from April 2007, gives preference to the assumption that people have the ability to make decisions about their health and social care. A two-stage test is advocated that considers, firstly, whether a person has any impairment or dysfunction of their mind or brain and, secondly, whether a problem affects their decision-making ability (Department of Health 2005). Cognitive impairment is very common in MS (Rao et al. 1991). However, rather than necessarily presenting as an overall global cognitive decline, it often presents as specific impairment of attention, working memory, speed of thought processing, verbal and visuospatial memory and executive function. Such impairments need careful consideration, and sometimes specialist assessment of applied cognitive abilities for specific decisions should be sought from a psychologist.

Practice Point 11.7

How would you determine if Mr X was experiencing depression?

Is it important to determine whether the family members are feeling strained in providing care for Mr X?

If Mr X was depressed and the family experiencing carer strain, what could be done to support them?

Commentary:

Best practice for the clinical assessment of depression has been described in national guidelines (NICE 2004). International consensus describes the characteristic symptoms of depression where the number of symptoms is considered to be indicative of the severity of an episode. The symptoms should be present for at least 2 weeks. It is possible that people with MS may well experience an increased prevalence of individual symptoms such as anger, irritability, discouragement and sadness or loss, but not necessarily clustered together in the way typical of depression. Equally fatigue and sleep disturbance due to other symptoms of MS are common. Given this it may be prudent to acknowledge the vegetative features but to focus more on disturbances in features of mood for the person with advanced MS (Feinstein 1999).

The quality of life for the person with advanced MS can be lowered when their informal carer feels that the burden of care is high even though they may feel that they remain an effective carer (Khan et al. 2007). Such a situation needs to be addressed with sensitivity. The most important perceived needs for people with advanced MS are non-professional social care, adaptation of the environment and rehabilitation (Forbes et al. 2007). The perspectives on care and what might constitute good care may well differ between the person with MS and their informal carer. The informal carer is likely to be their partner (spouse) or close family member, so the dynamic of the current relationship is likely to reflect the inherent values of the relationship before the need to provide care (Lobchuk 2006). It is sometimes possible to enable partners to accept formal provision of care as a method of reinstating lost pursuits. I am aware of patients and informal carers who have used the formal provision of care to pursue interests outside of the caring environment. This can enrich the relationship with new conversations and interest whilst still keeping the patient at the centre of decision-making. People with advance disease may need assistance with negotiating the myriad of social care provision but their desire to remain at home and be in control of their situation is paramount (Department of Health 2005 and McIlfatrick 2007).

Summary

This section has introduced the reader to key issues associated with MS and palliative care. It is important that health care professionals are sensitive to the phemonology of mental health issues and how they impact upon quality of life and a person's sense of well-being. It is important to maximise the clinical management of symptoms for people with MS who have complex neurological impairment. However, it is always necessary to recognise that here may be other issues that are negatively impacting upon the person's quality of life. These issues can be addressed through the provision of sensitive and compassionate health care.

Parkinson's disease

George Kernohan, Felicity Hasson and Dorothy Hardyway

Introduction

This sub-section aims to provide an overview of the palliative care needs and issues facing people with Parkinson's disease, their carers and the health profes-sionals who also provide care for them. It provides an overview of the palliative care needs throughout the illness trajectory, aiming to challenge some misconceptions about the disease within current models of caring practice.

Learning outcomes

Once you have read this section and completed the associated practice points you will be able to:

- Explain the aetiology and progression of Parkinson's disease
- Have a broad understanding of the four stages of Parkinson's disease and how the palliative phase can affect at each stage.
- Discuss the problems that may arise in managing people with Parkinson's disease and their palliative care needs and identify the importance of the role of the patient and carer in the management of the disease
- Understand that a shared care approach between palliative and Parkinson's disease teams is beneficial

What is Parkinson's disease?

Parkinson's disease (PD) is a progressive neurological condition, for which, at the time of writing, there is no cure. PD rarely causes death directly but it does shorten the lifespan and people in the later stages of the disease may have symptoms that exacerbate other fatal illnesses (Parkinson's Disease Society 2004). The cause or causes of PD are unknown, but genetic and environmental factors may be implicated (Calne 2000). Studies indicate that prevalence of the disease varies worldwide; however, this may be due, in part, to a lack of uniformity in diagnostic criteria and differing study methods (Mutch 1995). Globally, PD affects 6.3 million people (Baker and Graham 2004) and in the UK it is estimated that it affects around 2 people per 1000 (NICE 2006). A similar number of carers are directly affected by the course of the disease (Thomas (no date)). With the concentration in middle age, around one in ten people in their 40s and 50s are affected by the disease (Baker and Graham 2004). However, the mean age of onset is between 55 and 60 years (O'Brien 2002) with most people with PD being over 60 years of age (Hogstel 2001). The number of cases rises with age: in people in their 70s and 80s there is a prevalence of 1–3% (Tanner and Ben-Shlomo 1999). It is anticipated that the widely anticipated ageing population will cause a dramatic increase in the numbers of people diagnosed with the disease (Lillienfeld and Perl 1994; Scott 2002). The disease has a variable rate of progression although it is estimated that the average length of time a person will live with classic idiopathic Parkinson's is 15 years. Where the disease can be traced to trauma, tumour or use of drugs, it is known as atypical or Parkinsonism and the average survival is 10 years (Thomas and MacMahon 2004a).

The disease can present and progress very differently in individuals, resulting in no two cases of Parkinson's disease being alike; thus, each patient's trajectory is unique which adds to the uncertainty for the patient, care and health care professional. The major symptoms of Parkinson's include resting tremor, rigidity and bradykinesia (slower movement and speech) and as the disease progresses balance and gait become more affected and disability increases (Bunting-Perry 2006; Hudson et al. 2006). Tremor is present in 75% of cases (Hogstel 2001), with muscle weaknesses and instability also characteristic (Stephenson 2001), yet symptoms appear slowly and develop in no particular order. MacMahon and Thomas (1998) have defined four stages of Parkinson's disease: diagnosis, maintenance, complex and palliative care. These are described in the following sections, with activities in each case inviting the reader to reflect on learning points.

Four stages of Parkinson's disease

Diagnosis

There is often a long period of uncertainty as symptoms emerge. Gaining initial diagnosis is difficult and this process is compounded by the lack of a specific marker for the disease (Bhatia et al. 1998). Other conditions such as vascular pseudo-Parkinsonism and the Parkinsonian syndromes such as multiple systems atrophy and progressive supranuclear palsy create difficulties in diagnosing the disease (Findley et al. 2004). Indeed, the condition is mistaken for other neurodegenerative illnesses in up to 20% of cases (Hughes et al. 1992). Understandably a misdiagnosis of Parkinson's disease can cause considerable distress especially if the diagnosis is later reserved. At this early stage symptoms may have limited impact and the aim is to facilitate acceptance of the disease through the provision of information and psychological support (Lee et al. 2004, p. 51). Consider the case of Mr Brown:

Case 1 – diagnosis. The activities in this section are based on experiences of a PD Nurse Specialist in Palliative Care. All patients' names and identifying features have been changed to protect the identity of the participant. Each case is accompanied by a couple of practice points to ponder. Expert commentaries will follow each case.

Mr Alex Brown is a 55-year-old architect, married, with two teenage children. He attended his GP complaining of a painful right shoulder, which he feels is also affecting his handwriting which has become small and illegible. This worries him because it is impacting on his job. He also states that his sleep pattern is disturbed because he feels stiff and sore at night and unable to turn over in bed. His GP explains that he might have Parkinson's disease, and explains what it is and then makes a referral to a neurologist.

Because Mr Brown and his family are worried about the possible diagnosis, he books a private appointment with a neurologist to reduce the waiting time. The neurologist confirms that he may have Parkinson's disease and after discussion with Mr Brown decides to commence him on a dopamine agonist, and arranges to review him in 3 months.

Practice Point 11.8

Why is it decided he may have Parkinson's disease, and why is it not confirmed? Can you identify possible palliative care needs of Mr Brown at this stage? Discuss the role of the Parkinson Disease Nurse Specialist. To whom, within the multidisciplinary team, might she consider referring Mr Brown?

Commentary:

Mr Brown, the architect who was just diagnosed, had a preliminary diagnosis of PD made on his uncertain clinical picture and it was confirmed after several visits to the neurologist who observed his symptoms and his reaction to medication before making a definitive diagnosis of PD.

Even at diagnosis, Mr Brown had palliative care needs. At this early stage, these are information, education and support in accepting the diagnosis. He would also need basic information on prescribed medication to provide him with the opportunity to make informed choices. Knowing more about therapy will improve his compliance.

The PD Nurse Specialist will provide support for Mr Brown and his family, education and information and signposting to the appropriate health profession, local support group and PD Society. The nurse may be the main point of contact for any queries which may arise and might make referrals to the physiotherapist to allow for a baseline physical assessment, education and exercise and/or the OT to inform him about aids for work and how to manage in the workplace.

Maintenance

The second stage begins when symptoms and potential complications can be controlled with drug treatment, through a multidisciplinary approach (Lee et al. 2004; Thomas and MacMahon 1999). The objective is to ensure that the patient is able to live as normal a life as possible. However, Ward and Robertson (2004) claim that, at this stage, low expectations on the part of the patient, carer and health professional can lead to under treatment and too much acceptance of functional problems in this stage. If there is a poor awareness of the evolving needs of the patient, appropriate referrals and therapy are delayed, often until avoidable problems have already occurred. Mrs Suzi Watters is in this stage of disease:

Case 2 – the maintenance stage. Mrs Suzi Watters is a 38-year-old self-employed hairdresser, married, with two young children, a boy aged 6 and a girl aged 4 years.

Suzi was diagnosed with PD 4 years ago and has been able to work full time because her symptoms were well controlled with her medication, a dopamine agonist. But recently she has arranged an appointment with her GP as her situation has changed. Her symptoms are not as well controlled and have become more noticeable; she finds she has developed anxiety and the simplest of challenges increases her anxiety and her tremor, which then becomes more noticeable.

She has problems communicating with her clients because they do not seem to understand her as her voice always sounds hoarse and has become lower in tone.

Due to these changes Suzi has become quite self-conscious and no longer wants to socialise as much, especially with strangers. She tells her GP that she tires much easier and after a day's work she has no energy to play or interact with the children and she believes this is affecting her relationship with them.

Practice Point 11.9

What are the main quality of life issues here? What support could you suggest for her and her family, especially the children? Discuss which members of the multidisciplinary team should be involved at this stage and why.

Commentary:

Suzi was diagnosed with PD 4 years ago. Her quality of life issues are her ability to maintain full time work; she needs to be shown strategies to help her manage at work and to manage her fatigue. She is having problems with her speech: the speech and language therapist can teach her techniques to address these problems.

Her anxiety is exacerbating her symptoms; coping strategies can be taught by the Community Psychiatric Nurse who may use of cognitive behaviour therapy to gain control over negative thoughts.

In the maintenance stage, the family will require support and further education about Suzi's developing symptoms. Her husband can be encouraged to be more involved in care of the children and daily tasks, thus reducing Suzi's stress and fatigue. As a couple they need to maintain good communication, discussing issues as they arise and seeking help if necessary, and should be encouraged to join the local PD support group.

The PD Society has produced fun and easy to read booklets for children which help them to understand the illness. Suzi could help them read these and discuss issues which may trouble Suzi or the children.

The occupational therapist will teach Suzi coping strategies for her fatigue and discuss issues around her work.

A speech therapist can assess Suzi's speech and teach her techniques to manage these difficulties

The neurologist will review her medication and may provide some coordination of the other professionals.

Complex

In the third stage, the patient experiences diminished benefits from medication and an accumulation of disabilities and complications requiring more input from various members of the multidisciplinary team. Where available, a specialist PD team can play a major role in managing the symptoms. The patient at this complex stage will begin to rely on the assistance of others especially the informal carer, normally a family member, for complex and challenging care tasks such as medication administration, liaison with health care professionals, symptom assessment and dressing patients, as well as assisting with activities of daily living such as cooking, feeding and dressing (Aranda and Hayman-White 2001; Barg et al. 1998). Most informal carers take on these supportive caregiving role with little or no training (Oldham and Kristjanson 2004) and consequently experience psychological and physical distress (Higgingson et al. 1990; Seamark et al. 2007). The complex stage represents a further psychological milestone for both the patient and the carer (Ward and Robertson 2004) as the deterioration often results in significant change of roles and relationships (Brown et al. 1990; MacMahon and Thomas 1998; Nanton 1985). Not all complex cases benefit from informal care (see Paula's case below) so all members of the multidisciplinary team need to be aware of the physical and psychological needs of the patient (Bunting-Perry 2006; Lee et al. 2004). This is an issue for Paula; consider her case:

Case 3 – the complex stage. Paula is a 60-year-old lady who lives on her own. She was diagnosed with PD 8 years ago. She now relies on polypharmacy to control her symptoms. She is on a maximum dose of madopar four times a day, and also takes a dopamine agonist and takes entacapone to help make it work more effectively.

Despite this she is having dyskinesias (involuntary movements which are a side effect of madopar) and morning dystonias (painful cramping due to medication 'wearing off') of her toes. These dystonias sometimes last all morning and make it difficult for her to mobilise, so she no longer socialises in the morning.

She is feeling depressed about her symptoms and is finding it difficult to manage the timing and number of tablets she has to consume daily.

She now finds it more difficult to manage daily living tasks; having been very independent she now has to ask friends for help, which as a very independent lady she finds quite difficult to accept.

Practice Point 11.10

What strategies can be used to help Paula manage her medication and make it more effective? What palliative care issues would Paula have, and which issues would we need to discuss with her?

Commentary:

Paula is a more complex case. We might encourage her to keep a diary of her symptoms and to note the times she takes her medication and to do this over a week. We can use this diary to adjust the timing of her medication and determine if she requires to take the medication more often now (3 hourly).

To keep things right, we could provide her with a pill timer, which she can set for the times her medication is due and it will alarm to remind her. It is pocket size and unobtrusive. We will involve the social worker who would be able to establish a care package for Paula to help her manage at home.

Paula requires counselling to help her to come to terms with this stage of her illness. If you think Paula would be open to discussing her future, now might be the time to discuss future issues such as preferred place of care, appointing a person as a representative who is aware of her desired future care arrangements. These include sensitive discussions about artificial feeding, decisions about resuscitation in the event of organ failure and making an advanced directive. If left unresolved, these issues continue into the next phase; they do not 'go away' as noted in the fourth commentary, below.

Advanced disease

MacMahon and Thomas (1998) define a fourth stage as when the patient is unable to tolerate dopaminergic therapy, unsuitable for surgery, and is experiencing advanced co-morbidity. Here, emphasis is placed upon the quality of life, ensuring relief of symptoms and distress, aiming to ensure dignity at all times. Protection of the patient's autonomy is a particular challenge: it can seem easier to be guided by the informal carer and professional opinion, forgetting who really has the authority to decide on life and death issues: the patient themselves. The Gilbert family story illustrates palliative care in the advanced stage of PD; consider their case:

Case 4 – the advanced disease stage. James Gilbert is an 82-year-old gentleman diagnosed with PD 15 years ago. He is married and lives with his 76-year-old wife who is also his main carer.

They have an extensive care package in place to help his wife manage as James does not want to go to a care home. He is wheelchair bound, needs help with activities of daily living, has a permanent in-dwelling catheter and has to be hoisted when he is moved.

Because he developed hallucinations his oral dopamine agonists were discontinued with good effect but his PD medication has been reduced to madopar 125 mg five times a day and madopar CR 125 mg at night. After a period in hospital he has been commenced on a minimum dose of rotigotine patch to help his stiffness.

James cannot be left on his own, so his wife can only leave the house when some member of her family will sit with James. He is quite depressed and can sometimes be verbally aggressive towards his wife, who is finding it very difficult to manage and has recently been admitted to hospital with an episode of angina.

Practice Point 11.11

What are the main palliative care needs of this couple? What strategies could improve James' mood or attitude to his wife? How could you help them to deal with the uncertain future?

Commentary:

As an older couple coping with advanced PD, Mr and Mrs Gilbert require all the palliative care mentioned in this section. The symptoms suffered by Mr Gilbert need constant monitoring and control. With very limited mobility, there is a high risk of pressure ulcers: special mattresses and cushions should be considered to reduce the risk. If ulcers do occur, referral to a tissue viability nurse is warranted.

The couple may benefit from separate counselling. Mrs Gilbert requires more frequent respite in the form of a sitting service to allow her to maintain her social activities. Mr Gilbert would benefit from a befriender service, and have the opportunity to be taken out; this might relieve some of his frustrations. The couple need to be encouraged to talk and share their true feelings. If Mr Gilbert is against respite, maybe the other family members should be encouraged to care for him in their own home to allow Mrs Gilbert to have an extended time of respite.

If not already addressed, the family needs to understand the priority of a discussion, with their father, about the need to appoint someone to represent his wishes and to instigate an advanced directive, which would include such issues as preferred place of care as he may be more comfortable with nursing home care. In the near future, he may benefit from artificial feeding and his opinion of this are needed, if we are to respect his autonomy. Above all, his deterioration will need careful symptom control. The options on resuscitation in the event of organ failure will need to be known and planned. Very special sensitivity and high quality nursing care are required to help Mr and Mrs Gilbert face the end of life with confidence and dignity.

Palliative care throughout the disease trajectory

Together, the stages listed above betray the progressive nature of the disease, with progression increasing the complexity of the care required. The four stages provide an over-simplified picture as PD rarely follows a linear trajectory from diagnosis to maintenance, to complex and palliative care. After diagnosis the patient may move between stages or even suffer the consequences of all three, that is the stages are somewhat arbitrary. As the condition is incurable, symptom palliation and support are core elements of care through the disease trajectory, not just at the end where palliative care is usually found, as if it was separate from the progression of the illness and its input isolated to the terminal phase of the disease. There are few publications which describe the palliative care needs of people with Parkinson's (Lee et al. (no date)). Consequently the role of palliative care in the management of PD has not been clearly defined (Rudkins and Aird 2006) and needs are often under-recognised and considered too late in the trajectory (NICE 2006). Lee et al. (2004) argue that this excludes patients and families who may benefit from palliative care at much earlier stages of disease. Palliative care should be considered throughout all phases of the disease, and some clinicians now recommend that involvement in palliative care services should occur early, anticipating a person's needs well in advance of deterioration and assisting with later stage symptoms and psychological issues (Kiernan 2003).

Accepting the four stages as a loose model, the time a patient spends in each of these stages can be long and protracted; the average time spent in the traditional palliative care advanced stage is 2.2 years. Clearly, palliative care does not equate with end of life care: it is certainly bigger (Thomas and MacMahon 2004a and b). The traditional association with end of life may help to explain why the role of palliative care in Parkinson's disease has not been clearly defined (Lee et al. 2004). A number of policy frameworks recommend the need for the principles of palliative care to be applied in neurological conditions throughout the illness trajectory (National Council for Hospices and Specialist Palliative Care Services (NCHSPCS) 2003; NICE 2006). Incorporating palliative care throughout the stages of PD will help the patient and their carer to cope with the condition.

Palliative care beyond the hospice: palliative care beyond cancer

Traditionally, the term palliative care is synonymous with cancer care, at the end of life and believed to be the sole responsibility of hospice to deliver. With less than 6% of UK hospice patients admitted with non-malignant diseases (Morris and Gonsalkorale 2004) such stereotypes continue to prevail. Yet various policy initiatives recommended the delivery of palliative care regardless of condition or care setting (Department of Health (DoH) 2000, 2001b). Indeed, the World Health Organization definition of palliative care also implies the inclusion of other diseases:

> 'palliative care is an approach that improves the quality of life of patients and their families facing the problems associated with life-threatening illness.'
>
> (Sepúlveda et al. 2002, p. 94)

As Parkinson's disease is a progressive incurable condition which impacts the patient and the wider family circle, there is a growing recognition of the need for palliative care (Kristjanson et al. 2003). In response the DoH (2005) *National Service Framework for Long-Term Medical Conditions* focused on the palliative care needs of patients with chronic conditions, including Parkinson's, with a specific reference to the provision of palliative care. More recently the National

Institute for Health and Clinical Excellence (NICE 2006) has issued guidelines on Parkinson's disease that have recommended that palliative care issues should be considered at all phases of the disease.

Despite these policy imperatives, most palliative care services are rarely offered to patients dying with non-cancer diseases (Addington-Hall and Higginson 2001; Luddington et al. 2001) and the complexity of their needs is frequently underestimated (Thomas and MacMahon and 2004a and b). This may be explained, in part, by the difficulty in identifying the terminal phase due to the lengthy and variable symptomatic course (Clough and Blockley 2004). Consequently palliative care specialists have not traditionally been involved in caring for patients with Parkinson's and few palliative care services provide care to people unless they have cancer, and only a small percentage provide care to patients with neurological conditions (Addington-Hall 1998; Field and Addington-Hall 1999). This is reinforced by Kendall (2004) in a review of statistics published by the NCHSPCS in 2003 which highlights the inequality of access to specialist palliative care services for non-cancer patients in the UK.

Many studies demonstrate a considerable unmet palliative care needs among people with non-malignant conditions (Barby and Leigh 1995; Field and Addington-Hall 1999; Luddington et al. 2001) including Parkinson's (Kernohan et al. 2008). The primary palliative care needs of patients and families are across the domains of physical, psychological, social, information and spiritual. Each of these will now be addressed.

Palliative care is physical symptom control

Many patients with neurological conditions, including PD have similar physical problems to patients with cancer. For example, the Regional Study of Care for the Dying (Addington-Hall and McCarthy 1995) found that patients with non-cancer diseases were as likely as patients with cancer to suffer pain. Indeed 40–50% of patients with Parkinson's experience pain (Chaudhuri 2002a). While frequently under-diagnosed, pain can be categorized into musculoskeletal, dystonic, neuritic, akathitic or central pain (Ford 1998; Thomas and MacMahon 2004b). Dyskinetic pain arises as a secondary problem to dyskinesia (abnormal involuntary movements), which can result from fluctuations in response to the standard drug regime (Thomas and MacMahon 2004b). This can result in painful cramps or dystonia. Akathisa (restlessness) may also cause discomfort causing sleep disturbance. As a result up to 90% of patients experience sleep disturbance (Chaudhuri 2002b). Other underlying conditions such as osteoarthritis can also cause pain. Palliative care requires an assessment of pain (Lee et al. 2004), as it has an impact on the patient's and family's physical, emotional and social life; therefore, it is important to assess if pain is treatment related, indirectly related and or non-Parkinson's related.

People with PD can also experience problems with pressure sores due to their immobility, affecting up to 61–73% (Korczyn 1989).

Dysphagia, a difficulty with eating and swallowing, makes it hard to maintain an adequate diet and can even lead to weight loss and malnutrition, itself a dangerous symptom which can cause physiological changes such as the inability to fight infections (Low et al. 2003). In addition, between 40 and 65% of Parkinson's patients experience fatigue; however, it often remains undetected in clinical practice (Herlofson and Larsen 2002; Shulman et al. 2002). Against this backdrop patients can also experience recurrent acute episodes of infections involving the urinary tract, lung or skin (Giladi et al. 2001; Low et al. 2003), all of which impact on the patient's and carers quality of life. Given this complex disease process, symptom control is a highly important aspect of care for people with PD.

Palliative care meets psychological need

People with PD have been found to be susceptible to dementia and psychosis. Indeed, it is estimated that 40–80% of patients diagnosed with PD develop dementia (Aarsland et al. 2003; European Parkinson's Disease Association 2003). Many more will develop behavioural problems such as hallucinations, anxiety, apathy and depression (Aarsland and Karlsen 1999). Hallucinations can become permanent in 80% of patients (Graham et al. 1997) and can be related to dopaminergic medication.

Depression is also a major symptom of PD associated with increased disability and reduced quality of life. The actual prevalence is unclear (Lee et al. 2004); however, frequencies that are quoted range from 40 to 80% (BBC 2006; Bunting-Perry 2006; Zesiewicz et al. 1999). However, an estimated 40% rarely or never discuss this with a health care professional (BBC 2006); therefore, depression often goes unrecognized and untreated (Henderson et al. 1992). Bunting-Perry (2006) suggests that slowness of movement and stooped posture features of Parkinson's make the recognition of depression difficult. Yet the early recognition and treatment of depression is essential to achieve optimum management of both motor and non-motor symptoms (Weintraub and Stren 2005).

Palliative care includes patient and carer information and education

Providing information for patients and carers is an essential element in delivering high-quality palliative care (Payne 2002). Communication skills are viewed as crucial when treating neurodegenerative diseases, as together with counselling and behavioural modification these contribute substantially to the results of any treatment programme (Findley and Baker 2002). For example, Jarman et al. (2002) found that PD specialist nurses helped to preserve patient's sense of well-being through the use of counselling and educating patients, even though health outcomes were unchanged. However, the nature and style of communication and information provision remain problematic (Buckman 1998) with evidence of considerable variability in disclosure of diagnosis between patients with cancer and those with non-malignant disease, the latter being less likely to be informed (Seale et al. 1997). Moreover, written information leaflets have been found to focus on medical aspects of their disease, rather than experiential aspects known by fellow patients (Dixon-Woods 2001). A key need for patients and families is for more information about the disease, medications, financial support and support networks available (Parkinson's Disease society UK 2005). Yet research highlights ongoing deficiencies, for example, Kernohan et al. (2008) found that communication skills and information giving were inadequate, with provision provided on an ad hoc basis, leading to high levels of anxiety.

Palliative care is social

Whilst Parkinson's disease has a neurological basis, it has a wide impact on patients and families only partly related to motor symptoms (Ellgring et al. 1993). According to the National Council for Hospice and Specialist Palliative Care Services (1997), psychosocial care encompasses the psychological and emo- tional well-being of the patient and their family/carer. It also includes practical aspects of care such as financial, housing and aids to daily living. Bunting-Perry (2006) highlights the importance of evaluating the psychosocial aspects of the patient's life, as the diagnosis and management of PD can affect self-esteem and relationships (Bunting-Perry 2006).

Previous research has demonstrated that many non-cancer patients who are dying have unmet psychosocial needs such as anxiety, social isolation, depen- dency on others and financial difficulties (Kernohan et al. 2008; Luddington et al. 2001; McIlfatrick 2007; Spence et al. 2008). Kernohan et al. (2008) found high levels of emotional distress, fears for the future due to the unpredictably progression of the disease, social isolation and poor quality of life among car- ers and people with Parkinson's. Shulman et al. (2001) also found that patients experience anger, frustration and anxiety or depression and sleep disturbance.

Service provision for people with PD involves many agencies across acute, community and social services, including home care, acute care, rehabilitation, respite, residential and palliative or supportive care services (Kristjanson et al. 2006). However, the majority of patients with neurological diseases are increas- ingly being cared for at home (Ahlstrom 2006). The need for support to enable the patient to remain in the home environment and for the carer to cope with their role requires social support to be available. Research indicates that carers and people with PD and other non-malignant conditions have social needs similar to other palliative care populations: for example, in the form of financial assistance, support to preserve social networks, provision of respite care and equipment (Hull 1990; Hudson 2003; Kernohan et al. 2008; Seymour and Clark 2001; Spence et al. 2008). Indeed, as the diseases progresses and increasing care provision is required, fewer social outings and contacts occur, resulting in isolation for both the patient and carer (Hudson et al. 2006; Kernohan et al. 2008; O'Reilly et al. 1996; Schrag et al. 2000). Many patients and carers do not experience a coherent integrated system of social support to address their needs (Clausen et al. 2005; Sutton 2006). For example, a UK-wide survey of patients' and carer's experiences of advanced stage PD reported that formal and informal support was patchy, with some reporting abandonment, with carers' needs rarely assessed and little respite or bereavement support offered (Parkinson's Disease Society 2005). Indeed Lloyd (2000) claims that health and social care management for people with PD has failed with many patients or carers not proceeding to receive either community health care or social care assessments or services. This resulted in patients and carers not getting access to much needed support and lowering their expectations of quality of life.

Palliative care is spiritual

Whilst spiritual needs are considered an important domain in the care of dying patients (Low et al. 2003), contributing to well-being and coping strategies (McClain et al. 2003; Thiel and Robinson 1997; Walsh et al. 2002), there exists a lack of consensus as to what spiritual care actually is (Mount et al. 2002). Spiritual health is commonly presented as the response to the human search for meaning (Carson 1989; Harrison and Burnard 1993; Speck 1997; Stoter 1995). However, spiritual belief and religious affiliation are terms which are used interchangeably; yet Speck et al. (2004) point out that 'spiritual belief may or may not be religious, but most religious people will be spiritual' (p. 123). Compounding this is the fact that spiritual needs are not static; instead they are subject to change over the duration of the illness trajectory (NICE 2004). Hence, members of the multidisciplinary team need to provide ongoing assessment of spiritual needs.

Usually the responsibility to address spiritual issues rests with chaplains or pastoral teams; however, all members of the health professional team play an important role (Clark et al. 2003). However, health care professionals often have little preparation or training to respond to patients' and carers' spiritual needs (Power and Sharp 1988; Wasner et al. 2005). Consequently, while research has identified that spiritual concerns were important for both patients and carers at all stages of the illness progression, many reported unmet spiritual needs (Kernohan et al. 2008; Murray et al. 2004; Spence et al. 2008).

Summary – palliative care is needed

Parkinson's disease is a complex and challenging condition within which symptoms appear slowly and in no particular order. Whilst four broad stages of the disease progression have been identified, including diagnosis, maintenance, complex and palliative care, they are somewhat arbitrary and lead to the misconception that palliative care is separate, delivered only at the very advanced stages of disease. However, as patients live with Parkinson's for many years with no prospect of a cure coming soon, there is a need to extend palliative care if only in terms of equity and individual need for a basic quality of life (Field and Addington-Hall 1999). There is convincing evidence that many carers and patients have unmet palliative care needs, with regards to symptom control, psychosocial, social and spiritual support at all stages of the disease process.

References

Aarsland D, Anderson K, Larsen JP, Lolk A and Kragh-Sorensen P (2003) Prevalence and characteristics of dementia in Parkinson disease: an 8-year prospective study. *Archives of Neurology*. 60:387–392.

Aarsland D and Karlsen K (1999) Neuropsychiatric aspects of Parkinson's disease. *Current Psychiatry Reports*. 1:61–68.

Aboussouan LS, Khan SU, Meeker DP, Stelmach K and Mitsumoto H (1997) Effect of non-invasive positive-pressure ventilation on survival in amyotrophic lateral sclerosis. *Annals of Internal Medicine*. 127(6):450–453.

Abraham SS and Yun PT (2002) Laryngopharyngeal dysmotility in multiple sclerosis. *Dysphagia*. 16:69–74.

Addington-Hall J (1998) *Reaching Out: Specialist Palliative Care for Adults with Nonmalignant Disease*. London: National Council for Hospices and Specialist Palliative Care Services.

Addington-Hall J and McCarthy M (1995) Regional study of care for the dying: methods and sample characteristics. *Palliative Medicine*. 9:27–35.

Addington-Hall JM and Higginson IJ (2001) *Palliative Care in Non-Cancer Patients*. New York: Oxford University Press.

Ahlstrom G (2006) Personal assistance for patients living with a severe neurological disorder. *Journal of Neuroscience Nursing*. 38(3):183–193.

Aranda K and Hayman-White K (2001) Home caregivers of the person with advanced cancer: an Australian perspective. *Cancer Nursing*. 24:1–7.

Atkin K (2000) Adults with disability who reported excellent or good quality of life had established a balance of body, mind and spirit. *Evidence-Based Nursing*. 3:1–31.

Aubeeluck A and Buchanan H (2006) Capturing the Huntington's disease spousal carer experience. *Dementia*. 5(1):95–116.

Aubeeluck A and Moscowitz CB (2008) Huntington's disease. Part 3: family aspects of HD. *British Journal of Nursing*. 17(5):328–331.

Baker M and Graham L (2004) The journey: Parkinson's disease. *British Medical Journal*. 329:611–614.

Barby TFM and Leigh PN (1995) Palliative care in mother neurone disease. *International Journal of Palliative Nursing*. 1(4):183–188.

Barg F, Pasacreta J, Nuamah, I, Robinson K, Angeletti K, Yasko J and McCorkle R (1998) A description of a psychoeducational intervention for family caregivers of cancer patients. *Journal of Family Nursing*. 44:394–413.

BBC (2006) Depression risk with Parkinson's. Available at http://news.bbc.co.uk/1/hi/health/5075576.stm. Accessed on 29 April 2008.

Bhatia K, Brooks D, Burn D, Clarke C, Playfer J, Sawle G, Schapira A, Stewart D and Williams A (1998) Guidelines for the management of Parkinson's disease. *Hospital Medicine*. 59(6):469–480.

Bourke SC and Gibson GL (2004) Non-invasive ventilation in ALS: current practice and future role. *Amyotrophic Lateral Sclerosis and Other Motor Neurone Disorders*. 5(2):67–71.

British Brain and Spine Foundation (2000) *Motor Neurone Disease: A Guide for Patients and Carers*. London: BBSF.

Brønnum-Hansen H, Koch-Henriksen N and Stenager E (2004) Trends in survival and cause of death in Danish patients with multiple sclerosis. *Brain*. 127:844–850.

Brown RG, Jahamshahi M, Quinn NP and Marsden CD (1990) Sexual function in patients with Parkinson's disease and their partners. *Journal of Neurology, Neurosurgery and Psychiatry*. 53:480–486.

Buckman R (1998) Communication in palliative care: a practical guide. In: Doyle D, Hanks GW and MacDonald N (Eds), *The Oxford Textbook of Palliative Medicine* (2nd edition). Oxford: Oxford University Press, pp. 141–158.

Bunting-Perry L (2006) Palliative care in Parkinson's disease: implications for neuroscience nursing. *Journal of Neuroscience Nursing*. 38(2):106–113.

Burgess M (2002) *Multiple Sclerosis: Theory and Practice for Nurses*. London: Whurr Publishers.

Calne DB (2000) Parkinson's disease is not one disease. Parkinsonism and Related Disorders. 7:3–7.

Carson VB (1989) *Spiritual Dimensions of Nursing Practice*. Philadelphia: WB Saunders.

Chaudhuri KR (2002a) Pain in Parkinson's. A PDS Information Leaflet, Number 37. London: Parkinson's Disease Society.

Chaudhuri KR (2002b). Sleep and nighttime problems in Parkinson's. A PDS Information Leaflet, Number 30. London: Parkinson's Disease Society.

Clark P, Drain M and Malone M (2003) Addressing patients' emotional and spiritual needs. *Journal on Quality and Safety*. 29(12):659–670.

Clausen H, Kendall M, Murray S, Worth A, Boyd K and Benton F (2005) Would palliative care patients benefit from social workers' retaining the traditional 'casework' role rather than working as care managers? A prospective serial qualitative interview. *British Journal of Social Work*. 35(2):277–285.

Clough C and Blockley A (2004) Parkinson's disease and related disorders, Chapter 5. In: Voltz R, Bernat JL, Borasio GD, Maddocks I, Oliver D and Porkeroy RR (Eds), *Palliative Care in Neurology: Contemporary Neurology Series*. Oxford: Oxford University Press, pp. 48–58

Cottrell DA, Kremenchutzky K, Rice GPA, Koopman WJ, Hader W, Baskerville J and Ebers GC (1999) The natural history of multiple sclerosis: a geographically based study. 5. The clinical features and natural history of primary progressive multiple sclerosis. *Brain*. 122:625–639.

Currie R (2001) Spasticity: a common symptom of multiple sclerosis. *Nursing Standard*. 15(33):47–55.

Dawson S, Kristjanson LJ, Toye CM and Flett P (2004) Living with Huntington's disease: need for supportive care. *Nursing and Health Sciences*. 6:123–130.

Department of Health (2000) *The NHS Cancer Plan: A Plan for Investment, a Plan for Reform*. London: DoH.

Department of Health (2001a) *Good Practice in Consent and Implementation Guide: Consent to Examination or Treatment*. London: DoH.

Department of Health (2001b) *National Service Framework for Older People*. London: DoH.

Department of Health (2005a) *Mental Capacity Act 2005: Acute Hospital Training Set*. London: DoH.

Department of Health (2005b) *The National Service Framework for Long-term Conditions*. London: DoH.

Dixon-Woods M (2001) Writing wrongs? An analysis of published discourses about the use of patient information leaflets. *Social Science and Medicine.* 52:1417–1432.

Ellershaw J and Wilkinson S (2003) *Care of the Dying: A Pathway to Excellence.* Oxford: Oxford University Press.

Ellgring H, Seiler S, Perleth B, Frings E, Gasser T and Oetel W (1993) Psychosocial aspects of Parkinson's disease. *Neurology.* 43(12 Suppl 6):S41–S44.

European Parkinson's Disease Association (2003) Global Declaration on Parkinson's Disease. Available at http://epda.eu.com. Accessed on 28 April 2008.

Feinstein A (1999) *The Clinical Neuropsychiatry of Multiple Sclerosis.* Cambridge: Cambridge University Press.

Feinstein A (2002) An examination of suicidal intent in patients with multiple sclerosis. *Neurology.* 59:674–678.

Field D and Addington-Hall J (1999) Extending specialist palliative care to all? *Social Science and Medicine.* 48:1271–1280.

Findley L and Baker M (2002) Editorial treating neurodegenerative diseases: what patients want is not what doctors focus on. *British Medical Journal.* 324:1466–1467.

Findley L, Hurwitz B and Miles A (2004) The Effective Management of Parkinson's Disease. London: Aesculapius Medical Press.

Forbes A, While A and Taylor M (2007) What people with MS perceive to be important to meeting their needs. *Journal of Advanced Nursing.* 58(1):11–22.

Ford B (1998) Pain in Parkinson's disease. *Clinical Neuroscience.* 5:63–72.

General Medical Council (2002) *Withholding and Withdrawing Life Prolonging Treatment: Good Practice in Decision-Making.* London: GMC.

Ghaffer O and Feinstein A (2007) The neuropsychiatry of multiple sclerosis: a review of recent developments. *Current Opinion in Psychiatry.* 20(3):278–285.

Giladi N, Treves TA, Simon ES, Shabtai H, Orlov Y, Kandinov B, Paleacu D and Korczyn AD (2001) Freezing of gait in patients with advanced Parkinson's disease. *Journal of Neural Transmission.* 108:53–61.

Goldstein L (2006) Control of symptoms: cognitive dysfunction. In: Oliver D, Barasio GD and Walsh D (Eds), *Palliative Care in Amyotrophic Lateral Sclerosis: From Diagnosis to Bereavement* (2nd edition). Oxford: Oxford University, Chapter 4c, pp. 111–128.

Graham JM, Grunewald RA and Sagar HJ (1997) Hallucinations in idiopathic Parkinson's disease. *Journal of Neurology, Neurosurgery and Psychiatry.* 63:434–440.

Gregory S, Siderowf A, Golaszewski AL and McCluskey L (2002) Gastrostomy insertion in ALS patients with low vital capacity: respiratory support and survival. *Neurology.* 58(3):485–487.

Harrison J and Burnard P (1993) *Spirituality and Nursing Practice.* Aldershot: Averbury.

Henderson R, Kurlan R and Kersun JM (1992) Preliminary examination of the comorbidity of anxiety and depression in Parkinson's disease. *Journal of Neuropsychiatry and Clinical Neurosciences.* 4:257–264.

Herlofson K and Larsen JP (2002) Measuring fatigue in patients with Parkinson's disease – the Fatigue severity scale. *European Journal of Neurology.* 9:595–600.

Higginson I, Wade A and McCarthy M (1990) Palliative care: views of patients and their families. *British Medical Journal.* 301:277–281.

Hocking C, Brott T and Paddy A (2006) Caring for people with motor neurone disease. *International Journal of Therapy and Rehabilitation.* 13(8):351–356.

Hogstel MO (2001) *Gerontology: Nursing Care of the Older Adult.* Albany, NY: Delmar.

Hudson P (2003) Home-based support for palliative care families: challenges and recommendations. *The Medical Journal of Australia.* 179(Suppl 6):S35–S37.

Hudson P, Toye C and Kristjanson L (2006) Would people with Parkinson's disease benefit from palliative care? *Palliative Medicine*. 20:87–94.

Hughes AJ, Daniel SE, Kilford L and Leas AJ (1992) Accuracy of clinical diagnosis of idiopathic Parkinson's disease: a clinico-pathological study of 100 cases. *Journal of Neurology, Neurosurgery and Psychiatry*. 55:181–184.

Hull MM (1990) Family need and supportive nursing behaviours during terminal cancer: a review. *Oncology Nursing Forum*. 16:787–792.

Jarman B, Hurwitz B, Cook A, Bajekal M and Lee A (2002) Effects of community based nurses specialising in Parkinson's disease on health outcome and costs: a randomised controlled trial. *British Medical Journal*. 324:1072–1075.

Jones BJM (2007) Nutritional support at the end of life: the relevant ethical issues. *European Journal of Gastroenterology*. 19(5):383–388.

Keenan K, Miedzybrodzka Z, van Teijlingen E, McKee L and Simpson SA (2007) Young people's experience of growing up in a family affected by Huntington's disease. *Clinical Genetics*. 71(2):120–129.

Kendall M (2004) The changing face of palliative care. *Nurse2Nurse Magazine*. 4(4):54–56.

Kent A (2004) Huntington's disease. *Nursing Standard*. 18(32):45–51.

Kernohan WG, Hasson F, McLaughlin M, McLaughlin D, Cochrane B and Chambers H (2008) Do people with Parkinson's disease need palliative care? University of Ulster (in press).

Khan F, McPhail T, Brand C, Turner-Stokes L and Kilpatrick T (2006) Multiple sclerosis: disability profile and quality of life in an Australian community cohort. *International Journal of Rehabilitation Research*. 29(2):87–96.

Khan F, Pallant J and Brand C (2007) Caregiver strain and factors associated with caregiver self-efficacy and quality of life in a community cohort with multiple sclerosis. *Disability and Rehabilitation*. 29(16):1241–1250.

Kiernan MC (2003) Motor neuron disease: a Pandora's box. *The Medical Journal of Australia*. 178:311–312.

Korczyn AD (1989) Autonomic nervous system screening in patients with early PD. In: Pruntek H and Riederer P (Eds), *Early Diagnosis and Preventative Therapy in Parkinson's Disease*. New York: Springer.

Kristjanson LJ, Aoun S and Yates P (2006a) Are supportive services meeting the needs of Australians with neurodegenerative conditions and their families? *Journal of Palliative Care*. 22(3):151–157.

Kristjanson LJ, Aoun SM and Oldham L (2006b) Palliative care and support for people with neurodegenerative conditions and their carers. *International Journal of Palliative Nursing*. 12(8):368–377.

Kristjanson LJ, Toye C and Dawson S (2003) New dimensions in palliative care: a palliative approach to neurodegenerative diseases and final illness in older people. *The Medical Journal of Australia*. 179:S41–S43.

Lee M, Prentice WM and Walker RW (no date). Defining palliative care needs in Parkinson's disease? Poster Presentation.

Lee M, Walker R and Prentice W (2004) The role of palliative care in Parkinson's disease. *Geriatric Medicine*. 34(4): 51–54.

Lilinfeld DE and Perl DP (1994) Mortality from parkinsonism in the United States 1990–200. *Neurodegeneration*. 3:21–34.

Lloyd M (2000) Where has all the care management gone? The challenge of Parkinson's disease to the Health and Social Care Interface. *British Journal of Social Work*. 30:737–754.

Lobchuk MM (2006) Concept analysis of perspective taking: meeting informal caregivers needs for communication competence and accurate perception. *Journal of Advanced Nursing.* 54:(3):330–341.

Low JA, Pang WS and Chan DKY (2003) A palliative care approach to end-stage neurodegenerative conditions. *Annals of Academy of Medicine Singapore.* 32:778–784.

Luddington L, Cox S, Higginson I and Livesley B (2001) The need for palliative care for patients with non-cancer diseases: a review of the evidence. *International Journal of Palliative Nursing.* 7(5):221–226.

MacGill M (2003) Scottish Huntington's Association Annual Report 2002/2003. Elderslie: SHA.

MacMahon DG and Thomas S (1998) Practical approach to quality of life in Parkinson's disease. *Journal of Neurology.* 245:13.

Mallet D and Chekroud H (2001) A focus on hereditary disease. *European Journal of Palliative Care.* 8(4):147–149.

McClain CS, Rosenfeld B and Breitbart W (2003) Effect of spiritual well-being on end-of-life despair in terminally-ill cancer patients. *Lancet.* 361:1603–1607.

McDermott C and Shaw P (2008) Diagnosis and management of motor neurone disease. *British Medical Journal.* 336:658–662.

McGuire V and Nelson LM (2006) Epidemiology of ALS. In: Mitsumoto H, Przedborski S and Gordon P (Eds), *Amyotrophic Lateral Sclerosis.* New York: Taylor & Francis, pp. 17–21.

McIlfatrick S (2007) Assessing palliative care needs: views of patients, informal carers and healthcare professionals. *Journal of Advanced Nursing.* 57(1):77–86.

McIntyre R and Lugton J (2005) Supporting family and carers. In: Lugton J and McIntyre R (Eds), *Palliative Care: The Nursing Role* (2nd edition). Edinburgh: Elsevier, pp. 261–302.

Midgard R, Albrektsen G, Riise T, Kvale G and Nyland H (1995) Prognostic factors for survival in multiple sclerosis: a longitudinal, population based study in More and Romsdal Norway. *Journal of Neurology, Neurosurgery and Psychiatry.* 58(4):417–421.

Miller RG, Mitchell JD, Lyon M and Moore DH (2007) Riluzole for Amyotrophic Lateral Sclerosis (ALS)/Motor Neurone Disease (MND). Cochrane Database Systematic Review; Issue 1, CD001447.

Miller RG, Rosenberg JA, Gelina DF, Mitsumoto H, Newman D and Suril R (1999) Practice parameter: the care of the patient with amyotrophic lateral sclerosis (an evidence based review). *Neurology.* 52(7):1311–1323.

Minden SL, Orav J and Reich P (1987) Depression in multiple sclerosis. *General Hospital Psychiatry.* 9:426–434.

Mitsumoto H, Przedborski S and Gordon PH (2006) *Amyotrophic Lateral Sclerosis.* London: Taylor and Francis. Table 1, p. 18.

Morris C and Gonsalkorale M (2004) Palliative care and Parkinson's disease. *European Parkinson's Nurses Network (EPNN) Journal.* 3:11–12.

Moskowitz CB and Marder K (2001) Palliative care for people with late stage Huntington's disease. *Neurologic Clinics.* 19(4):849–865.

Motor Neurone Disease (MND) Association (2001) A Problem-Solving Approach for GPs and the Primary Health Care Team. MND Association. Available at http://www.mndassociation.org/life_with_mnd/getting_more_information/publications/publications_1.html. Accessed on 2 December 2008.

Mount BM, Lawlor W and Cassell EJ (2002) Spirituality and health: developing a shared vocabulary. *Annals of the Royal College of Physicians and Surgeons of Canada.* 35:303–307.

Murray S, Kendall M, Boyd K, Worth A and Benton T (2004) Exploring the spiritual needs of people dying of lung cancer or heart failure: a prospective qualitative interview study of patients and their carers. *Palliative Medicine.* 18(1):39–45.

Mutch WJ (1995) Parkinson's disease. *Journal of Neurology, Neurosurgery and Psychiatry.* 57:672–681.

Nance MA and Westphal B (2002) Comprehensive care in Huntington's disease. In: Bates GP, Harper PS and Jones L (Eds), *Huntington's Disease.* Oxford: Oxford University Press, pp. 475–500.

Nanton V (1985) The consequences of Parkinson's disease – needs, provisions and initiatives. *Journal of the Royal Society of Health.* 105(2):52–54.

National Collaborating Centre for Chronic Conditions (2003) *Multiple Sclerosis: Management of Multiple Sclerosis in Primary and Secondary Care.* London: NICE.

National Council for Hospice and Specialist Palliative Care Services (1997) Feeling better: psychosocial care in specialist palliative care. Occasional Paper No. 13. London: National Council for Hospice and Specialist Palliative Care Services.

The National Council for Hospice and Specialist Palliative Care Services (2003) Palliative care for adults with non-malignant disease: developing a national policy. Available at www.hospice-spc-council.org.uk. Accessed on 25 April 2008.

National Institute of Clinical Excellence (NICE) (2003) *Multiple Sclerosis: Management of Multiple Sclerosis in Primary and Secondary Care.* London: NICE.

National Institute for Clinical Excellence (2004) *Guidance on Improving Supportive and Palliative Care for Adults with Cancer.* London: NICE.

National Institute for Clinical Excellence (2006) Parkinson's disease: national clinical guideline for diagnosis and management in primary and secondary care. London: NICE. Available at http://www.nice.org.uk/nicemedia/pdf/cg035fullguideline.pdf. Accessed on 18 April 2008.

Neary D, Snowden JS and Mann DM (2000) Cognitive change in motor neurone disease/amyotrophic lateral sclerosis (MND/ALS). *Journal of the Neurological Sciences.* 180:15–20.

Nursing & Midwifery Council (2008) The Code – Standards of conduct, performance and ethics for nurses and midwives. NMC London

O'Brien T (2002) Neurodegenerative disease. In: Addington-Hall J and Higginson I (Eds), *Palliative Care for Non-Cancer Patients.* Oxford: Oxford University Press, pp. 44–95.

O'Connor P, Lee L, Ng PT and Wolinsky JS (2001) Determinates of overall quality of life in secondary progressive MS: a longitudinal study. *Neurology.* 57(5):889–891.

O'Reilly F, Finnan F, Allwright S, Davey-Smith G and Ben-Shlomo Y (1996) The effects of caring for a spouse with Parkinson's disease on social, psychological and physical well-being. *British Journal of General Practice.* 46:507–512.

Oldham L and Kristjanson LJ (2004) Development of a pain management programme for family carers of advanced cancer patients. *International Journal of Palliative Nursing.* 10:91–99.

Oliver D (2002) Palliative care for motor neurone disease. *Practical Neurology.* 2:68–79.

Oliver DC (2006) What will the doctor do? Chapter 2. *Motor Neurone Disease a Family Affair* (2nd edition). London: Sheldon Press, pp. 221–267.

Oliver D, Bell J, Gallagher D, Newton J, Rackham C, Swannick J and Thompson S (2007) Development of a pathway to facilitate gastrostomy insertion for patients with MND. *International Journal of Palliative Nursing.* 13(9):426–429.

Parkinson's Disease Society (2004) Will I die from Parkinson's? Available at http://www.parkinsons.org.uk/default.aspx?page=7002. Accessed on 28 November 2008.

Parkinson's Disease Society (2005) *Just Invisible: The Advanced Parkinson's Project*. London: Parkinson's Disease Society.

Paulsen A (1999) *Understanding Behaviour in Huntington's Disease* (2nd edition). New York: Huntington's Disease Society of America.

Payne S (2002) Information needs of patients and families. *European Journal of Palliative Care*. 9(3):112–114.

Pickett T Jr, Altmaier E and Paulsen JS (2007) Caregiver burden in Huntington's disease. *Rehabilitation Psychology*. 52(3):311–318.

Power KG and Sharp GR (1988) A comparison of sources of nursing stress and job satisfaction among mental handicap and hospice nursing staff. *Journal of Advanced Nursing*. 13:726–732.

Quarrell O (1999) *Huntington's Disease: The Facts*. New York: Oxford University Press.

Quinn A (2006) Evaluation of a new post: the West Berkshire clinical nurse specialist for rare neurological conditions. Reading, University of Reading. Available at http://www.wbna.org.uk/. Accessed on 2 December 2008.

Rabeneck L, McCoullough LB and Wray NP (1997) Ethically justified, clinically comprehensive guidelines for percutaneous endoscopic gastrostomy tube placement. *The Lancet*. 349(9050): 496–498.

Rao SM, Leo GJ, Bernardin L and Unverzagt F (1991) Cognitive dysfunction in multiple sclerosis: frequency, patterns, and prediction. *Neurology*. 41:685–691.

Ream E (2008) Fatigue. In: Stevens E and Edwards J (Eds), *Palliative Care: Learning in Practice*. Exeter: Reflect Press. pp. 221–267

Riudavets MA, Colegial C, Rubio A, Fowler D, Pardo C and Troncoso JC (2005) Causes of unexpected death in patients with multiple sclerosis: a forensic study of cases. *The American Journal of Forensic Medicine*. 26(3):244–249.

Robins Whalin T-B (2007) To know or not to know: a review of behaviour and suicide ideation in preclinical Huntington's disease. *Patient Education and Counselling*. 65(3):279–287.

Robins Whalin T-B, Backman L, Lundin A, Haegermark A, Winblad B and Anvret M (2000) High suicidal ideation in persons testing for Huntington's disease. *Acta Neurologica Scandinavica*. 102(3):150–161.

Rosenblatt A, Ranen NG, Nance MJ and Paulsen JS (2004) *A Physician's Guide to the Management of Huntington's Disease* (2nd edition). Ontario: Huntington Society of Canada.

Rudkins H and Aird T (2006) The importance of early consideration of palliative care in Parkinson's disease. *British Journal of Neuroscience Nursing*. 2(1):10–16.

Schrag A, Jahanshahi M and Quinn N (2000) How does Parkinson's disease affect quality of life? A comparison with quality of life in the general population. *Movement Disorders*. 15(6):112–118.

Scott S (2002) Understanding the challenge of Parkinson's disease. *Nursing Standard*. 16(41):48–52.

Scott A and Foulsom M (2000) Speech and language therapy. In: Oliver D, Barasio GD and Walsh D (Eds), *Palliative Care in Amyotrophic Lateral Sclerosis*. Oxford: Oxford University Press, Chapter 6.3.

Scottish Huntington's Association (2006) Draft care pathway. Elderslie: SHA. Available at http://www.hdscotland.org/Downloads/Library/Care%20Pathway.pdf. Accessed on 10 January 2009.

Scottish Motor Neurone Disease Association (2004) A Problem Solving Approach for General Practitioners and Social Care Professionals. 1st edition. Available at www.elib.scot.nhs.uk. Accessed on 2 December 2008.

Scottish Motor Neurone Disease Register (1992) A prospective study of adult onset motor neurone disease in Scotland. Methodology, demography and clinical features of incident cases in 1989. *Journal of Neurology, Neurosurgery, Psychiatry.* 55:536–541.

Seale CF, Addington-Hall JM and McCarthy M (1997) Awareness of dying: prevalence, cause and consequences. *Social Science Medicine.* 45:477–484.

Seamark DA, Seamark C and Halpin D (2007) Palliative care in chronic obstructive pulmonary disease: a review for clinicians. *Journal of the Royal Society of Medicine.* 100(5):225–233.

Sepúlveda C, Marlin A, Yoshida T and Ullrich A (2002) Palliative care: the World Health Organization's global perspective. *Journal of Pain and Symptom Management.* 24:91–96.

Seymour J and Clark D (2001) Palliative care and geriatric medicine: shared concerns, shared challenges. *Palliative Medicine.* 15(4):269–270.

Shakespeare DT, Boggild M and Young C (2000) Anti-spasticity agents for multiple sclerosis. *Cochrane Database of Systematic Reviews.* Issue 4. Art. No.: CD001332.

Shakespeare J and Anderson J (1993) Huntington's disease – falling through the net. *Health Trends (England).* 25(1):9–23.

Shulman LM, Taback RL, Bean J and Weiner WJ (2001) Comorbidity of the non-motor symptoms of Parkinson's disease. *Movement Disorders.* 16:507–510.

Shulman LM, Taback RL, Rabinstein AA and Weiner WJ (2002) Non-recognition of depression and other non-motor symptoms in Parkinson's disease. *Parkinsonism and Related Disorders.* 9:193–197.

Simpson SA (2006) Late stage care in Huntington's disease. *Brain Research Bulletin.* 72(2–3):179–181.

Speck P (1997) Spiritual issues in palliative care. In: Doyle D, Hanks G and MacDonald M (Eds), *The Oxford Textbook of Palliative Medicine.* Oxford: Oxford University Press, pp. 805–814.

Speck P, Higginson I and Adddington-Hall J (2004) Editorial spiritual needs in health care. *British Medical Journal.* 329:123–124.

Spence A, McLaughlin D, Watson B, Cochrane B, Kernihan G, Hasson F and Waldon M (2008) A study of palliative care needs and services available in advanced COPD. Northern Ireland Hospice Care, Northern Ireland (in press).

Squires N (2006) Dysphagia management for progressive neurological conditions. *Nursing Standard.* 20(29):53–57.

Stephenson C (2001) Major diseases: an overview. In: Hogstel MO (Ed), *Gerontology: Nursing Care of the Older Adult.* Albany, NY: Delmar.

Storey L, Callagher P, Mitchell D, Addison Jones R and Bennett W (2006) Extending choice over where with motor neurone disease receive end of life care. *British Journal of Neuroscience Nursing.* 2(10):493–498.

Storey L and Pemberton C (2002) The preferred place of care plan and why it was developed. Available at www.cancerlancashire.org.uk/ppc.html. Accessed on 21 April 2008.

Stoter D (1995) *Spiritual Aspects of Health Care.* London: Mosby.

Sulaiman S (2007) *Learning to Live with Huntington's Disease.* London: Jessica Kingsley.

Sutton L (2006) Developing palliative care support for people with Parkinson's disease: moving forward together. The National Council for Palliative Care, United Kingdom. Available at http://www.bjhm.co.uk/ppts/(21-09-2006)parkinsons2006/developing-palliative-care-support.ppt. Accessed on 7 May 2008.

Tanner CM and Ben-Shlomo Y (1999) Epidemiology of Parkinson's disease. *Advances in Neurology.* 80:152–159.

Thiel MM and Robinson MR (1997) Physician's collaboration with chaplains. Difficulties and benefits. *Journal of Clinical Ethics*. 8:94–103.

Thomas K (2003) *Caring for the Dying at Home: Companions on the Journey*. Oxford: Radcliffe Medical Press.

Thomas S (no date). Palliative care for neurological conditions: an introduction. Royal College of Nursing, London. Available at http://www.ncpc.org.uk/download/events/Neuro/Sue_Thomas_090207.pdf. Accessed on 18 April 2008.

Thomas S and MacMahon D (1999) The challenge of Parkinson's disease. *Journal of Community Nursing*. 13:18–22.

Thomas S and MacMahon DG (2004a). Parkinson's disease, palliative care and older people: part 1. *Nursing Older People*. 16(1):22–26.

Thomas S and MacMahon DG (2004b). Parkinson's disease, palliative care and older people: part 2. *Nursing Older People*. 16(2):22–26.

Travers E, Jones K and Nicol J (2007) Palliative care provision in Huntington's disease. *International Journal of Palliative Nursing*. 13(3):125–130.

Traynor BJ, Alexander M, Corr B, Frost E and Hardiman O (2003) An outcome study of riluzole in amyotrophic lateral sclerosis. A population-based study in Ireland, 1996–2000. *Journal of Neurology*. 250(4):473–479.

Turner AP, Williams RM, Bowen JD (2006) Suicidal ideation in multiple sclerosis. *Archives of Physical and Medical Rehabilitation*. 87:1073–1078.

van Broekhoven-Grutters E, Gaasbeek D and Veninga-Verbaas M (2000) *Nutrition and Huntington's Disease, A Practical Guide: A Multidisciplinary Approach*. Apeldoorn Beekbergen, The Netherlands: Atlant Zorggroep.

Vucic S, Burke D and Kiernan MC (2007) Diagnosis of motor neurone disease, chapter 6. In: *The Motor Neurone Disease Handbook*. Australia: Australasian Medical Publishing Company Limited.

Wagner-Sonntag E and Prosiegel M (2006) Dysphagia. In: Oliver D, Borasio GD and Walsh D (Eds), *Palliative Care in Amyotrophic Lateral Sclerosis*. Oxford: Oxford University Press, pp. 62–71.

Walsh K, King M, Jones L, Tookman A and Blizard R (2002) Spiritual beliefs may affect outcome of bereavement: prospective study. *British Medical Journal*. 324:1551–1556.

Ward C and Robertson D (2004) Rehabilitation in Parkinson's disease. *Review in Clinical Gerontology*. 13:223–239.

Warner R (2006) Understanding fatigue in multiple sclerosis: a case study inquiry. *British Journal of Neuroscience Nursing*. 2(9):462–469.

Wasner M, Longaker C, Johannes Fegg M and Domenico Borasio G (2005) Effects of spiritual care training for palliative care professionals. *Palliative Medicine*. 19:99–104.

Weintraub D and Stern MB (2005) Psychiatric complications in Parkinson's disease. *American Journal of Geriatric Psychiatry*. 13:844–851.

Wollin J, Yates P and Kristjanson L (2006) Supportive and palliative care needs identified by multiple sclerosis patients and their families. *International Journal of Palliative Nursing*. 12 (1):20–26.

Zesiewicz TA, Gold M, Chari G and Hauser RA (1999) Current issues in depression in Parkinson's disease. *American Journal of Geriatric Psychiatry*. 7:110–118.

Useful websites

www.hdscotland.org (Scottish Huntington's Association).

www.hda.org.uk (Huntington's Disease Association).

www.huntingtonsociety.ca/ (Huntington Society of Canada).

www.hsc-ca.org (Huntington Society of Canada).

www.hdlighthouse.org (Huntington's Disease Lighthouse).

www.euro-hd.net (European Huntington's Disease Network).

www.huntingtonproject.org (Huntington Project).

www.huntington-assoc.com (International Huntington Association).

www.stanford.edu/group/hopes/basics/timeline/r2.html (Huntington's Outreach Project for Education at Stanford).

www.geneticseducation.nhs.uk (National Genetics Education and Development Centre).

www.scotGEN.org (Scottish Genetics Education Network).

Chapter 12

Palliative care for people with end stage renal disease

Helen Noble

Introduction

This chapter offers a description of two distinct groups of terminally ill renal patients – those who opt not to commence dialysis to treat their renal failure and those who decide to withdraw from dialysis therapy. It not only includes an overview of the needs of those dying with renal failure but also highlights the lack of research in this area and emphasises the lack of supportive and palliative care that many of these patients have received in the past.

Learning outcomes

Once you have read this chapter and completed the associated practice points you will be able to:

- Discuss the nature of renal disease and the particular problems that may ensue in the renal population when end stage renal disease is reached
- Describe the needs of those renal patients who opt not to commence dialysis and those who decide to withdraw from dialysis
- Explain the urgent need for research to offer greater understanding of the needs, experiences and trajectory to death of renal patients coming to the end of life

Background

Five million individuals worldwide have some form of chronic kidney disease (CKD) and approximately 1.5 million people must be kept alive with dialysis (ISN and IFKF 2007). In recent years the number of patients developing CKD has increased and the dialysis population is becoming increasingly elderly with the median age of new patients in 2002 at 65 years. In the last 20 years the prevalence rate of patients 75 years and over has doubled and in addition to being older, patients with CKD often have a substantial number of co-morbid

Table 12.1 Stages of kidney disease.

Stage	Description	GFR* mL/min/1.73 m²
1	Slight kidney damage with normal or increased filtration	More than 90
2	Mild decrease in kidney function	60–89
3	Moderate decrease in kidney function	30–59
4	Severe decrease in kidney function	15–29
5	Kidney failure; requiring dialysis or transplantation	Less than 15

*GFR is the estimated glomerular filtration rate and is a test used to determine how well the kidneys are working with 100 mL/min being a normal reading and less than 15 mL/min indicating end stage renal disease requiring dialysis.

conditions including diabetes mellitus, congestive heart failure and malignancy. It is not surprising then that CKD patients have a shortened life expectancy and carry a high symptom burden (Cohen et al. 2006). Involvement of palliative care teams in patients with renal failure has increased over the last decade as it becomes clearer that this group of patients have specific health care needs especially towards the end of life (Rich et al. 2001).

Chronic kidney disease is characterised by gradual and usually permanent loss of kidney function over a variable period of time, usually months to years. Five stages are recognised, increasing in severity from Stage 1 to Stage 5 (Table 12.1). Stage 5 CKD is also referred to as end stage renal disease (ESRD), where there is total or near-total loss of kidney function and patients need dialysis or transplantation to stay alive.

Which renal patients need palliative care?

Patients with Stage 5 CKD need to be considered for palliative and supportive care input and include those who:

- make a personal decision not to embark on renal replacement therapy (RRT).
- are advised against embarking on RRT because the burden of frequent dialysis may outweigh likely survival and quality of life benefits. This is an extremely complex and difficult decision and is likely to apply more often to those with poorer prognoses (Murtagh 2007).
- after receiving dialysis decide that they would like to withdraw from treatment. These patients often require additional support as the decision to withdraw is being made, because again it is a complex process and can be emotionally fraught. The patient may have received dialysis treatment for some time but experienced an increase in suffering on dialysis and reduced quality of life, and may have taken some time to decide that they would like to discontinue treatment (Ashby et al. 2005).

- are already receiving dialysis but have a poor prognosis, often because of co-morbid conditions such as cardiac disease (Murtagh 2007). The chronicity and co-morbidity associated with ESRD make palliative and supportive care natural accompaniments to its management.

Renal supportive and palliative care services

Renal supportive care services (RSCS) are being developed in response to patients deciding not to commence or to withdraw from dialysis, and the higher profile being afforded to these patients nationally (Chan et al. 2007; Murtagh et al. 2006; Noble et al. 2007). In particular, the *National Service Framework for Renal Services: Part Two* includes a specific section on end of life care and encourages the integration of palliative care and renal skills to provide and develop services (DoH 2005). It is important to recognise that dialysis and renal transplantation are treatments rather than cures for ESRD. Chronic renal dysfunction can therefore be viewed as a progressive and incurable disease, and supportive and palliative care should ideally commence at the time of diagnosis, and increase in importance as time goes on (Chambers et al. 2004). Unfortunately the renal community is some way from reaching this goal and services need to continue developing as they attempt to extrapolate the meaning of renal disease for patients and carers and identify palliative care needs throughout the patient journey, ultimately until death.

In common with other non-cancer conditions, it is important to understand survival and illness trajectories in ESRD and how these differ from cancer. Where possible it is important to estimate the best timing for, and triggers into, palliative care (general, renal and specialist palliative care, as needed) and the resources needed for palliative and end of life provision, and to facilitate advance care planning where possible. Patients may be clear about their preferred place of care (PPC), for example, and may wish to die at home, but if this is not discussed and documented in a timely fashion it may not be possible to abide by the patient's wishes. It is also important to understand other palliative care needs such as symptom burden, psychological issues, social and spiritual needs and even more importantly the interventions which may be most effective (Murtagh 2007). Unfortunately we know little about the needs of this group of patients, especially those opting not to commence dialysis, so further research and development in this area is critical to ensure that services are managed appropriately and in a patient-centred fashion (Noble et al. 2005).

Withdrawing and withholding dialysis

In the early days of dialysis therapy, withdrawal from dialysis was viewed with distaste and regarded as tantamount to suicide. Several authors have debated the issues around young people deciding to withdraw from dialysis, and have drawn the conclusion that to forgo a life-saving treatment such as dialysis is a decision that should be questioned (Moon and Graber 1985; Viederman and Burke 1974). The assumption is that no one who is able to make clear and competent decisions would be likely to take this route.

Although it would appear that during the 1970s and 1980s withdrawal from dialysis was an unusual occurrence, a seminal paper by Neu and Kjellstrand (1986) revealed that withdrawal of dialysis was in fact a common phenomenon in many renal units. Their study in The Regional Kidney Disease Center, the largest centre for long-term dialysis in Minnesota USA, began with 1766 patients who entered a dialysis programme between 1966 and 1983. All patients were observed for a minimum of 1 year or until their death. Dialysis was discontinued in 155 (9%) of the 1766 patients studied and this accounted for 22% of all deaths. Sixty-six patients were competent when the decision to withdraw from dialysis was made and 39% of this group had no new medical complications.

The patients in the study broadly fell into three groups: half of the patients were deemed incompetent (23 were comatose, 37 had advanced dementia and 6 had severe intellectual deficits due to previous strokes) and could not comprehend the benefits, or not, of dialysis. They often experienced considerable side effects. The competent patients fell into the other two groups: those who had no obvious medical complication at the time they made the decision to withdraw from dialysis and those who made the decision following the development of a complication. As the authors state, however, it is difficult to evaluate the role of complications in influencing withdrawal decisions because they are so common in populations on dialysis.

This study was retrospective and relied on gathering data from patients' case notes. Unfortunately it is not apparent why and how patients made the decision to discontinue dialysis treatment (although it is clear that many patients were incompetent and therefore the decision was made for them). Patients who were competent participated in long discussions with the health care team and fully understood that death would result following cessation of dialysis. The competent patients opting to discontinue dialysis appeared to have made deliberate decisions having spent several years on dialysis before treatment was stopped.

Whether or not a patient should be allowed to discontinue life-supporting treatment had been a matter of intense debate for some time, although most major religions were in agreement that if treatment was burdensome a patient might withdraw from it and that such withdrawal was not suicide (Sacred Congregation for the Doctrine of the Faith 1980). Interestingly, Neu and Kjellstrand (1986) affirm that:

'Patients, physicians, and families should . . . be willing to consider discontinuing treatment when its main effects are only discomfort and pain. However such a decision is obviously to be regarded as a deeply regrettable step, taken only as a last resort, at the request of the competent patient or, if the patient is incompetent, at the family's behest. Paradoxically the trend in the United States is to do just the opposite.' (Neu and Kjellstrand 1986, p. 19)

They go on to state, perhaps controversially, that some physicians believe that decisions are not always made in the patient's best interests, and are often subjective depending on culture and personnel perspectives. They imply that some patients are encouraged to dialyse when it may not be to their benefit. As opposing views are heard in relation to the difficult topic of withdrawing and withholding dialysis they make the interesting point:

> 'If these trends continue, they will force patients and their families to fight both for access to, and relief from, the medical system.' (Neu and Kjellstrand 1986, p. 19)

Throughout the 1990s, several published papers addressed the issue of not initiating dialysis (Kilner 1990; Rutecki et al. 1994) and others focused on decision-making, but decision-making by the renal doctor with little reference to the patient (Noble 2007). Other papers originating from the United States offer guidelines to help physicians help their patients make decisions (Galla 2000; Moss et al. 1993; Moss 2001). Again, however, the voice of the patient seems hardly to be heard.

International perspectives

Very little can be found in the literature from countries outside the US and the UK, but two international papers give an indication of the situation regarding dialysis abatement in Italy and Israel. Rombola (2002) makes a very significant point that in Italy every year, 1250 million euros (2% of the total health expenditure) is spent to maintain approximately 41 000 patients on chronic dialysis. He argues that in terms of balanced health policy, no ethical principles can justify the utilisation of such a huge quantity of resources by such a small number of patients. Rombola goes on to say that rules need to be established which ensure that those who receive dialysis are 'able to maintain the essential characteristics of human beings' and that 'doctors cannot presume that the best solution coincides with the extension of patients' life' (p. 33).

A paper by Steinberg (2003) reveals that within the health care system of Israel, there is no clear consensus on practice when caring for the dying patient. His investigation of 'Do not Resuscitate' (DNR) orders in the terminally ill concluded that terminally ill patients never took part in the decision-making process and were never consulted on their wishes. Families were not involved in decision-making and in some cases decisions were made by a single medical professional. Steinberg concluded that:

> 'This approach represents an extreme form of unethical paternalism and it requires an urgent societal intervention to establish an ethically sound decision-making process.' (Steinberg 2003, p. 672)

Since this study, a national committee known as the 'Steinberg Committee' has formulated a legislative proposal which takes into account the issues related to the dying patient and is based on a balance between opposing views such as autonomy, beneficence and non-maleficence. It relates to various treatment modes (including dialysis), establishes a clear position on withdrawing and withholding treatment and validates advanced directives. It also promotes concepts of modern palliative care, something that seems to be missing from the renal arena.

Practice Point 12.1

Working on a general surgical ward you care for a patient undergoing a total hip replacement who is also receiving haemodialysis therapy three times per week. One morning while nursing this patient she tells you that she hates dialysis and wants to stop treatment. She becomes more distressed and tells you that she is constantly in pain, feels sick and tired after every dialysis treatment and feels she is reaching the end of her life. How do you respond to her concerns and who might you contact to ensure she receives appropriate input and support?

Commentary:

It will be important to take this woman's concerns seriously and ensure that she feels comfortable talking her fears through with you. Your listening skills will be of paramount importance and being empathetic to her situation will help her feel safe and cared for. Once she has been given time to discuss her situation, the hospital renal team could be asked to offer psychological support in the form of a renal counsellor or social worker. The next stage may take some time as options are discussed and feelings expressed. However, if this patient does eventually make the decision to withdraw from dialysis she will need to be supported through this, and her preferred priorities of care should be discussed. If she wishes to die at home or in a hospice, and this is possible, arrangements for discharge should be made as a matter of urgency as death may ensue within two weeks or even less. If she decides to die in hospital, she may wish to be transferred to the renal unit if she is already familiar with members of the renal team. If transfer is not possible or appropriate, the renal team should visit her regularly and palliative care input should be sought.

Symptom management

Murtagh et al. (2006) undertook a systematic review of the literature on symptom prevalence in ESRD. As expected many symptoms are similar to those experienced by people receiving dialysis. The symptoms identified are detailed in Table 12.2.

Symptom prevalence was found to be similar to or greater than that of other patient populations (cancer and non-cancer) nearing the end of life. Some symptoms (including pruritus, sleep disturbances and depression) have

Table 12.2 Symptoms identified in Stage 5 CKD.

Symptom	% of patients
Fatigue/tiredness	71
Pruritus	55
Constipation	53
Anorexia	49
Pain	47
Sleep disturbance	44
Anxiety	38
Dyspnoea	35
Nausea	33
Restless legs	30
Depression	27

Adapted from Murtagh et al. (2006).

been well studied in the renal population, but others (principally pain) have been covered only rarely. This may be because pain is not considered problematic for renal patients, or because pain is commonly due to co-morbid conditions rather than the renal disease itself (Davison 2003). Interestingly, all the identified studies are related to patients on or approaching dialysis. Since then, only one paper (Murtagh et al. 2006) has added to the knowledge base by addressing symptoms encountered by those who opt not to embark on dialysis.

It is increasingly being recognised that poor symptom control in the CKD Stage 5 population is at least partly due to a focus on the disease itself, and not the symptoms (Ferro et al. 2004; Murtagh et al. 2006). Symptoms may be related to co-morbid conditions rather than the renal disease, and renal teams may consider these the responsibility of other health professionals. However, as these patients have an eGFR < 15 mL/min, non-renal health professionals may lack both the skills and the confidence to manage their symptoms appropriately. Good symptom control needs to be proactive and include detailed and thorough symptom assessment at regular intervals (Murtagh et al. 2006).

Pain

The causes of pain in a patient with CKD Stage 5 are often due to co-morbid conditions as well as the renal disease itself, and can include ischaemic pain from peripheral vascular disease, neuropathic pain related to diabetes mellitus and bony pain from osteoporosis (Davison 2003; Ferro et al. 2004).

It has been suggested that the World Health Organization (WHO) analgesic ladder approach to managing pain is appropriate for those with CKD Stage 5 (Ferro et al. 2004; Murtagh et al. 2006). Combined with reviews of opioid use in renal failure and expert clinical opinion, Murtagh et al. (2006) use the guidelines summarised in Table 12.3.

Table 12.3 Pain relief in those with CKD Stage 5.

Step 1	Paracetamol 1 g four times daily
Step 2	Tramadol 50–100 mg four times daily (reduce dose depending on creatinine clearance). AVOID codeine, dihydrocodeine and dextropropoxyphene.
Step 3	Moderate pain and outpatient/at home – buprenorphine, oxycodone, hydromorphone or fentanyl. Transfer to fentanyl transdermal patches once the pain is controlled (fentanyl is considered the safest drug to use in CKD Stage 5).
	Severe pain and inpatient – fentanyl (25 μm starting dose) subcutaneously as required, then in a continuous subcutaneous infusion if necessary.

Adapted from Murtagh et al. (2006).

Pruritis (Itch)

Itch is a common problem for those with renal failure but the evidence supporting pharmacological treatments is limited. Management includes:

- Exclusion of other causes of itch including systemic or dermatological causes
- Correction of calcium, phosphate, and parathyroid levels
- Identification of xerosis (dry skin), and if identified the use of liberal emollients
- Use of cetirizine, which is non-sedating, if the itch is widespread
- Use of more sedating antihistamines such as chlorpheniramine if the itch is widespread and poor sleep reported

Other measures to be used with caution include thalidomideamine and ondansetron but as stated, itch is difficult to treat and agreeing a management plan with the patient and a trial of medication to identify benefit may be helpful (Murtagh et al. 2006).

Anaemia

Anaemia develops in the early stages of renal disease and is primarily due to a decrease in the production of erythropoietin by the kidney. Symptoms of anaemia can include weakness, chronic fatigue, breathlessness and a reduction in libido. Recombinant human erythropoietin therapy in the form of an injection for those with CKD can lead to a correction of the anaemia and improved quality of life (Shirani and Finkelstein 2004). Treatment is similar for those on RRT and those who have opted not to commence treatment. It is recommended that all anaemic renal patients who have decided not to embark on dialysis be offered an appropriate dose of erythropoietin therapy to reduce lethargy and fatigue and thereby improve quality of life.

Fluid overload

Patients with ESRD not managed by dialysis will ultimately retain fluid not removed by the kidneys. Diuretics including frusemide (up to 250–500 mg/day

$+/-$ metolazone 2.5 mg daily) can be used. However some patients, especially those not being managed with dialysis, may require hospital admission for intravenous diuretics. Fluid overload becoming more difficult to manage is an indication that the patient is deteriorating, and at this stage the comfort of the patient takes priority.

Nausea, vomiting and anorexia

Nausea and vomiting are common side effects of uraemia, so an increase in these symptoms is likely as kidney function decreases. It is important that antiemetics are prescribed, and these might include levomepromazine (5 mg as required) or haloperidol (0.5–1.5 mg as required).

Nutrition can be problematic for dialysis patients and those who have decided not to have dialysis, and anorexia is common. Sometimes poor nutrition is due to depression or anaemia and both should be treated appropriately. Taste disorders have been reported and zinc deficiency should be considered as a possible cause. A trial of oral zinc (220 mg daily) may be useful (Germain and McCarthy 2004).

Insomnia

Problems of sleep disturbance have been reported in 50–90% of dialysis patients (Germain and McCarthy 2004) and also in patients who opt not to dialyse (although the evidence in this population is limited to one paper by Murtagh et al. 2006). Insomnia can be related to pain and other symptoms but research has also demonstrated a high incidence of specific primary sleep disorders in end stage renal disease (Cohen et al. 2006). Management should begin by examining and instituting appropriate changes in lifestyle including avoiding caffeinated beverages late in the day, cutting out alcoholic beverages in the evening, and refraining from daytime naps (although this last point is very difficult for some patients and may impact on their quality of life).

Hypnotics with a short duration of action may be considered and include zolpidem (5–10 mg) or temazepam (7.5–30 mg) at bedtime (Germain and McCarthy 2004).

Fatigue and lethargy

Renal disease causes lethargy, which can be extremely debilitating and is difficult to manage successfully. Haemoglobin should be maintained between 11 and 12 g/dL (Renal Association 2003). Immobility can lead to further lethargy so activity should be encouraged if possible. Treatment of depression and the encouragement of good nutrition may help (Germain and McCarthy 2004). Simple achievable goals can be identified with the patient which may improve their sense of well-being once accomplished.

Symptom management at the end of life

Many patients will withdraw from dialysis because of the burden of symptoms that they experience, and additional distressing symptoms may appear as the end of life is approached. Fainsinger et al. (2003) found significant symptom distress related to pain, immobility and pruritus in more than a quarter of the 532 patients included in their study. Once withdrawal of dialysis takes place, symptoms related to dialysis procedures will cease but others will remain and those associated with uraemia and fluid overload may well become worse. Although little is known about the symptom prevalence of those who decide not to have dialysis at the end of life, it is assumed that many symptoms may be similar and the author's experience verifies this. To ensure the appropriate treatment of symptoms, anticipatory prescribing is essential.

Pain may not be a feature of dying but is likely to continue in those for whom it is already present and new discomforts can occur from joint and skin pressure due to reduced mobility (Levy et al. 2004). Fear of a painful death is a concern of patients and families and acknowledgement of this is an important part of its management. When the oral route is lost, paracetamol and NSAIDs may be administered rectally. If an alternative route is required, the least painful option is probably to administer analgesia via continuous subcutaneous infusion, following the principles of the WHO analgesic ladder discussed earlier in this section.

Breathlessness is common after dialysis ceases because of fluid retention, symptomatic acidosis and related air hunger. Occasionally the former may be relieved by ultrafiltration (Levy et al. 2004), but this is unusual and commoner management strategies include non-pharmacological methods such as ensuring a comfortable position, fanning with cool air, the use of oxygen and reassurance from staff. A benzodiazepine such as midazolam may contribute to relief of breathlessness, particularly where there is accompanying agitation or distress (Levy et al. 2004).

If nausea and vomiting are present during the terminal phase and the patient is unable to swallow, antiemetics can be administered by continuous subcutaneous infusion. Other symptoms that may arise as the patient becomes more uraemic include thirst, hiccoughs and itching, and each needs to be actively managed. Good mouth care can relieve thirst and patients can suck small pieces of ice as able.

Psychological care

Skilled communication on the part of professionals is required to facilitate a 'not for dialysis' decision if patients are making the decision not to embark on dialysis. Full explanation of possible outcomes, disease progression and prognosis is necessary. The facilitation of future management decisions, in accordance with the patient's information preferences, is of paramount importance.

For those on dialysis a review of dialysis and its impact on the patient should be carried out at appropriate intervals. There is general agreement that dialysis can be withdrawn or withheld for patients with ESRD in the following situations (Cohen and Germain 2005):

- Patients with the ability to make decisions and of sound mind, who being fully informed and making voluntary choices, refuse dialysis or request dialysis be discontinued
- Patients who no longer possess decision-making capacity, who have previously indicated a wish to not receive dialysis in an oral or written advance directive
- Patients who no longer possess decision-making capacity and whose carer refuses dialysis or requests that it be discontinued
- Patients with irreversible, neurological impairment

A time-limited trial of dialysis may be offered if the patient wishes to commence dialysis for a set time period and then review the situation and decide whether it is appropriate to continue. Although this is an option, stopping dialysis is usually a more difficult concept for a patient and their carers than not starting it, and in such circumstances it may be better never to start at all. In reality time-limited trials of dialysis are usually terminated by the onset of a complication or another illness that makes continuing dialysis unachievable (Chesser 2005).

Advance care planning as illness progresses can be a useful tool in dialysis units. A study by Davison and Simpson (2006) highlighted the fact that the discussing of advance care planning was not a major concern to renal dialysis patients, but patients often felt that doctors and nurses experienced in the treatment of ESRD were barriers to hope when they did not discuss end of life issues. Also, despite patient awareness of the inherent uncertainty associated with prognosis, this information was still actively sought and helped patients feel empowered.

Achieving these goals requires a shift from a predominantly disease-focused approach towards more patient-centred management. The renal disease itself, while it cannot be neglected, is often less important than overall quality of life, and the patient themselves should be encouraged to decide what treatment they can or cannot tolerate as the illness progresses.

Social support

There is only one paper which alludes to the impact on families or carers when a patient does not commence dialysis (Ashby et al. 2005) and little is known about the long-term psychological impact of stopping life support treatments on surviving loved ones. Carers of those opting not to dialyse found prognostic uncertainty difficult and felt abandoned as they attempted to manage difficult medication regimes and dietary modifications. They felt that if they made any change to medication or diet they might cause harm to the patient and their misdemeanour would be identified in routine blood tests used to assess renal function and therefore deterioration in health. Little else is known about these carers.

Phillips et al. (2005) sought to determine if there was an increase in pathologic grief in family members after deaths that followed dialysis discontinuation. They carried out telephone interviews to collect data on demographics, attitudes, and families' comfort levels with the decision to withdraw dialysis. It was important to reflect the intensity of any post-traumatic phenomena which resulted from withdrawal of dialysis. There-fore, the Impact of Event Scale (Horowitz et al. 1979), a 15-item ques-tionnaire used to evaluate experiences of avoidance and intrusion, was administered.

Twenty-six family members were interviewed approximately 55 months after patients had died. A low overall level of distress was found and in-trusiveness was highest for spouses and primary caregivers. Only one re-spondent remembered the death as having been 'bad' although 62% of pa-tients were recalled as having suffered distressing symptoms in the last days of life. Almost all of the families reported becoming more comfort-able with the decision to hasten death than originally when the decision had first been made to withdraw dialysis. Clearly there is an urgent need for more research which highlights the impact of withholding or withdraw-ing dialysis on those who are caring for these patients and ultimately left behind.

Practice Point 12.2

A 70-year-old man who has made the decision not to have dialysis is admitted to your ward with a diagnosis of fluid overload and non-specific pain. Discuss the care you would offer this man and options for managing his symptoms.

Commentary:

This man would require a full nursing assessment to determine the severity of his presenting symptoms and to identify other symptoms that might require treat-ment. Fluid overload should be treated with appropriate intravenous diuretics and analgesia should be adequate to relieve pain, following the WHO analgesic ladder. Once his symptoms are under control the patient should be discharged to his preferred place of care if possible, in consultation with his carer/s, ensuring that follow-up is arranged by renal or palliative care teams. This man may well be reaching the end of life and appropriate discussions related to this will be required.

The terminal phase

A patient opting not to dialyse will live for an average of 6.3 months (Smith et al. 2003). In those who withdraw from dialysis the average time to death is 8 days. Research aimed at understanding what constitutes a 'good death' for a renal patient has found that patients and families consider it to be free of pain, peaceful, brief, with loved ones present and where the patient has chosen to die. Moderate satisfaction has been found in relation to the actual death on the part of the relatives but they also report that patients suffer an unacceptable degree of pain and suffering (Cohen and Germain 2004).

Detailed and expert end of life care in the final days or weeks of these patients' lives is essential, which may involve extensive liaison between renal specialists and other care providers in the community, hospices, or hospitals. There are many barriers to good end of life care in this population. It is not unusual to find patients being dialysed till death even though they are not for resuscitation and families are aware they are very sick, but a discussion concerning their actual death has not taken place (Noble and Rees 2006). This may be due to poor communication between professionals and patients and their families and a fear that talking about dying will upset those it affects.

A good death for someone with ESRD is similar to that for someone dying with another disease and includes the maintenance of dignity, choice over where death occurs, easy access to palliative care, a brief death, time to say goodbye and bereavement services for those left behind (Germain et al. 2007). Symptoms in these patients at the end of life can include retained secretions, shortness of breath, agitation, nausea and vomiting, pain, pruritus and thirst. Each symptom can be managed, whether in a hospital ward, a hospice, a nursing home or the community using a multidisciplinary approach. Individualised care is essential as each patient will have his or her unique trajectory to death with its own specific requirements.

Summary

There continues to be growing recognition within the nephrology and palliative care communities that many patients with ESRD have unmet palliative care needs, especially as this population ages and many present with numerous co-morbid conditions. Fortunately this is starting to be recognised with the recent publication of the textbook *Supportive Care for the Renal Patient* (Chambers et al. 2004), the *National Service Framework for Renal Diseases* (DoH 2005) (highlighting the need for appropriate end of life care) and the Royal College of Physicians report on the *Changing Face of Renal Medicine* (The Royal College of Physicians 2007). Unfortunately, reference to renal supportive and palliative care in these last two documents is very brief and offers little in the way of evidence to improve practice. More helpfully, a renal version of the Liverpool Care Pathway, an integrated care pathway to be used with those dying of renal failure in primary and secondary care setting, has recently been developed (Douglas et al. 2007; Marie Curie Palliative Care Institute 2008). It would appear that clinical and research practice in this area is improving (Murtagh 2007) and it is hoped that resources and evidence will continue to swiftly evolve.

References

Ashby M, op't Hoog C, Kellehear A, Kerr PG, Brooks D, Nicholls K and Forrest M (2005) Renal dialysis abatement: lessons from a social study. *Palliative Medicine.* 19(5):389–396.

Chambers EJ, Germain MJ and Brown E (Eds) (2004) *Supportive Care for the Renal Patient.* Oxford: Oxford University Press.

Chan CH, Noble H, Lo SH, Kwan TH, Lee SL and Sze WK (2007) Palliative care for patients with end-stage renal disease: experiences from Hong Kong. *International Journal of Palliative Nursing.* 13(7):310–314.

Chesser A (2005) Palliative care in advanced renal disease. In: Faull C, Carter Y and Daniels L (Eds), *Handbook of Palliative Care* (2nd edition). Oxford: Blackwell Publishing.

Cohen LM and Germain MJ (2004) Measuring quality of dying in end-stage renal disease. *Seminars in Dialysis.* 17(5):376–379.

Cohen LM and Germain MJ (2005) The psychiatric landscape of withdrawal. *Seminars in Dialysis.* 18(2):147–153.

Cohen LM, Moss AH, Weisbord SD and Germain MJ (2006) Renal palliative care. *Journal of Palliative Medicine.* 9(4):977–992.

Davison SN (2003) Pain in hemodialysis patients: prevalence, cause, severity, and management. *American Journal of Kidney Diseases.* 42(6):1239–1247.

Davison SN and Simpson C (2006) Hope and advance care planning in patients with end stage renal disease: qualitative interview study. *British Medical Journal.* 333(7574):886.

DoH (2005) *National Service Framework for Renal Services: Part Two.* London: The Stationery Office.

Douglas C, Murtagh F and Ellershaw J (2007) Symptom control for the patient dying with ESRD – development of evidence based guidelines based on the LCP. Abstract accepted at the 10th EAPC Conference, 2007. Available at http://www.eapcnet.org/budapest2007/pdf/thursday_poster.pdf. Accessed on 22 November 2008.

Fainsinger RL, Davison SN and Brennis C (2003) A supportive care model for dialysis patients. *Palliative Medicine.* 17(1):81–82.

Ferro CJ, Chambers J and Davison SN (2004) Management of pain in renal failure. In: Chambers EJ, Germain M and Brown E (Eds), *Supportive Care for the Renal Patient.* Oxford: Oxford University Press.

Galla J (2000) Clinical practice guideline on shared decision-making in the appropriate initiation of and withdrawal from dialysis. *Journal of the American Society of Nephrology.* 11(7):1340–1342.

Germain M and McCarthy S (2004) Symptoms of renal disease: dialysis-related problems. In: Chambers EJ, Germain M and Brown E (Eds), *Supportive Care for the Renal Patient.* Oxford: Oxford University Press.

Germain MJ, Cohen LM and Davison SN (2007) Withholding and withdrawal from dialysis: what we know about how our patients die. *Seminars in Dialysis.* 20(3):195–199.

Horowitz M, Wilner N and Alvarez W (1979) Impact of event scale: a measure of subjective stress. *Psychosomatic Medicine.* 41(3):209–218.

International Society of Nephrology and International Federation of Kidney Foundations (2007) World Kidney Day. Available at http://www.worldkidneyday.org/pages/why.php. Accessed on 22 November 2008.

Kilner JF (1990) Ethical issues in the initiation and termination of treatment. *American Journal of Kidney Diseases*. 15(3):218–227.

Levy JB, Chambers EJ and Brown EA (2004) Supportive care for the renal patient. *Nephrology Dialysis and Transplantation*. 19(6):1357–1360.

Marie Curie Palliative Care Institute (2008) Guidelines for LCP drug prescribing in advanced chronic kidney disease. Liverpool: Marie Curie Palliative Care Institute. Available at http://www.dh.gov.uk/en/Publicationsandstatistics/Publications/PublicationsPolicyAndGuidance/DH_085320?IdcService=GET_FILE&dID=166616&Rendition=Web. Accessed on 22 November 2008.

Moon JB and Graber GC (1985) When Danny said no! Refusal of treatment by a patient of questionable competence. *Journal of Medical Humanities and Bioethics*. 6(1):12–27.

Moss AH (2001) Recommendations regarding conflict resolution and forgoing dialysis in special patient populations. *Nephrology News and Issues*. 15(13):51–54.

Moss AH, Rettig RA and Cassel CK (1993) A proposal for guidelines for patient acceptance to and withdrawal from dialysis: a follow-up to the IOM report. *Anna Journal*. 20(5):557–561.

Murtagh F (2007) Introduction to end-stage renal disease in palliative and supportive care. NHS National Library for Health. Available at http://www.library.nhs.uk/palliative/ViewResource.aspx?resID=267423&tabID=290. Accessed on 22 November 2008.

Murtagh FE, Addington-Hall JM, Donohue P and Higginson IJ (2006) Symptom management in patients with established renal failure managed without dialysis. *European Dialysis and Transplant Nurses Association/European Renal Care Association Journal*. 32(2):93–98.

Murtagh FEM, Murphy E, Shepherd KA, Donohoe P and Edmonds PM (2006) End-of-life care in end-stage renal disease: renal and palliative care collaboration. *British Journal of Nursing*. 15(1):8–11.

Neu S and Kjellstrand CM (1986) Stopping long-term dialysis. An empirical study of withdrawal of life-supporting treatment. *New England Journal of Medicine*. 314(1):14–20.

Noble H (2007) Dialysis decision-making and advance planning – an evidence guide for palliative professionals. NHS National Library for Health. Available at http://www.library.nhs.uk/palliative/ViewResource.aspx?resID=271069&tabID=289. Accessed on 22 November 2008.

Noble H, Chesser A and Go J (2007) Developing a Renal Supportive Care Service for patients opting not to dialyse. *End of Life Journal*. 1(3):51–55.

Noble H, Chesser A and Kelly D (2005) The cessation of dialysis in patients with end-stage renal disease: developing an appropriate evidence base for practice. *European Dialysis and Transplant Nurses Association/European Renal Care Association Journal*. 31(4):208–211.

Noble H and Rees K (2006) Caring for people who are dying on renal wards: a retrospective study. *European Dialysis and Transplant Nurses Association/European Renal Care Association Journal*. 32(2):89–92.

Phillips JM, Brennan M, Schwartz CE, and Cohen LM (2005) The long-term impact of dialysis discontinuation on families. *Journal of Palliative Medicine*. 8(1):79–85.

Renal Association (2003) *Treatment of Patients with Renal Failure: Recommended Standards and Audit Measures*. London: Renal Association and Royal College of Physicians.

Rich A, Ellershaw J and Ahmad R (2001) Palliative care involvement in patients stopping haemodialysis. *Palliative Medicine*. 15(6):513–514.

Rombola G (2002) Dialysis for everybody? At any cost? *Journal of Nephrology*. 15(6):S33–S42.

Rutecki GW, Rodriguez L, Cugino A, Jarjoura D, Hastings F and Whittier FC (1994) End of life issues in ESRD. A study of three decision variables that affect patient attitudes. *American Society of Artificial Internal Organs Journal*. 40(3):M798–M802.

Sacred Congregation for the Doctrine of the Faith (1980) Declaration on Euthanasia. *Canadian Conference of Catholic Bishops*. Ottawa: Publications Service.

Shirani S and Finkelstein F (2004) Sexual dysfunction in patients with chronic kidney disease. In: Chambers EJ, Germain M and Brown E (Eds), *Supportive Care for the Renal Patient*. Oxford: Oxford University Press.

Smith C, Da Silva-Gane M, Chandna S, Warwicker P, Greenwood R and Farrington K (2003) Choosing not to dialyse: evaluation of planned non-dialytic management in a cohort of patients with end-stage renal failure. *Nephron Clinical Practice*. 95(2):c40–c46.

Steinberg A (2003) End-of-life decision making process. *Harefuah*. 142(10):672–673.

The Royal College of Physicians (2007) The changing face of renal medicine in the UK: the future of the speciality. *Report of a Working Party 2007*. London: RCP.

Viederman M and Burke D (1974) Case studies in bioethics. Saying 'no' to haemodialysis. Should a minor's decision be respected? *Hastings Center Report*. 4(4):8–10.

Chapter 13

Palliative care issues for people with cancer

Susan Jackson

Introduction

This chapter has a dual focus. It begins by discussing the diversity of cancer as a disease and highlights some of the common difficulties patients with cancer may experience during their illness trajectory. It then explores some of the professional challenges that nurses can face while trying to deliver holistic care to this often vulnerable group of patients.

Learning outcomes

Once you have read the chapter and completed the associated activities, you will be able to:

- Gain a greater understanding of the diversity of cancer as a disease
- Appreciate how palliative care can contribute to care at different points of the patient's illness trajectory
- Explore the challenges of providing palliative and end of life care for patients with certain site-specific cancers

Cancer – an illness of many

Despite the changing focus over the past few years towards non-malignant illnesses, cancer remains at the heart of palliative care. It is a diverse illness in both number and type and poses many professional challenges on a daily basis for nurses and other health care professionals. Treatments for cancer can vary from aggressive and curative with a very positive prognosis for patients, to palliative and supportive with a very guarded outlook for others. This can often make it difficult to determine when and how to implement palliative care to different groups of patients.

It is estimated that there are over 200 different types of cancer with approximately 300 000 people being diagnosed with the illness in the UK on a yearly basis (Cancer Research UK 2008a). Of the 200 types, breast, lung, large bowel and prostate remain the most common, accounting for over half of all new cases of cancer. These statistics support the belief that by the age of 74 one in three people in the UK will develop some form of the disease (Cancer Research UK 2008a). This represents a commonality with the global picture where there are an estimated 10 million new cases of cancer diagnosed annually in people throughout the world (Parkin et al. 2001). The incidence of cancer has risen by 22% in the last 15–20 years and according to the World Cancer Report this could rise further to affect up to 15 million people by the year 2020. On a more positive note, however, there is strong support that with government-led health promotion, early detection and screening strategies it is suggested that this alarming number could be decreased by one third (Stewart and Kleihues 2003). Mortality statistics show that approximately 25% of all deaths within the UK and Europe are caused by cancer and 12% on a global level (Cancer Research UK 2005; Parkin et al. 2001). Considering these stark statistics it is not surprising that many people are adversely affected by the disease and its associated treatments.

Palliative and end of life care is an integral part of the care given to people with advanced cancer; however, improved treatments and survival for many cancers means that palliative care can also be of great benefit to people at other junctions of their cancer journey. Many women with metastatic breast cancer can now be expected to live for several years due to improved local and systemic treatments (Peto et al. 2000) and are a prime example of a cohort of patients who can gain from the inter-professional partnership of palliative care and oncology teams working together. A relatively high number of people with a diagnosis of Hodgkin's disease or non-Hodgkin's lymphoma can also expect to live for many years and can in fact be cured (Bowles and Marcus 2003). Nevertheless there can be times during the treatment phase where their general well-being and quality of life will be severely affected but their care can be positively influenced by good palliative care practices. At the other end of the spectrum, survival rates for lung cancer have changed little over the past 25 years (Gregor and Milroy 2001), with less than 10% of patients being alive 5 years after diagnosis (National Institute Clinical Excellence (NICE) 2005; Scottish Intercollegiate Guidelines Network (SIGN) 2005a). One Scottish analysis claimed that 50% of patients would be dead within four months of their initial diagnosis of lung cancer (Scottish Executive Health Department 2001) which underlines the necessity to have palliative care as an integral part of the care package for this group of people.

The above points emphasise the diversity of cancer as a disease and highlight some of the challenges that health care practitioners face in the delivery of effective palliative care to a large number of people with different needs.

Cancer as a chronic disease

A chronic illness is one which is of longstanding duration that is managed rather than cured and often requires patients and their carers to participate in self-management strategies to meet some of their long-term health care needs (Greenstreet 2006). It is also widely recognised that a chronic illness can adversely affect a person's quality of life and have a negative impact on their sense of identity and control. One of the fundamental principles of palliative care is to consider the person as a whole, taking cognisance of their physical, psychological and spiritual needs, a principle which is mirrored in the management of chronic illnesses where the emotional dimensions of the disease are recognised and addressed while working in partnership with the patient and their carer throughout the duration of the disease (Davis et al. 2000). Cancer is increasingly being categorised as a chronic illness and indeed the above points could easily be related to a great number of people who are living with cancer. A recent study in Australia examining the concerns of women with breast cancer described how a small number of women felt they were often faced by a pessimistic outlook from others regarding their future. This was deemed to be an unhelpful approach and they preferred to think more positively, considering themselves to be living with a chronic illness as opposed to dying of breast cancer (Oxlad et al. 2008). The enormous task of ensuring an equitable palliative care service to patients with life-limiting illnesses other than cancer has been embraced by health and social care providers throughout the UK in recent years; however, it is also vital to explore the challenges the diversity and distinctiveness of cancer poses for palliative care providers. Thinking of cancer as a chronic illness, as well as an acute illness which many people die from, may contribute to this concept.

Practice Point 13.1

Categorising cancer as a chronic illness may encourage health care professionals to think about different aspects and approaches to care; however, what do you think may be the difficulties associated with this point of view? It may be helpful to consider:

The diversity of cancer as an illness
The involvement of the patient and the carers in the management of their illness
The general negative perceptions of a diagnosis of cancer

Commentary:

One of the major differences between cancer and other chronic illnesses is the fact that there are over 200 types which are categorised as one illness. Within this collective identity lie very distinctive incidence, mortality, individual treatment plans and clinical outcomes (Tritter and Calnan 2002). This can be demonstrated by considering a person with a diagnosis of pancreatic cancer compared to a child with an acute leukaemia. Although individually distinctive illnesses, with very different expected outcomes, they are both nevertheless categorised as cancer. This alone highlights one of the main difficulties of classifying cancer as a chronic illness.

Chronically ill people have long-term health problems and very often a definitive diagnosis is made after a period of time. During this time they have had to deal with a succession of losses; however it could be argued that they have also had the opportunity and time to come to terms with their illness and revise or adapt their lifestyles to compensate (Greenstreet 2006). Many chronic illnesses are capable of being managed by the person themselves in the course of everyday life; therefore, much of the care provided is through monitoring and advice. Although this could also be true for some people with cancer, the acuteness of a diagnosis of cancer, the complexity of subsequent multidisciplinary treatments and ensuing uncertainty make it difficult for the person in this situation to be fully involved in the self-management of their illness (Tritter and Calnan 2002).

A final issue to discuss when considering cancer as a chronic illness is the general public's negative perceptions surrounding the illness. It is an illness believed to be associated with suffering and death and can lead to social isolation and difficulties with family communication. This perception could be closely linked to the fear often displayed by patients and their carers when the concept of palliative care or hospice support is raised.

Palliative care for specific cancers

This section examines the contribution palliative care can make along the cancer trajectory and explores some issues relating to a selection of specific tumour sites. It is outwith the scope of the chapter to discuss in depth all the problems that patients may face; however, a range of both challenging and common situations will be discussed to demonstrate the diversity of palliative care needs of people with cancer.

Advanced breast cancer – an overview

Breast cancer is the most common cancer within the UK and Europe and its incidence has increased by over 50% in the last 20 years (Cancer Research UK 2008b). Despite this, more women are surviving longer than before, with eight out of ten expected to live for greater than 5 years. Nevertheless approximately 10% of women with breast cancer will present with advanced disease which has implications for them in terms of long-term survival and symptom burden. On a more positive note, due to advances in management and treatment, many women in this category are also leading relatively active lives with supportive and palliative care enabling them to live with a chronic illness. It should also be remembered however that a number of women will experience significant physical and psychological symptoms which have a profound effect on their quality of life; therefore, it would be wrong to think that all women with advanced breast cancer live well with a chronic illness.

Whether at initial presentation or recurrence at a later date, metastatic breast cancer is incurable and it has been suggested that a recognised aim of treatment at this stage is to keep the patient as well as possible for as long as possible

(Iddawela et al. 2006). By using this statement as the benchmark for treatment of advanced disease, the focus of care remains on the well-being of the patient and should always take the impact of any treatments on quality of life into consideration. One of the biggest challenges for nurses and health care professionals caring for this group of patients is appreciating the need for 'active' palliative care. To achieve stabilisation of advanced breast cancer, a combination of treatments are employed either singularly or in combination to achieve the best possible outcome. These commonly include endocrine therapy, chemotherapy and targeted therapy (Herceptin), bisphosphonates and, less commonly, surgery (British Association Surgical Oncology 2005; Harmer 2005; SIGN 2005b). This approach to care requires input from oncology, palliative and primary care professionals and its success depends on effective inter-departmental and inter-professional communication and cross-boundary working.

Common symptoms

Effective symptom control is a key component of effective palliative care and is one of the cornerstones of improving quality of life for patients with advanced breast cancer; it is therefore important to discuss the impact and management of common symptoms.

Pain

It has been estimated that approximately 70% of women with metastatic breast cancer will suffer pain originating from multiple sites and causes (Rosenfield and Stahl 2006); however the vast majority of pain is caused by bone metastases. Direct involvement of adjacent structures by either the primary or metastatic lesion can also be the cause of pain, for instance if the tumour becomes fixed to the underlying muscle in the chest wall or with further progression causes rib erosion (Bentley and Fallon 2006). In addition malignant infiltration of the skin, fungating lesions, lymphoedema and neuropathic pain are also all sources of pain for patients with locally advanced breast cancer.

The concept of 'total pain' as described in 1978 by Cecily Saunders is particularly relevant to women with advanced breast cancer. Many patients associate their pain with tumour progression and advancing disease, and hence experience high levels of fear, hopelessness and distress, all of which can exacerbate their levels of pain (Breitbart et al. 2004). Due to the complexity of pain, it should be managed by a multi-professional team including nurses, oncologists, surgeons, physiotherapists and palliative care specialists and assessment must consider any contributing physical, social, psychological and spiritual factors. Due to the often knowing and therapeutic relationships nurses build with women in this situation they are in a prime position to play a key role in the assessment of pain; therefore they should be confident in asking the 'right' questions. According to the SIGN Guidelines (2008) a comprehensive review of pain should include the following points:

- Site and number of pains
- Intensity/severity of pains

- Any radiation?
- Timing
- Quality – i.e. nagging, burning, sharp
- Does anything aggravate it or relieve it?
- Type
- Pain relief history
- Impact of daily living activities

It is also recommended by SIGN (2008) that a simple formal assessment tool should be used to assess and monitor pain. There are various scales available, ranging from basic descriptions of the pain to visual analogue scales and their use will differ in different clinical areas; however, it is now recognised best practice in all palliative and oncology care settings to utilise a validated pain assessment chart for patients who are being treated for cancer-related pain (NHS Quality Improvement Scotland 2004; SIGN 2008).

Practice Point 13.2

What pain assessment tool is utilised to assess and monitor cancer-related pain within your own area of practice? Consider how its use contributes to the effective management of the patient's pain?

Commentary:

Following effective assessment, decisions have to be made as to the best management plan to relieve the pain. This is where the multi-dimensional approach is essential as depending on the cause of the pain the woman may benefit from a primary therapy such as chemotherapy, radiotherapy or a course of antibiotics; nevertheless in almost all cases, it will be necessary to prescribe analgesia in addition to these primary treatments. The World Health Organization (WHO) recommends the use of a three-step pain ladder to effectively manage cancer-related pain using a combination of opioid, non-opioid and adjuvant analgesia (World Health Organization 1996) and best practice guidelines within palliative and cancer care use this as the basis for recommended practice (Quality Improvement Scotland 2004; SIGN 2008). A diagram of the WHO three-step pain ladder can be seen in Chapter 8 (heart failure).

It should be remembered that this analgesic matrix acts as a baseline for cancer pain management and other drugs and approaches will be used to complement this depending on the source and type of pain present. The use of ongoing pain assessment is particularly useful in determining the adequacy of the prescribed analgesia and will guide the health care professional to consider the need to change or add drugs to the regime.

Antidepressants, anticonvulsants and corticosteroids have all been shown to be useful as adjuvants to analgesics in the management of neuropathic pain in patients with advanced breast cancer, for example brachial plexopathy (Bentley and Fallon 2006).

There is some evidence to suggest that the use of topical opioids applied to malignant ulcerating lesions can help relieve localised pain (Flock 2003); however, there is only anecdotal evidence to support their use in the management of fungating breast lesions. Nevertheless their use is advocated by many palliative care specialists on a named patient basis (Grocott 2007).

Specially trained physiotherapists and some clinical nurse specialists play a pivotal role in the effective management of lymphoedema for women with advanced breast cancer and contribute greatly to effective pain management. Many women may also find relaxation, distraction techniques and some complementary therapies useful. The presence and effect of a therapeutic relationship between the nurse or physiotherapist and the patient cannot be underestimated in the management of lymphoedema-related pain.

Using a pain assessment tool and involving the woman in the monitoring of her pain can not only be used as an indicator of progress towards a pain-free (or less pain) experience, but can also offer the patient a degree of control and decision-making in her own treatment and care.

Fatigue

Cancer-related fatigue is a complex symptom with social, psychological and physical components, and women with advanced breast cancer are commonly beset by the problem. It has been found to be a major obstacle to normal functioning and has a negative effect on a patient's quality of life (De Santo-Madeya et al. 2007; Gualandi et al. 2003). Like pain, it is a subjective and individual experience and effective management is based on careful evaluation of the severity of the symptom and the effects the fatigue is having on the woman's quality of life. As stated earlier in the chapter many women with metastatic breast cancer can live full and active lives; however the overwhelming exhaustion which occurs after even the most simple of tasks can have a profound effect on many others.

According to Sweeney (2006), the underlying principles of effective management of cancer-related fatigue can be based on the answers gained from answering the following questions:

- Are there any underlying causes of fatigue? (reversible and non reversible)
  - Anaemia
  - Underlying infection
  - Anxiety and/or depression
  - Pain
  - Dehydration
  - Opiod toxicity
  - Anorexia/cachexia
- To what extent is the fatigue affecting the patient's life?
- Are there any therapeutic measures available with a reasonable cost/benefit ratio?

Implementing a robust multi-dimensional approach using both pharmacological and non-pharmacological interventions can have a positive effect on the quality of life of a woman with advanced breast cancer; therefore it is imperative that nurses and health care professionals appreciate the significance of cancer-related fatigue on women at this stage of their illness.

Skeletal complications of bone metastases
It is estimated that as many as 75% of women with advanced breast cancer will have bone metastases, and in addition to pain may experience other skeletal complications which can have a major impact on their quality of life (Harvey and Cream 2007). These potential problems add to the challenge for health care professionals to provide a care plan which will offer this group of patients a combination of active and palliative treatments which will enable them to 'live as well as possible for as long as possible'.

Hypercalcaemia is a common metabolic disorder which occurs frequently in patients with advanced breast cancer causing a range of gastrointestinal, renal and neurological disturbances. It is important for nurses to be aware of the symptoms and have knowledge of the recommended forms of treatment. According to Reyna and Bruera (2006) there are four main aims of treatment for malignant hypercalcaemia:

- Correction of dehydration
- Inhibition of bone resorption (bisphosphonates)
- Increasing renal excretion of calcium
- The treatment of the underlying malignancy

Consideration should also be given to the anxiety and fear levels that women may be experiencing, as hypercalcaemia is often associated with disease progression.

Pathological fractures take place spontaneously when the affected bone has been considerably weakened by the metastases. This can happen to patients who have established metastases or it may be the first indication that bone secondaries are present; either way this skeletal complication can be a source of great pain and distress and will again require multi-professional management to achieve the best outcome for the patient.

Spinal cord compression is classified as a palliative care or oncological emergency and is yet another complication which can affect women with advanced breast cancer, occurring when a metastatic tumour either encroaches on the epidural space or causes vertebral collapse, propelling pieces of bone into the dura (Bucholtz 1999). It is imperative that this condition is detected at an early stage, before any neurological impairment takes place to prevent major complications such as paraplegia. If paralysis occurs this can have a devastating effect on the patient's quality of life and is closely linked to high levels of distress and anxiety. Nurses have a dual responsibility: to have the ability to identify at-risk patients and be aware of the early signs of spinal cord compression and also to ensure honest, effective communication and support for both the patient and the family during what can be an extremely distressing event (Drudge-Coates and Rajbubu 2008a).

The main clinical signs of spinal cord compression include severe pain, sensory impairment, motor weakness and autonomic dysfunction, affecting bladder and bowel function and mobility and feeling of the lower extremities (Drudge-Coates and Rajbubu 2008b). As previously emphasised, early diagnosis is vital and should be confirmed by the 'gold standard' diagnostic tool of a Magnetic Resonance Imaging (MRI) scan. Subsequent management will be multi-dimensional and may include combinations of steroid therapy, radiotherapy, chemotherapy, pain control, bisphosphonates and possibly decompression surgery (Reyna and Bruera (2006). Again this treatment plan highlights the active palliative care approach which is necessary for women with advanced disease.

It is outwith the scope of this chapter to provide in-depth information regarding spinal cord compression; however readers can access full guidelines written by the West of Scotland Cancer Managed Clinical Network (WoSCAN 2006) which present an excellent overview of early detection, diagnosis and management of malignant spinal cord compression.

Psychosocial support and communication issues

Women with advanced breast cancer are known to be at high risk of psychological morbidity and the multitude of physical symptoms, the uncertain future, loss of control and negative body image perception all contribute. The incidence of clinically significant anxiety or depression has been quoted as being as high as 25% in women with advanced breast cancer (Grunfield 2006); it is therefore essential that women have access to appropriately trained health care professionals in order to address their psychological needs at all points of their cancer journey (NICE 2004). Psycho-social support and open and honest communication are central to good palliative care and should be integrated into the treatment plan for this group of women which will allow them to be as involved as they can be in decisions regarding their treatment and care. Doing so can facilitate a return of some control, feelings of empowerment and reclaimed independence.

Summary

Advanced breast cancer is a highly complex disease which for many will be regarded as a chronic illness with long-term health effects but for countless others will be a terminal illness with multiple distressing and emotional issues. The challenge for nurses and other health care professionals is to provide holistic but sometimes active palliative care to meet the varied physical, social, psychological and spiritual needs of this vulnerable group of women.

Table 13.1 Summary of cellular disruption.

Disease	Mechanism of Cellular Disruption
Leukaemia	**Early** stages of blood cell development within the bone marrow where malignant cells replace what would become erythrocytes, leucocytes and platelets.
Lymphoma	Malignant changes in **mature** blood cells which have moved from the bone marrow into the lymph nodes and other parts of the immune system.
Myeloma	Malignant changes in plasma cells which have returned to the bone marrow in the **final stages** of their life. Excessive numbers of abnormal plasma cells destroy surrounding bone.

Haematological malignancies – an overview

Haematological cancers together represent the fifth most common type of cancer in the UK, accounting for 7% of all cancers, and are divided into three main disease groups of leukaemia, lymphoma and myeloma (NICE 2003). The underlying cause of all three classifications of illnesses is a genetic change in a particular group of blood cells at different stages of maturation. To increase understanding, the mechanisms of cellular disruption for the individual illnesses are summarised in Table 13.1.

Despite the underlying common denominator, haematological malignancies are a diverse group of illnesses which differ in symptoms, illness trajectory and outcomes (Ansell et al. 2007). According to relatively recent statistics, the overall prevalence of haematological cancer would appear to be rising, with the greatest increase in the number of people with non-Hodgkin's lymphoma. Although no seemingly clear reason for this is apparent, some studies suggest it may be partly due to improved diagnostic techniques over the past 20 years (Cartwright et al. 2005).

Integrating two different philosophies of care

Haematology oncology is associated with intensive and longstanding therapy where advances in treatments are common and fast paced – the emphasis is on cure.

Palliative care is associated with quality of life and support – the emphasis is on comfort and end of life care.

Both are very sweeping and general statements but however highlight the different philosophies of care and the challenges of combining both to deliver effective and high-quality care to patients with haematological malignancies. It has been suggested that there is little integration between palliative care and haematology services within the UK; however there would appear to be little evidence to support this train of thought (Ansell et al. 2007). Work has however been carried out in Australia on this topic and it has been found that patients with haematological malignancies do not receive timely and appropriate referrals to specialist palliative care services (McGrath and Holewa 2006; McGrath and Holewa 2007a and b). Despite the limited evidence from the UK, NICE produced guidelines for care for patients within haemato-oncology and recommended that palliative care and haematology services should work closer together to provide a more integrated approach to care (NICE 2003).

One of the main challenges within this speciality is deciding when palliative care should be introduced, and this can unfortunately be a source of conflict between different groups of professionals (Balsdon 2006). Many patients who are diagnosed with a haematological malignancy can be acutely ill and require intensive nursing and medical support over a long period of time. For example a young adult with acute leukaemia will undergo several intensive courses of chemotherapy and may then proceed to either stem cell or bone marrow transplant. During this time he or she will receive care from an established multi-professional haematology team and possibly the support of high-dependency/intensive therapy specialists. Although there will be a number of treatment- and disease-related toxicities and complications for the patient to endure during this treatment phase, the ultimate outcome is often cure. Other situations can include patients who unfortunately reach an end of life situation suddenly and unexpectedly with others living with their illness for many months or years, coping with treatments and regular blood product support. All are complex situations where the need for skilled care interventions and effective, honest communication is essential. Multi-professional haematology teams provide ongoing physical and psychological support during this time and build up extremely good relationships with patients and their families and it could be argued that the palliative care philosophy forms the basis for haematology–oncology practice. Nevertheless a study recently completed in Australia examining a best-practice model for end of life care for patients with haematological malignancies identified certain core elements which were seen to contribute to the difficulties of integrating the two philosophies of palliative care and haemato-oncology, some of which are listed below:

- The 'high tech' and invasive nature of treatments
- The speed of change to a terminal event
- Prolonged treatments
- Close relationships with haematology team
- Clinical optimism
- Patients often show signs of positive recovery close to death
- No clear distinction between curative and palliative phase

McGrath and Holewa (2006)

Nurses working within the haematology–oncology setting will be familiar with many of the above situations which can lead to frustrations if the appropriate model of care is not fully implemented to the benefit of patients and their families.

Practice Point 13.3

You are caring for a young man with acute leukaemia who is undergoing a stem cell transplant. He is experiencing various distressing symptoms, his mood is low and he is anxious about his future. You suggest that someone from the hospital palliative care team may be able to help, but when you suggest this he says:

'I thought palliative care doctors were just for people who are dying?'

Consider how best you can approach this situation to alleviate his fears and facilitate the input of a palliative care specialist.

Commentary:

The above practice point is a typical example of a challenging situation for nurses who care for patients with an acute 'curative' illness. Public and some professional attitudes are still of the opinion that palliative care services are purely for patients who are terminally ill with an often reluctance to involve them in the care of a patient with an acute haematological illness. It would also be fair to suggest that there has been a failure of some within the palliative care profession to recognise the contribution that active treatment and support from the haematology team can make towards symptomatic relief (Boyce et al. 2003). Nevertheless, recent changes in attitudes are seeing more and more palliative care specialists being involved with patients with a haematological cancer from the point of diagnosis, (Booth and Bruera 2003) and doctors and nurses are finding this particularly helpful for patients who are undergoing intensive chemotherapy. This approach mirrors one of the underlying principles of palliative care advocated by the World Health Organization.

'Palliative care is applicable early in the course of the illness, in conjunction with other therapeutics that are intended to prolong life, such as chemotherapy and radiation therapy and includes those investigations needed to better understand and manage distressing clinical complications.'

(Sepulveda et al. 2002)

The multi-professional composition of a clinical team looking after patients with haematological malignancies should increase the likelihood that patients are offered the most appropriate treatment for their condition, utilising a broad range of expert knowledge from the start. As stated earlier, nurses working within haematology–oncology practice invariably build good therapeutic relationships with their patients because of the duration and complexities of treatments. They are therefore in a prime position to introduce the positive aspects of palliative care specialists to their patients, particularly in relation to providing relief for distressing symptoms. Furthermore reassurance and a clear explanation that this speciality does not solely become involved at the end of life are also advantageous. Good inter-disciplinary and inter-departmental working, with all professionals recognising the skills and responsibilities of each other, can also go some way to facilitating joint working, ultimately benefiting the patient. According to Fleissig et al. (2006) all patients with cancer should feel reassured that the specialists involved in their care are working together and will carefully consider treatment options from different perspectives.

Common clinical problems

Patients with haematological malignancies will have physical symptoms as a result of both the underlying disease and the associated treatments, however despite the prevalence and intensity of some of these symptoms there is a paucity of evidence available relating specifically to symptom control within haemato-oncology (Spathis 2003). It is recommended that the basic principles of symptom control which are regularly practiced within palliative care are used to achieve the best outcome for the patient, including assessing the cause of the symptom, being proactive and observing, treating promptly and regularly and most importantly reassessing regularly and repeatedly (Twycross and Wilcock 2003). These used in conjunction with some basic principles of palliative care, which are noted below will give the best chance of successful symptom relief for the patient:

- Consider psychosocial and spiritual factors
- Effective communication
- Multi-professional approach to care
- Attention to detail
- Never say 'there is nothing more to be done'

Twycross and Wilcock (2003)

Consideration has to be given to the need to provide what is considered to be 'active' treatments to provide effective symptom control in this group of patients and indeed in the preface of a book discussing palliative care in haematology patients the editors make the following comment:

'it is now increasingly understood that excellent palliative care may involve treatment with blood and blood products, intravenous drugs and other inter-ventions once thought alien to giving holistic patient centred care.'

Booth and Bruera (2003)

As stated earlier, treatments for leukaemia, lymphoma and myeloma can be complex and protracted; it is therefore essential for all members of the health care team to be aware of how to achieve good symptom control. There is anecdotal evidence to suggest that nurses practicing within acute haemato-oncology units may have a lack of confidence in their knowledge of complex symptom control and do benefit from the knowledge and skills of their spe-cialist palliative care colleagues, and it could be argued that this situation has improved with the increasing presence of hospital palliative care teams. It has also been suggested that nurses working within palliative care units have a lack of confidence in their knowledge and understanding of haematology–oncology practice, one of the reasons being that very few patients with a haematological malignancy are cared for within the hospice or palliative care setting. This situation again highlights the need for cross-boundary and inter-departmental working to achieve the best possible outcome for the patient and their family.

Specific issues at the end of life

The dying phase for many patients with cancer is predictable and is recognised by a gradual decline in function over a period of time (Ellershaw and Ward 2003); however there are some issues with terminal care in haematology which create specific challenges. According to Hicks (2003) patients with haematological cancers fall into two broad categories at the end of life: those who die during the phase of active treatment and those who die from advanced progressive disease. Those who die during the active phase of their treatment, may do so unexpectedly or suddenly as a result of treatment-related toxicities, haemorrhage, infection or treatment failure. This can cause major emotional upset for all involved as there has been no gradual deterioration and therefore no time to come to terms with the gravity of the situation. The focus of care can change very quickly and unexpectedly from cure to end of life.

Although patients within the other category may show signs of gradual deterioration and disease progression, they may still be undergoing active interventions such as blood product support and chemotherapy for symptom control and it can be difficult for the patient and the family to understand that the focus of care has changed. It has been suggested that nurses within haematology recognise when their patients reach the dying phase before their medical colleagues, leading to conflict within the team and sometimes ethical and moral dilemmas for the staff (McGrath 2001). Recognising the dying phase has been described as an important clinical skill that requires experience and although difficult and finely balanced with this population of patients it can be achieved (Ellershaw and Ward 2003; Hicks 2003). Open, honest and sensitive communication with the patient and the family is key to achieving this outcome, as is effective communication between members of the multi-professional team. Acknowledging when possible that the patient has reached or may reach the dying phase reduces the risk that the family will face regret and unresolved issues after death.

Due to the prolonged treatments and active support haematology patients receive from the hospital-based haematology teams during their illness they can lose contact with their primary care teams and community palliative care services which can have ramifications for end of life care at home. This had been identified by nursing staff within a haematology day unit in England where a project was undertaken to try to resolve some of the problems this situation posed for the patient and the health care professionals (Boyce et al.

2003). It had been recognised that because of frequent visits to the day unit for treatments it was difficult for the patients to access their local Macmillan Clinical Nurse Specialists and other members of the local palliative care team; consequently some symptom control issues were being left unaddressed and psychosocial support was deemed inadequate. By working closely together, the community palliative care team and the nursing staff from the haematology day unit produced a model of care to address these concerns, resulting in a much improved palliative care service for a group of patients with haematological malignancies who prior to this readjustment of care would not have had access to this support (Boyce et al. 2003). This is a good example of how palliative care and haematology can successfully integrate for the benefit of the patient.

The majority of patients with haematological malignancies will die within an acute setting rather than at home or in a hospice; however this does not mean that good end of life care cannot take place. Many clinical areas have implemented the Liverpool Care Pathway (LCP) (Ellershaw 2007) as a tool to help them achieve good end of life care for their patients and despite the specific challenges within haematology–oncology there is anecdotal evidence to suggest that the LCP can help facilitate good end of life care within haematology and bone marrow transplant units. Ellershaw (2007) in fact stated that the LCP is a powerful lever for all clinical settings to reach one of the goals declared within the National Cancer Plan (DoH 2000) which was to improve the care of the dying to the level of the best.

Summary

Patients with haematological malignancies have a profound hope for cure and they show an incredible ability to endure the intensive and prolonged treatments that are the 'gold standard' of care within this speciality. Even when their illness shows signs of relapse or progression few patients show resistance to continuing medical interventions. It is therefore imperative that multi-disciplinary teams from both specialities of haematology and palliative care continue to work together to maintain the fast-paced advances in treatment and the provision of holistic care for this group of patients. It may be that the underlying philosophies of both specialities are not as dissimilar as was once thought.

Lung cancer

The statistics regarding lung cancer which were discussed earlier in the chapter emphasise the prevalence of this illness and make it one of the most common cancers that nurses and health care professionals will encounter in clinical practice. Approximately 85% of patients will be diagnosed with either locally advanced or metastatic disease and the general prognosis for patients is poor (Corner et al. 2005). The World Health Organization suggests that palliative care is the total care of the patient whose illness is not responsive to treatment

(Sepulveda et al. 2002) and this philosophy is a particularly predominant feature of treatment for patients with lung cancer. It could be argued that despite the widespread recognition in clinical practice that palliative care is an integral part of lung cancer treatment, specific difficulties remain for patients.

A heavy symptomatic burden can be experienced with dyspnoea and fatigue commonly featuring as major contributors to impaired quality of life. Quality of life has been defined as a sense of well-being concerning physical, psychological social and spiritual dimensions (Ferrell 1996). There are evidence-based strategies and guidelines used widely within palliative and lung cancer care to help patients cope with the distress these symptoms cause, for example nursing- or physiotherapist-led interventions using a combination of specific breathing techniques, relaxation therapy and psychosocial support (Connors et al. 2007; Hately et al. 2003). There is a great deal of fear and anxiety related to both symptoms and experience by patients and carers alike; hence a major component of treatment is the provision of openness, honesty and continuity of care, all of which will contribute enormously to the quality of life for this population.

As well as the physical issues, patients with lung cancer also experience high levels of anxiety and depression (Lloyd-Williams et al. 2004) and often feel socially isolated. It has been suggested that this may be related to the negative public perception of lung cancer, where people are thought in some way to be to blame for their own illness due to the link with tobacco and smoking. This can cause many patients to have feelings of guilt, shame and low self-esteem and some may feel they have no right to look for extra support and help (Chapple 2004). These factors can result in the social withdrawal of the person from many of their everyday activities which can further affect quality of life.

An interesting but harsh fact was listed recently by the editor of a lung cancer journal which summarised the negativity and poor perception of lung cancer when he stated:

'In the United Kingdom there is one charity solely committed to lung cancer – The Roy Castle Foundation. There are over 200 charities devoted to breast cancer. More women die from lung cancer than breast cancer.'

Peake (2007)

Nurses have the responsibility of reassuring patients and their carers that although smoking may have contributed to their illness this should not affect the care they justly deserve to receive.

Many patients with lung cancer will reach the terminal stages of their illness relatively soon after diagnosis and although it may be clinically easier to identify when patients reach this stage than in some other forms of cancer, it remains a challenge to provide good end of life care. As stated earlier in the chapter, the knowledge to effectively diagnose dying and the use of the LCP can have a major impact on the delivery of care at this stage of the illness (Ellershaw and Ward 2003), and as well as improving the quality of care for the patient and the family it can lead to greater job satisfaction for the health care team.

Dealing with patients and families affected by lung cancer includes specific physical, psychological, social and spiritual aspects of concern relating to negative public perception, poor prognosis and heavy symptom burden. This section has provided a very brief overview of the difficulties faced by patients and the real challenge is to confront the issues and ensure that everyone affected by this disease has access to good palliative care.

Conclusion

This chapter has discussed the diversity of cancer as a disease and has used three very different site specific groups of cancers to demonstrate the complexities and challenges that are facing health care professionals in the delivery of effective palliative care. It has been outwith the scope of the chapter to discuss individual physical and psychological issues in any depth, and it is suggested that readers should find such information within sources recommended in the further reading section.

The underlying principle of palliative care is to improve the quality of life for patients and this closely matches the underlying philosophy of nursing where people are treated individually with dignity and respect and with a high standard of care (Nursing and Midwifery Council 2008). By considering some of the issues raised in the chapter, nurses should be able to broaden their thinking and challenge practice to embrace different approaches to care for patients with cancer.

The perception of cancer as a terminal disease is changing with many people now thinking of it in terms of a chronic illness. Palliative care is also changing with the emphasis being geared towards non-malignant illnesses. Despite the changes the origins of palliative care should not be forgotten. Those who are living and dying with the disease can carry an enormous burden in terms of physical, social, psychological and spiritual concerns; therefore ensuring palliative care is available to people in terms of need and not life expectancy can make a huge difference to the lives of a person with cancer. Cancer should remain at the heart of palliative care.

References

Ansell P, Howell D, Garry A, Kite S, Munro J, Roman E and Harvard M (2007) What determines referral of UK patients with haematological malignancies to palliative care services? An exploratory study using hospital records. *Palliative Medicine*. 21:487–492.

Balsdon H (2006) Palliative care, Chapter 26. In: Grundy M (Ed), *Nursing in Haematological Oncology* (2nd edition). Edinburgh: Bailliere Tindall.

Bentley A and Fallon M (2006) Pain control in advanced local disease, Chapter 2. In: Booth S and Earl H (Eds), *Palliative Care Consultations – Advanced Breast Cancer*. New York: Oxford University Press.

Booth S and Bruera E (Eds) (2003) *Palliative Care Consultations – Haemato-Oncology*. New York: Oxford University Press.

Bowles K and Marcus R (2003) Management of lymphoma, Chapter 2. In: Booth S and Bruera E (Eds), *Palliative Care Consultations – Haemato-Oncology*. New York: Oxford University Press, pp. 11–28.

Boyce A, McHugh M and Lyon P (2003) Proactive palliative care choices for haematology day unit patients. *International Journal of Palliative Nursing*. 9(12):544–550.

Breitbart W, Payne D and Passik S (2004) Psychological and psychiatric interventions in pain control. In: Doyle D, Hanks G, Cherney N and Calman K (Eds), *Oxford Textbook of Palliative Medicine* (3rd edition). Oxford: Oxford University Press.

British Association of Surgical Oncology (2005) Guidelines for the management of symptomatic breast disease. London, Royal College of Surgeons. Available at http://www.baso.org/content/Abs-Guidelines.asp. Accessed on 9 May 2008.

Bucholtz J (1999) Metastatic epidural spinal cord compression. *Seminars in Oncology Nursing*. 15(3):150–159.

Cancer Research UK (2005) Cancer stats – worldwide cancer (factsheet). Cancer Research UK. Available at http://info.cancerresearchuk.org/cancerstats/. Accessed on 17 April 2008.

Cancer Research UK (2008a) Cancer stats – incidence UK (factsheet). Cancer Research UK. Available at http://info.cancerresearchuk.org/cancerstats/. Accessed on 17 April 2008.

Cancer Research UK (2008b) Cancer stats: key facts – breast cancer. Available at http://publications.cancerresearchuk.org/WebRoot/crukstoredb/CRUK_PDFs/BRSUMSTAT07.pdf. Accessed on 17 April 2008.

Cartwright R, Wood H and Quin M (2005) Non-Hodgkins lymphoma, Chapter 16. In: Quin M, Wood H, Cooper N, and Rowan S (Eds) *Cancer Atlas of the UK and Ireland 1991–2000*. London: Office National Statistics. Available at http://www.statistics.gov.uk/statbase/Product.asp?vlnk=14059. Accessed on 17 April 2008.

Chapple A (2004) Stigma, shame and blame experienced by patients with lung cancer: a qualitative study. *British Medical Journal*. 328(7454):1470.

Connors S, Graham S and Peel T (2007) An evaluation of physiotherapist led non-pharmacological breathlessness programme for patients with intra-thoracic malignancy. *Palliative Medicine*. 21(4):285–287.

Corner J, Hopkinson J, Fitzimmons D et al. (2005) Is late diagnosis of lung cancer inevitable: interview study of patient's recollections of symptoms before diagnosis. *Thorax*. 60:314–319.

Davis R, Wagner E and Groves T (2000) Advances in managing chronic disease. *British Medical Journal*. 320(7234):525–527.

Department of Health. (2000) *The NHS Cancer Plan: A Plan for Investment, a Plan for Reform*. London: Department of Health.

DeSanto-Madeya S, Bauer Wu S and Gross A (2007) Activities of daily living in women with advanced breast cancer. *Oncology Nursing Forum*. 34(4):841–846.

Drudge-Coates L and Rajbubu K (2008a) Diagnosis and management of spinal cord compression – Part 2. *International Journal of Palliative Nursing*. 14(4):175–180.

Drudge-Coates L and Rajbubu K (2008b) Diagnosis and management of spinal cord compression – Part 1. *International Journal of Palliative Nursing*. 14(3):110–116.

Ellershaw J (2007) Care of the dying: what a difference the LCP makes. *Palliative Medicine*. 21:365–368.

Ellershaw J and Ward C (2003) The care of the dying patient: the last days and hours of life. *British Medical Journal*. 326:30–34.

Ferrell B (1996) The quality of lives: 1525 voices of cancer. *Oncology Nursing Forum.* 23:909–916.

Fleissig A, Jenkins V, Catt S and Fallowfield L (2006) Multidisciplinary teams in cancer care: are they effective in the UK. *The Lancet Oncology.* 7(11):935–943. Available at http://oncology.thelancet.com. Accessed on 11 April 2008..

Flock P (2003) Pilot study to determine the effectiveness of diamorphine gel to control pressure ulcer pain. *Journal of Pain and Symptom Management.* 25(6):547–554.

Greenstreet W (2006) From spirituality to coping strategy: making sense of chronic illness. *British Journal of Nursing.* 15(17):938–942.

Gregor A and Milroy R (2001) Lung cancer, Chapter 4. In: *Cancer Scenarios – An Aid to Planning Cancer Services.* Edinburgh: Scottish Executive, pp. 64–81.

Grocott P (2007) Care of patients with malignant wounds. *Nursing Standard.* 21(24):57–66.

Grunfield E (2006) Psychological and social issues for patients with advanced breast cancer, Chapter 3. In: Booth S and Earl H (Eds), *Palliative Care Consultations – Advanced Breast Cancer.* New York: Oxford University Press, pp. 33–44.

Gualandi R, Rocci L, Vincenzi B, Romiti A, Tomao S, Tonnini G, De Marinis M and Santini D (2003) Fatigue after primary treatment in breast cancer survivors: a preliminary prospective study. *International Nursing Perspective.* 3:137–144.

Harmer V (2005) Breast cancer – new treatments, new strategies. *British Journal of Nursing.* 14(16):844–845.

Harvey H and Cream L (2007) Biology of bone metastases: causes and consequences. *Clinical Breast Cancer.* 7(Suppl 1):S7–S13.

Hately J, Laurence V, Scott A, Baker R and Thomas P (2003) Breathlessness clinics within specialist palliative care settings can improve quality of life and functional capacity of patients with lung cancer. *Palliative Medicine.* 17:410–417.

Hicks F (2003) The last days of life, Chapter 15. In: Booth S and Bruera E (Eds), *Palliative Care Consultations Haemato-Oncology.* New York: Oxford University Press, pp. 237–248.

Iddawela M, Ahmad A, McAdam K and Earl H (2006) Current management of advanced breast disease, Chapter 1. In: Booth S and Earl H (Eds), *Palliative Care Consultations – Advanced Breast Cancer.* New York: Oxford University Press, pp. 1–15.

Lloyd-Williams M, Dennis M and Taylor F (2004) A perspective study to determine the association between physical symptoms and depression in patients with advanced cancer. *Palliative Medicine.* 18:558–563.

McGrath P (2001) Caregivers' insights on the dying trajectory in hematology oncology. *Cancer Nursing.* 24(5):413–421.

McGrath P and Holewa H (2006) Missed opportunities: nursing insights on end of life care for haematology patients. *International Journal of Nursing Practice.* 12:295–301.

McGrath P and Holewa H (2007a) Description of an Australian model for end of life care in patients with haematologic malignancies. *Oncology Nursing Forum.* 34(1):79–85.

McGrath P and Holewa H (2007b) Special considerations for haematology patients in relation to end-of-life care: Australian findings. *European Journal of Cancer Care.* 16:164–171.

National Institute Clinical Excellence (NICE) (2003) *Improving Outcomes in Haematological Cancers: The Manual.* London: NICE.

National Institute Clinical Excellence (NICE) (2004) *Improving Supportive and Palliative Care for Adults with Cancer.* London: NICE.

National Institute Clinical Excellence (NICE) (2005) *The Diagnosis and Treatment of Lung Cancer: Methods, Evidence and Guidance*. London: NICE.

NHS Quality Improvement Scotland (2004) *The Management of Pain in Patients with Cancer – Best Practice Statement*. Edinburgh: NHSQIS.

Nursing and Midwifery Council (NMC) (2008) *The Code: Standards of Conduct, Performance and Ethics for Nurses and Midwives*. London: NMC.

Oxlad M, Wade T, Hallsworth L and Koczwara B (2008) 'I'm living with a chronic illness, not . . . dying with cancer' a qualitative study of Australian women's self-identified concerns and needs following primary treatment for breast cancer. *European Journal of Cancer Care*. 17:157–166.

Parkin D, Bray F, Ferlay J and Pisani P (2001) Estimating the world cancer burden: Globescan 2000. *International Journal of Cancer*. 94:153–156.

Peake M (2007) Raising the public and political profile of lung cancer. *Lung Cancer in Practice*. 4(1):1–5.

Peto R, Boreham J and Clarke M (2000) UK and USA breast cancer deaths down 25% in year 2000 at ages 20–69 years. *Lancet*. 355(9217):1822.

Reyna Z and Bruera E (2006) The management of pain and other complications from bone metastases, Chapter 9. In: Booth S and Earl H (Eds), *Palliative Care Consultations – Advanced Breast Cancer*. New York: Oxford University Press.

Rosenfield R and Stahl D (2006) Pain management of bone metastases in breast cancer. *Journal of Hospice and Palliative Nursing*. 8(4):233–245.

Saunders C (1978) *The Management of Terminal Disease*. London: Edward Arnold.

Scottish Executive Health Department (2001) *Cancer Scenarios: An Aid to Planning Cancer Services in Scotland in the Next Decade*. Edinburgh: Scottish Executive.

Scottish Intercollegiate Guidelines Network (2008) Control of pain in adults with cancer – a national clinical guideline No 106. Edinburgh: NHS Quality Improvement Scotland. Available at http://www.sign.ac.uk/pdf/SIGN106.pdf. Accessed on 8 January 2009.

Scottish Intercollegiate Guidelines Network (2005a) Management of patients with lung cancer – a national clinical guideline No 80. Edinburgh: NHS Quality Improvement Scotland. Available at http://www.sign.ac.uk/pdf/sign84.pdf. Accessed on 6 May 2008.

Scottish Intercollegiate Guidelines Network (2005b) Management of women with breast cancer – a national clinical guideline No 84. Edinburgh: NHS Quality Improvement Scotland. Available at http://www.sign.ac.uk/pdf/sign80.pdf. Accessed on 9 May 2008.

Sepulveda C, Malin A, Yoshida T and Ullrich A (2002) Palliative care: the World Health Organization's global perspective. *Journal of Pain and Symptom Management*. 24(2):91–96.

Spathis A (2003) The essentials of symptom control in haemato-oncology, Chapter 8. In: Booth S and Bruera E (Eds), *Palliative Care Consultations Haemato-Oncology*. New York: Oxford University Press, pp. 111–136.

Stewart B and Kleihues P (2003) *World Cancer Report*. International Agency for Research on Cancer. Geneva: World Health Organization.

Sweeney C (2006) The management of fatigue in breast cancer, Chapter 7. In: Booth S and Earl H (Eds), *Palliative Care Consultations – Advanced Breast Cancer*. New York: Oxford University Press, pp. 77–90.

Tritter J and Calnan M (2002) Cancer as a chronic illness. *European Journal of Cancer Care*. 11:161–165.

Twycross R and Wilcock A (2003) *Symptom Management in Advanced Cancer* (3rd edition). Oxon: Radcliffe Publishing.

West of Scotland Cancer Managed Clinical Network (WoSCAN) (2006) Malignant spinal cord guidelines. Available at http://www.palliativecareglasgow.info/Professional%20Resources/woscan_mscc_guidelines.asp. Accessed on 11 May 2008.

World Health Organization (1996) *Cancer Pain Relief* (2nd edition). Geneva: World Health Organization.

Further reading

Booth S and Bruera E (2003) *Palliative Care Consultations – Haemato-oncology*. New York: Oxford University Press.

Booth S and Earl H (2006) *Palliative Care Consultations – Advanced Breast Cancer*. New York: Oxford University Press.

Grundy M (2006) *Nursing in Haematological Cancer* (2nd edition). Edinburgh: Bailliere Tindall.

Harmer V (2003) *Breast Cancer: Nursing Care and Management*. London: Whurr Publishers.

Kearney N and Richardson A (2006) *Nursing Patients with Cancer*. Edinburgh: Churchill Livingston.

West of Scotland Cancer Managed Clinical Network (WoSCAN) (2006) Malignant spinal cord guidelines. Available at http://www.palliativecareglasgow.info/Professional%20Resources/woscan_mscc_guidelines.asp. Accessed on 11 May 2008.

Chapter 14

Palliative nursing care for people with human immunodeficiency virus (HIV) and acquired immunodeficiency syndrome (AIDS)

May McCreaddie

Introduction

This chapter focuses on the issues relating to the provision of palliative nursing care for people who have been diagnosed with HIV/AIDS. It begins by providing a background to HIV/AIDS before reviewing the impact of the disease on the international community. The chapter then reviews the drug therapies currently available before discussing the notion that HIV/AIDS has become a chronic illness. Following this the chapter reviews the challenges of providing palliative care for this group, examining current issues in pain management, HIV-related dementia, depression and complex co-morbidities. The chapter finishes with a case study to show how the disease affected one individual.

Learning outcomes

Once you have read this chapter and completed the associated practice points, you will be able to:

- Discuss the history of HIV/AIDS
- Describe the global impact of HIV/AIDS
- Analyse the challenges facing nurses when caring for this client group
- Discuss the local needlestick injury policy that is in place in your clinical area

Background

Five cases of PCP (pneumocystic carrini pneumonia) in previously healthy young men were reported by the Centre for Disease Control (CDC) in the US in the summer of 1981 (CDC 1981). These cases signified the first public portent of AIDS and laid the foundations for the subsequent discovery of HIV in 1983. HIV – the virus that causes AIDS – was later isolated from a blood sample taken from a man in the Congo in 1959, demonstrating that HIV was not a 'new' virus but had in fact been present in other countries for some considerable time (Zhu et al. 1998).

The five cases in the US were all young, gay men prompting this disease of immune deficiency to be initially labelled GRIDS – gay-related immune deficiency syndrome. Subsequent diagnoses in the broader community soon put paid to that misnomer although AIDS and HIV remained and to a certain extent remains firmly embedded in the public's perception as a 'Gay' disease. The reality is, however, that approximately 75% of the world's HIV infected are heterosexual (United Nations Joint Programme on HIV/AIDS (UNAIDS)/World Health Organization (WHO) 2007). HIV may be a disease that the disenfranchised, poor, or uneducated are particularly vulnerable to, but a virus with a predilection for homosexual men it is not.

Unlike people, HIV – the virus – does not discriminate against potential hosts: it is not who you are but rather what you do that makes infection possible. A virus, in an infectious fluid, that enters into a susceptible host *may* result in infection.

It is known that the factors essential to infection are:

1. an infectious agent
2. a mode of transmission
3. a susceptible host

'All three must be present in order for infection to *potentially* occur.'

(Day 2000)

Despite the somewhat hysterical history of HIV the virus is, with regards to the factors essential to infection, just like any other pathogen. Once inside the host however, HIV has the potential to create a disease process of myriad and fluctuating symptoms and diseases.

Over 20 years on from its emergence in the western world in the early 1980s over 65 million people have been infected with HIV (UNAIDS/WHO 2007). HIV remains a major public health issue, a significant disease burden and a focus for care and treatment interventions across both wealthy and resource-poor countries. It also presents an ongoing challenge and font of knowledge for nurses, nursing and palliative care.

International impact of HIV and AIDS

HIV and AIDS may appear to be less visibly present in terms of public awareness; nonetheless it remains arguably the most significant infectious disease in the world and infects millions of individuals across the five continents.

In addition to the above figures, the numbers of new infections in 2007 totalled 2.5 million (1.8–4.1) with numbers of AIDS deaths estimated at 2.1 million (1.9–2.4). These figures have decreased somewhat from initial projections; however, the diagnostic and reporting methodology has become more refined and robust across disparate countries and health services, making current figures more accurate (See Table 14.1).

Approximately 6800 people become infected every day with 5700 deaths reported; thus global prevalence is currently relatively stable. There are local reductions across countries with a decrease in new infections. Sub-Saharan Africa, however, accounts for nearly a third of the new HIV infections with a 29% prevalence rate in pregnant women reported in South Africa. In some African villages, for example, 1 in 4 adults are known to be infected making HIV a significant social and economic threat. In contrast the Western World, that is the rest of the world outwith Asia and Africa, including Eastern Europe continues to see the pandemic maintained in specific populations such as injecting drug users and men who have sex with men. Current drug therapy offers the opportunity to turn a terminal disease into a chronic illness; however, therapies are not universally available and resource-poor countries (ironically those with the greatest HIV prevalence) are least likely to have access to those therapies (UNAIDS 2007).

Practice Point 14.1

What is the prevalence of HIV and AIDS in your local area?
How does it compare with the national (UK) picture?
What is the distribution of infections across groups?

Commentary:

The figures for HIV in the UK and elsewhere can be obtained from www.hpa.org.uk and/or any of the sites below. Look at how the figures are presented, by which groups (MSM, heterosexuals, injecting drug users, others). Look at how the figures have changed over the years and how these figures in the UK in the various groups compare with similar figures elsewhere, for example Africa.

Drug therapy

Anti-retroviral therapy (ART) has developed considerably since AZT or zidovudine monotherapy was licensed in 1987. Over 20 drugs are now currently

Table 14.1 Numbers living with HIV in 2007.

Estimated Total	Parameters of estimation 33.2 million	30.6–36.1 million
Adults	30.8	28.2–33. 6
Females	15.4	13.9–16.6
Children (under 15)	2.5	2.2–2.6

Adapted from UNAIDS/WHO (2007).

Table 14.2 Drugs and their actions.

Drug type and name	Action
Entry inhibitors (T-20*, CCR5)	Blocks viral attachment to cell
Nucleoside analogues (NAs) (AZT, DDI)	Prevents HIV RNA changing into cell DNA
Non-nucleoside analogues (efavirenz, nevirapine)	Prevents HIV RNA changing into cell DNA
Integrase inhibitors (raltegravir†)	Blocks HIV integration into cell DNA
Protease inhibitors (lopinavir, nelfinavir)	Blocks 'new' HIV being assembled

*Injections given twice daily, all other medications capsules/tablet based.
†Not licensed in Europe; currently two nucleoside analogues (NA) with a non-nucleoside analogue reverse transcriptase inhibitor (NNRTI) or a protease inhibitor (PI) are the preferred option.
‡Anti-retroviral data is based on BHIVA 2006 guidelines. 2008 guidelines are available based on the most recent studies. Adapted from BHIVA (2006).

available. ART or HAART (highly active anti-retroviral therapy] involves using two or more classes of drugs in combination (British HIV Association – BHIVA 2006). There are five different types of drugs that work at different stages of the HIV life cycle, seen here in Table 14.2.

A separate class of drug called fusion inhibitors (FI) will also be available to patients who have run out of all (effective) options or combinations of NAs (nucleoside analogues] and NNRTIs (non-nucleoside analogue reverse transcriptase inhibitors). Integrase inhibitors, CCR5 inhibitors and vaccine development all demonstrate that HIV remains a potent area for drug development. The prospect of 'cure' per se, however, remains a long-term hope rather than a short- to medium-term possibility.

HIV may have been discovered over 20 years ago, but it is the way in which it 'hijacks' the immune system and causes disease that makes cure a longer term prospect. The CD4 cell is the main cell in the immune system: the collection of cells and organs that work together to fight disease and tumour (Playfair 1995). HIV attaches and enters the CD4 cell effectively turning it into a virus factory. Drug therapy primarily seeks to prevent the virus replicating within the CD4 cell, thereby reducing the amount of circulating virus and the destruction of CD4 cells. This allows the CD4 cells and immune system to re-constitute and confer a more vigorous defence against infections and/or tumour. A patient with advanced HIV disease is likely to have a low CD4 count and a high viral load. Opportunistic infections (OIs – infections that take the opportunity to cause problems] emerge where previously a robust immune system would have sufficed. In advanced stages of the disease, therefore, an individual can have a plethora of infections and/or tumours requiring symptomatic treatment in addition to the cause (virus) being similarly treated with ART.

A chronic illness?

While ART has seen a considerable increase in longevity and quality of life for patients with HIV since it became fully established in 1996, it is not a panacea.

Indeed ART has increased life expectancy to the point of a re-configuration of HIV as a chronic illness rather than a terminal one (BHIVA 2007). ART however, like most drug therapies, is not without complications. Firstly, ART remains a preserve of the Western World. Resource-poor countries have extremely limited, if any, access to pharmaceutical therapies (Harding et al. 2005; O'Neill and Marconi 2003). Secondly, while adult drug regimes are relatively advanced, paediatric ART is constrained by ethical issues and limited clinical trials. Thirdly, encouraging adherence to ART is necessary to increase the potential for a successful outcome and this remains a challenging issue (BHIVA 2001). Fourthly, ART can cause toxicity, interactions and side effects leading to a variety of distressing problems. Lastly, but not the least virological failure is still possible (BHIVA 2006).

Despite the tremendous advances of ART, AIDS and associated co-morbidities remain an important cause of death in HIV. A diagnosis of advanced HIV disease may currently offer longer life expectancy, better quality of life with greater therapeutic options (Brechtl et al. 2001); nonetheless these issues increase the challenges to palliative nurses rather than negate them (Cochrane 2003).

The challenge of palliative care in HIV disease

Seroconversion is the interval of time between exposure to infection and the development of a marker that denotes actual infection. In HIV infection this is the development of an antibody 3 weeks to 3 months following exposure. The individual is therefore said to be antibody positive, that is, infected with the virus. People who are currently diagnosed HIV positive may face a future that is relatively symptom-free for ten years plus depending upon their existing CD4 count and viral load. CD4 is a marker on the T4 lymphocyte, the main cell in the immune system and a normal CD4 count is one in excess of $600 \, \text{mm}/\text{L}^3$. Patients will have their CD4 and/or viral load monitored regularly depending upon their current state of health. A CD4 count approaching $350 \, \text{mm}/\text{L}^3$ or less will initiate discussions on the appropriateness or otherwise of commencing ART (BHIVA 2006). A CD4 count of $200 \, \text{mm}/\text{L}^3$ or less is likely to lead to increasing symptoms and/or disease, necessitating further drug therapies (antibiotics, antivirals, etc.) thereby complicating treatments.

In the past patients with decreasing CD4 counts were likely to find themselves admitted to infectious disease (ID) wards with stringent infection control precautions implemented. Universal precautions are of course universal, but patients today on failing therapies and/or decreasing CD4 counts are more likely to be nursed at home and in a variety of other settings (hospice, medical wards, drug treatment centres) rather than in the more stereotypical setting of an infectious diseases unit. Consequently, a broader spectrum of nurses is likely to provide palliative care for patients with advanced HIV disease (Easterbrook and Meadway 2001).

In such instances the aims of palliative care for patients with advanced HIV disease is no different to those of a patient with a (non-HIV) cancer diagnosis. There are three AIDS defining tumours: Kaposi's sarcoma, high grade B-cell non-Hodgkin's lymphoma and invasive cervical carcinoma in addition to non-AIDS defining tumours (non-small cell lung cancer and hepatocellular carcinoma). Firstly HIV differs from a cancer diagnosis in that it presents a distinctly uncertain and myriad disease process that varies from person to person (BHIVA 2007). There is therefore no one prescriptive care package format. Secondly, HIV is a condition primarily afflicting the disenfranchised and often most challenging of individuals or groups. It therefore requires an approach from nurses that enhances the likelihood of successful engagement and palliation. Ultimately an all-inclusive holistic and affirmative approach to both life and death, balanced with freedom from pain and suffering, are the central tenets of palliation in HIV as they are in other conditions (O'Neill and Fallon 1997).

Pain and symptom management

Early indications of managing advanced HIV infection or AIDS denote the importance of pain and symptom management (Newshan and Sherman 1999) Pain can arise from the numerous infections or tumours that attempt to overpower the immune system. From headache with cryptococcal meningitis to abdominal pain from mycobacterium avium complex or dysphagia due to oesophageal candidiasis, pain is numerous and diverse in its presentation in HIV disease. Pain may be directly related to HIV, due to the consequences of immune suppression, HIV disease therapies or another unknown reason.

Pain can also have a significant psychological and functional impact and it is useful to establish the type of pain, for example nociceptive or neuropathic pain in order to provide appropriate management. Unfortunately, despite the recent advances in drug therapies the management of pain in HIV patients remains sub-optimal (Coughlan 2003). Clearly the varied presentation of pain and pain sites in HIV disease complicates this process; nevertheless there is no excuse for a patient in pain particularly when under-medicated. Addicted patients (and ex-addicted patients) can suffer most from under-medication as providers may make a series of ill-informed judgements regarding appropriate treatment strategies (McCreaddie and Davison 2002; Peretti-Watel et al. 2004).

Evidenced-based, non-judgemental care

There is also an assumption that patients receiving treatment in specialist settings, such as ID, will be given high-quality, non-judgmental care. Experience has shown however that discrimination and/or lack of knowledge are no respecter of boundaries or specialties. Nurses should always seek to ensure that palliative care, particularly in this area, is based on evidence, not opinion or ill-informed hearsay (McCreaddie 2004; Pratt 2003). Thus, pain and symptom management in HIV disease is similarly no different from that of a patient with (non-HIV related) cancer. Assessment is key and safe and effective analgesia free from unwanted side effects the primary outcome (Portenoy and Lesage 1999).

Practice Point 14.2

Given that HIV is a communicable disease and that many patients may require parenteral analgesia, what is your local policy, guideline and/or procedure on needlestick injury? Specifically, what does it say with regard to post-exposure prophylaxis?

Commentary:

You should have been able to obtain your needlestick injury procedures, etc. from your local occupational health department and/or your local health authority. Consider how difficult this may have been to get a hold of? Do you think that professionals are well aware of them? Did they have a policy on post-exposure prophylaxis (PEP)? Is PEP available at your local Accident and Emergency department? Remember PEP is only an option if the factors essential to infection (e.g. virus, in an infectious fluid and entry to host) are evident. Thus, it is really only if the patient is a known HIV patient that PEP should come into play. Remember that all body fluids should be treated as infectious, that is why there are universal precautions in place.

More than just physical care

Like good palliative care in other settings HIV palliation is more than just attending to an individual's physical needs or symptoms. Sexuality or sexuality needs, for example, are often touted as a key aspect of holistic palliative care yet it is invariably consigned to a single sentence with little light shed on what exactly that may entail. People with HIV disease have a range of contagion and non-contagion-related sexuality needs that are integral to them as individuals as well as perhaps their partners (McCreaddie 2006). A disease that may have been acquired sexually can ravage both body image and libido. It is important therefore that nurses acknowledge patients as sexual beings with concomitant feelings and desires as psychological difficulties may present if problems are left unaddressed (BHIVA –BASHH-FFP-UK 2007; Shover and Jensen 1988).

HIV dementia

Mental health issues generally are highly prevalent in this population group and as with other conditions mental health problems are more likely to manifest in palliative care situations (Karus et al. 2004).

HIV dementia, for example, is a sub-cortical dementia that tends to present initially with slowed information processing, cognitive or psychomotor capabilities, verbal memory and difficulties with new learning is a diagnosis of exclusion. Thankfully HIV dementia is less prevalent now thanks to ART (McKeogh 1995); nevertheless it may still present with patients on 'salvage therapy' or no therapy. ART has generally poor penetration of the blood–brain barrier (BBB) while HIV crosses the BBB and replicates presenting as an infectious as opposed to organic dementia.

'Young' patients with HIV dementia are notoriously difficult to place as appropriate facilities tend to house the over 65 age group. HIV dementia patients can be managed in the community with appropriate assistance from psychiatric colleagues or specialist services. Key issues such as ensuring adherence to ART and other medication plus managing social and behavioural manifestations of the dementia can prove particularly challenging (Stephenson et al. 2000).

Depression and complex co-morbidities

Depression is a highly prevalent condition in HIV and may be a pre-existing or subsequent diagnosis relating either to the disease or as a consequence of therapies (Israelski et al. 2007). Substance use and co-morbid mental health problems are also highly prevalent and (Draper et al. 2005) in tandem with HIV dementia or any other co-morbidities or disease presentations make HIV palliative care a complex challenge and balancing act. Thus, specialist support for these complex conditions is crucial especially when palliation is the focus. Equally, it is important for nurses not to be caught up in a 'referral' culture where problems are identified for another specialist to solve. Many of these patients are used to being passed from pillar to post, off-loaded onto another specialist under the guise of lack of experience or time. An established relationship with the patient founded on trust and respect at a time of uncertainty and declining health is likely to be more beneficial to their care than specialist referrals (Markowitz and Rabow 2004; Petrasch et al. 1998).

Nursing the broad spectrum of people with HIV disease

HIV disease presents a broad spectrum of patients, identities and groups. Whether caring for patients in resource-poor or resource-rich countries, marginalized or disenfranchised groups invariably predominate. Every country and society has its scapegoats or underclass who invariably suffer most from a disease that is ultimately undiscriminating. HIV positively thrives in the discriminated and dispossessed: from infected housewives in India or gypsy orphans in Romania to a roofless and rootless injecting drug user in the UK. Consequently, it requires a nursing response that is both dynamic and appropriate to the stage of HIV palliation.

Assessing complex needs

Patients may be, for example, injecting drug users, homeless, ex or current prisoners, gay men, refugees or asylum seekers. Tuberculosis is for example a significant co-morbidity for the asylum seeking population and requires specific management (BHIVA 2005). All of those individuals or groups have their own identities, culture and/or language and associated challenges. For some legal matters may prevail with issues of residency status or benefits taking precedence over adherence to ART. For others treatment matters may assume equal importance. Thus, preventing opiate and/or benzodiazepine withdrawal may go hand in hand with the management of PCP and associated symptoms. Inevitably HIV patients generally present with co-morbidities as a direct consequence of HIV (cancer, HIV dementia) or in addition to HIV (depression, HCV). Accordingly, it has to be stressed that managing complex co-morbidities is generally the rule in HIV palliation rather than the exception (BHIVA 2004a; BHIVA 2004b; Wood et al. 1997). Recognizing that the priority for the patient is also the 'priority' for the nurse is key to successful palliation.

Patient-provider partnership

Nurses also need to be flexible and innovative in their approach to palliation whatever the environment or client group. Disenfranchised clients or groups may anticipate negative care and treatment from health care professionals based on past experience (McCreaddie 2004). They will therefore be more difficult to engage with and maintain in treatment. Care and treatment approaches therefore may have to be somewhat 'opportunistic' and negotiation and compromise will feature strongly in the relationship. Patient autonomy is noted to be a key feature in palliation generally; however, patient autonomy and patient-provider partnership (as opposed to paternalism) is a long-standing feature of care and treatment in HIV (McCreaddie 2002; McCreaddie 2004; Pratt 2003). Nurses providing palliative care to HIV patients no matter the setting therefore need to be communicative, flexible, responsive and persistent.

Case study

The first patient I involved in teaching health care staff about HIV disease and other bloodborne viruses was an intelligent and articulate man who was committed to making staff aware of 'his side' of the story. So keen was Gerry (pseudonym used to protect identity) to challenge the stigma of HIV and open up the minds of resistant staff he even undertook one training session with oxygen to hand and his brother at his side, patiently taking questions no matter how intrusive. Gerry held the strong belief that HIV was not the problem, but rather it was individuals' (and society's) attitude and behaviour in response to it. He wanted it to be treated like another disease because it was another disease.

Certainly, HIV is a multi-system disease of immune dysfunction that primarily infects and affects the disenfranchised and as such it provides tremendous challenges, particularly with regard to palliation. As the health care workers who were lucky enough to talk with Gerry found out, it also provides tremendous learning opportunities and a chance to demonstrate palliative nursing care at its very best.

Summary

- HIV was first seen as a *disease* in 1981, identified as a *virus* in 1983 and the first anti-retroviral *therapy* (ART) became available as AZT in 1987
- Currently there are over 20 drugs available: two classes of drugs that work at four different stages of the virus lifecycle
- There are 33.2 million people currently living with HIV in the world, many in sub-Saharan Africa, the vast majority of whom do not have access to ART
- Although ART has the potential to turn a terminal disease into a chronic illness, palliative care presents particular challenges to nurses due to the uncertainty of the disease process and the broad spectrum of patients and patient groups
- Assessment is the key to all aspects of care specifically pain and symptom management, as is non-judgemental, evidenced-based care
- The broad spectrum of HIV in terms of identities, patients and groups requires an innovative, dynamic, non-judgemental and partnership approach to palliative care.

References

BHIVA (2001) *Adherence*. London: Mediscript Ltd.

BHIVA (2004a) *Hepatitis B Co-Infection*. London: Mediscript Ltd.

BHIVA (2004b) *Hepatitis C Co-Infection*. London: Mediscript Ltd.

BHIVA (2005) *TB/HIV Co-Infection*. London: Mediscript Ltd.

BHIVA (2006) *Treatment of HIV-Infected Adults with Anti-Retroviral Therapy*. London: Mediscript Ltd.

BHIVA (2007) *HIV-Associated Malignancies*. London: Mediscript Ltd.

BHIVA-BASHH-FPP UK (2007) *Sexual and Reproductive Health for People Living with HIV*. London: Mediscript Ltd.

Brechtl JR, Breitbart W, Galietta M, Krivo S and Rosenfeld B (2001) The use of highly active antiretroviral therapy (HAART) in patients with advanced HIV infection: impact on medical, palliative care, and quality of life outcomes. *Journal of Pain and Symptom Management*. 21(1):41–51.

Centers for Disease Control (CDC) (1981) Pneumocystis pneumonia – Los Angeles. *Morbidity and Mortality Weekly Report (MMWR)*. 30:250–252.

Cochrane J (2003) The experience of uncertainty for individuals with HIV/AIDS and the palliative care paradigm. *International Journal of Palliative Nursing*. 9(9):382–388.

Coughlan M (2003) Pain and palliative care for people living with HIV/AIDS in Asia. *Journal of Pain and Palliative Pharmacotherapy*. 17:91–104.

Day M (2000) Infection control. *Nursing Standard*. 14(28):52–57.

Draper JC, Elinore F and McCance-Katz T (2005) Medical illnesses and co-morbidities in drug users: implications for addiction pharmacotherapy treatment. *Substance Use and Misuse*. 40(13):1899–1921.

Easterbrook P and Meadway J (2001) The changing epidemiology of HIV infection: new challenges for HIV palliative care. *Journal of the Royal Society of Medicine*. 94(1): 442–448.

Harding R, Easterbrook P, Higginson IJ, Karus D, Raveis, VH and Marconi K (2005) Access and equity in HIV/AIDS palliative care: a review of the evidence and responses. *Palliative Medicine*. 19(3):251–258.

Israelski DM, Prentiss DE, Lubegas S, Blamas G, Garcia P, Muhammad M, Cummings S and Koopman C (2007) Psychiatric co-morbidities in vulnerable populations receiving primary care for HIV/AIDS. *AIDS Care*. 19(20):220–225.

Karus D, Raveis VH, Marconi K, Selwyn P, Alexander C, Hanna B and Higginson IJ (2004) Mental health status of clients from three HIV/AIDS palliative care projects. *Palliative and Supportive Care*. 2(2):125–138.

Markowitz AJ and Rabow MW (2004) Perspective on care at the close of life: coda. Over-coming the false dichotomy of 'curative' vs 'palliative' care for late-stage HIV/AIDS: 'let me live the way I want to live, until I can't'. *JAMA: Journal of the American Medical Association*. 291(4):492.

McCreaddie M (2002) Involving patients in teaching about bloodborne viruses. *Nursing Standard*. 16(44):33–36.

McCreaddie M (2004) *Sex, Drugs and Bloodborne Viruses: An Easy to Read Guide for Health and Social Care Workers*.Wiltshire: APS Publishing.

McCreaddie M (2006) Chronic illness and sexuality needs in HIV positive homosexual men. *HIV Nursing*. Spring:1–5.

McCreaddie M and Davison S (2002) Pain management in drug users. *Nursing Standard*. 16(19):45–51.

McKeogh M (1995) Dementia in HIV disease – a challenge for palliative care? *Journal of Palliative Care*. 11(2):30–33.

Newshan G and Sherman DW (1999) Palliative care: pain and symptom management in persons with HIV/AIDS. *Nursing Clinics of North America*. 34(1):131–145.

NHIVNA (2007) *National HIV Nursing Competencies*. London: Mediscript Ltd.

O'Neill B and Fallon M (1997) ABC of palliative care: principles of palliative care and pain control. *British Medical Journal*. 315:801–804.

O'Neill J and Marconi K (2003) Underserved populations, resource-poor settings, and HIV: innovative palliative care projects. *Journal of Palliative Medicine*. 6(3): 457–459.

Peretti-Watel P, Bendiane MK, Galinier A, Lapiana JM, Favre R, Pegliasco H and Obadia Y (2004) Opinions toward pain management and palliative care: comparison between HIV specialists and oncologists. *AIDS Care*. 16(5):619–627.

Petrasch S, Bauer M, Reinacher-Schick A, Sandmann M, Kissler M, Kuchler T, Kruskem-per G, Dorr T and Schmiegel W (1998) Assessment of satisfaction with the commu-nication process during consultation of cancer patients with potentially curable dis-ease, cancer patients on palliative care, and HIV-positive patients. *Wiener Medizinische Wochenschrift*. 148(2):491–499.

Playfair J (1995) *Infection and Immunity*. Oxford: Oxford University Press.

Portenoy RK and Lesage P (1999) Management of cancer pain. *The Lancet*. 353:1695–1700.

Pratt RJ (2003) *HIV and AIDS: A Foundation for Nursing and Healthcare Practice* (5th edition). London: Arnold Publishers.

Shover LR and Buus Jensen S (1988) *Sexuality and Chronic Illness*. London: Guildford Press.

Stephenson J, Woods S, Scott B and Meadway J (2000) HIV-related brain impairment from palliative care to rehabilitation. *International Journal of Palliative Nursing*. 6(1):6–11.

UNAIDS (2007) *Financial Resources Required to Achieve Universal Access to HIV Prevention, Treatment, Care and Support*. Available at http://data.unaids.org/pub/Report/2007/20070925_annex_iv_interventions_en.pdf. Accessed on 25 November 2008.

UNAIDS/WHO (2007) *AIDS Epidemic Update: Latest Developments in the Global AIDS Epidemic*. UNAIDS/WHO.

Wood CGA, Whittet S and Bradbeer CS (1997) ABC of palliative care: HIV infection and AIDS. *British Medical Journal*. 315:1433–1436.

Zhu T, Korber BT, Hanimias AJ, Hooper E, Sharp PM and Ho DD (1998) An African HIV-1 sequence from 1959 and implications for the origins of the epidemic. *Nature*. 391:584–597.

Further reading

McCreaddie M (2004) *Sex, Drugs and Bloodborne Viruses: An Easy to Read Guide for Health and Social Care Workers*. Wiltshire: APS Publishing.
As it says an easy to read guide, not palliative care specific but a broader guide to the topic.

Pratt RJ (2003) *HIV and AIDS: A Foundation for Nursing and Healthcare Practice* (5th edition). London: Arnold Publishers.
A comprehensive text on all HIV and AIDS nursing matters. Recommended.

NHIVNA (2007) *National HIV Nursing Competencies*. London: Mediscript Ltd. Available at www.nhivna.org.
Identifies the competencies for HIV nursing

Websites

www.aidsmap.com – This is the website of NAM

NAM is an award-winning, community-based organisation, which works from the UK. We deliver reliable and accurate HIV information across the world to HIV-positive people and to the professionals who treat, support and care for them.

www.bhiva.org – This is the website of The British HIV Association

BHIVA has become the leading UK professional association representing professionals in HIV care. Now 13 years old, it is a well-established and highly respected organisation with national influence committed to providing excellence in the care of those living with and affected by HIV.

www.i-Base.info – This is the website of i-Base

'HIV i-Base is a treatment activist group, HIV-positive led and committed to providing timely HIV treatment information both to positive people and to health care professionals . . . it is involved in several community networks, including the European AIDS Treatment Group (EATG), the European Community Advisory Board (ECAB) and the International Treatment Preparedness network.'

www.nhivna.org – This is the website of National HIV Nurses Association

'NHIVNA aims to provide an academic and educational forum for the dissemination of original nursing research in the field of HIV/AIDS. We also aim to address the communication and support needs of nurses working in this area. We hope that these activities will assist in the promotion of good practice in the care of people with HIV.'

www.unaids.org – This is the website of The United Nations Joint Programme on HIV/AIDS.

'UNAIDS, the Joint United Nations Programme on HIV/AIDS, is an innovative joint venture of the United Nations family, bringing together the efforts and resources of ten UN system organizations in the AIDS response to help the world prevent new HIV infections, care for people living with HIV, and mitigate the impact of the epidemic.'

www.who.int – This is the website of The World Health Organization.

'WHO is the directing and coordinating authority for health within the United Nations system. It is responsible for providing leadership on global health matters, shaping the health research agenda, setting norms and standards, articulating evidence-based policy options, providing technical support to countries and monitoring and assessing health trends.'

PART TWO

PALLIATIVE CARE FOR CHILDREN AND YOUNG PEOPLE

Chapter 15

The history and ethos of palliative care for children and young people

Shirley Potts

Introduction

This chapter focuses on the history and ethos of paediatric palliative care, that is palliative care for children and young people under the age of 18. It begins by providing definitions of this type of care before reviewing the history of childhood, the rights of children and the children's hospice movement. The chapter then discusses the differences in illness categories between children's and adult palliative care services. Moving on from this the chapter illustrates the issues relating to the dying child and education before discussing the psychosocial issues that are specific to palliative care for children and young people. The chapter finishes by defining the way forward for palliative care for this group which includes the important issue of transitional care into adult services.

Learning outcomes

Once you have read this chapter and completed the associated practice points, you will be able to:

- Discuss the history of palliative care for children and young people
- Describe the main psychosocial issues that are pertinent to this group
- Consider what requires to be done in the future to ensure all children and young people receive the palliative care they require

Background

'Palliative care for children and young people with life limiting conditions is an active and total approach to care, embracing physical, emotional, social and spiritual elements. It focuses on enhancement of quality of life for the child and support for the family and includes the management of distressing symptoms, provision of respite and care through death and bereavement.'
(Association for Children with Life-Threatening or Terminal Conditions/Royal College of Pediatrics and Child Health 2003)

End of life care for the elderly or for mature adults with a terminal illness is an issue that many can identify with. Most people will have known a hospice user or an elderly relative requiring palliation. There is also a personal identification in the sense that many of us would prefer such services to be in place for our own needs, should that situation arise. The death of a child, however, is still something of a social unmentionable. Death in childhood in the UK of the twenty-first century this is, thankfully, a rare occurrence. There is a benign assumption within society that childbearing and child raising can almost always be assumed to have a successful and healthy outcome. So those children and families for whom this is not the case may experience the isolation and indifference of a society unwilling to acknowledge that, sadly, there are instances where children will indeed die from their condition. For the medical profession, paediatric palliative care shares some of the history, and much of the ethos, of adult palliative services referred to in Part 1 of this book. There are, however, some significant differences and this chapter considers those in more depth.

A prominent difference in paediatric palliative care concerns the nature of childhood. Children are evolving and developing so their understanding of their situation may change through differing developmental stages. Children, including sick children, have certain rights and legal entitlements – such as involvement in education, child protection issues, family involvement in decision-making. As with adult palliative care, the hospice movement has made a considerable contribution to the field. The children's hospice movement is somewhat younger but no less active in generating innovative developments in the end of life care of children and young people encompassing their medical, social, emotional and spiritual needs. The breadth of holistic care offered within paediatric palliative care is further explored later in the chapter but let us first note the dramatic changes the past century has brought, concluding with very recent and continuing developments in the status of paediatric palliative care.

History

The conceptualisation of childhood and the rights of children have seen considerable change in recent times. At the beginning of the twentieth century the Edwardian child would be likely to have had first-hand experience of bereavement through siblings, contemporaries or older relatives and neighbours. Conditions such as diphtheria and tuberculosis were ubiquitous and often incurable. There was no National Health Service, so poverty was an obvious decisive factor in accessing health care; and nutritional understanding was limited, with the result that even children from more comfortable backgrounds were oft-times malnourished. Deaths from accidents were not unusual and the safety records of manufacturing industries, for example, left much to be desired. It is perhaps unsurprising that the Edwardian writer J. M. Barrie – himself a bereaved brother – should give his best-known character, Peter Pan, the line, 'to die will be an awfully big adventure' (Barrie 1993). Could Barrie have been offering some solace to a multitude of young people who would face either their own or a sibling's death in childhood? (His compassion was endorsed by his bequeathing of all royalties from Peter Pan to Great Ormond Street Hospital for Sick Children (GOSH). Even when copyright expired in 1987, 50 years after Barrie's death, a unique act of parliament ensured that GOSH will benefit from Barrie's gift for as long as the hospital exists). So, child death was relatively commonplace for the communities of a century ago but in the 1950s with the advent of the NHS, coupled with major advances in medical treatment and inoculation, the UK society rapidly adopted a complacence that heralded a widespread disregard of child death. It was sufficiently rare to be strategically ignored. Children with a terminal prognosis would be sent home to be with their family – perhaps eventually dying in hospital if nursing care requirements exceeded the family's capabilities. Many children with a congenital degenerative condition or disability would be institutionalised for the duration of their life and it is disquieting to recall that this was the accepted and considered medical directive until as recently as the 1960s. Bewildered parents whose newborn was given this stark prognosis acquiesced to the greater knowledge and experience of medical professionals. Fortunately, that 'out of sight; out of mind' perception has altered dramatically in recent times and children's needs have become far more prominent on the political agenda, with repercussions seen in medicine, education, social care and family life. The launch of the Every Child Matters agenda (2004) highlighted the concerted efforts of government and other agencies in valuing the earliest years of a child's development right through to adulthood. The irony of the five outcomes of ECM – be healthy, stay safe, enjoy and achieve, make a positive contribution, achieve economic well-being – was not lost on those caring for life-limited children and the Every Disabled Child Matters (EDCM) campaign was soon launched under the auspices of the National Children's Bureau. In 2007 EDCM launched its second Private Members Bill, the *Disabled Children (Family Support) Bill*, calling for statutory respite opportunities for families caring for a child with a disability or long-term life-limiting condition. The affinity of disability issues with childhood palliative care needs is understandable and the two have been mutually supportive in achieving improved status in government policy and law. In March 2008 EDCM celebrated 'as the House of Lords last night amended the Children and Young Persons Bill to create a new duty on local authorities to help parents caring for disabled children by giving them breaks from their caring responsibilities' (EDCM 2008). Respite care, sometimes in the course of a quite long-term, though life-limiting, illness, takes far greater predominance within paediatric units and children's hospices have emerged as services offering holistic care to children, some of whom may be considered to be disabled, with life-threatening or life-limiting conditions. *Life-threatening conditions* are those that may be cured, but where treatments may not be successful and a child could die. *Life-limiting conditions* are those that cannot be cured and where death in childhood is likely. The recent history of paediatric palliative care would suggest that children's hospices are offering expertise through their experience of pain control in children, rare conditions and longer-term involvement with their patient group (Goldman 1998). 'However, the contribution that children's hospices make in ensuring quality care for life-limited children and their families over many years is sometimes discounted by those who perceive the primary role of hospices as providing places where children go to die. Such a misapprehension is no doubt borne out of experience of adult in-hospice care which primarily focuses on the last days of a patient's life' (Brown and Warr 2007, p. 20). Such a focus on end stage care is far from the reality of children's hospice provision, as will be revealed in the rest of this chapter.

The children's hospice movement

Where the modern hospice service for adults is ascribed to the inspiration of Dame Cicely Saunders, the birth of the children's hospice movement can be attributed to Sister Frances Dominica.

Frances Dominica Ritchie was born in Scotland in 1942. She trained as a nurse at the Hospital for Sick Children, Great Ormond Street and at the Middlesex Hospital London but in the final stages of her nursing training became convinced that she was called to a vocation in religious community. In 1966 she joined the Society of All Saints, an Anglican Religious Community, becoming Mother Superior from 1977 to 1989. In 1979, Mother Frances encountered a young family whose first daughter, Helen, had been left profoundly disabled through a brain tumour. A friendship sprung up, and Mother Frances eventually offered to care for Helen while the family took a brief, much needed, long weekend in Devon. This compassionate and insightful nun had recognised the need for respite for a family walking a journey of unknown length with a very fragile and much loved child. 'The seed of Helen House had been sown.' (Worswick 2000, p. 52) Determined fund-raising and unshakeable vision resulted in Helen House children's hospice opening in Oxford in 1982. It was the first children's hospice in the world and heralded a new dimension in paediatric palliative care.

Children's hospices have since increased in number, though somewhat ran-domly situated around the UK, primarily because these voluntary-funded units have tended to spring up through the instigation of highly motivated bereaved families, so it has been impossible to plan demographically. Martin House in Yorkshire opened in 1987, Acorns in Birmingham in 1990, and Derian House in Lancashire in 1992. Twenty-two years after Helen House opened, Doyle wrote;

'In the UK in 2004, there were 30 with a total of 229 beds. Scotland's second unit will open in 2005. Most are freestanding, a few attached to adult palliative care units. There are 55 doctors staffing them and 2 consultants in paediatric palliative medicine in the UK. Both the University of Cardiff and King's College, London offer courses in paediatric palliative care.'

(Doyle 2005)

Today, there are around 40 services across the UK – only two in Scotland yet, unsurprisingly, a preponderance in the southeast of England. Despite this anomaly, interest in paediatric palliative care is growing steadily. Palliative care was recognised as a subspecialty in general medicine in 1987 – yet in 2007 there were still only six *Paediatric* Palliative Care Consultants in the UK (ACT 2007a). However, many more doctors such as general paediatricians, paediatricians in related specialist areas, adult palliative care doctors, and General Practitioners practising in children's hospices now see themselves as having a high interest in children's palliative care (ACT 2007b). Several children's units have commenced life as a home care service offering support for families in the community, epitomising the concept that hospice is a philosophy as much as a place.

While most major towns now have an adult hospice within their environs, families of terminally ill children may find themselves hundreds of miles from the respite facility of a children's hospice. It is difficult to conceive of a more evenly distributed service while children's hospice remains without substantial statutory funding support. The Association of Children's Hospices (ACH) estimated in 2000 that average children's hospice funding from the statutory sector, mostly local Primary Care Trusts, amounts to only 5% of income. For some, this erratic funding source is as little as 3% – and with the typical cost of maintaining an 8–10 bedded unit amounting to approximately £2 000 000 a year; it is clear that children's hospices have thus far been heavily dependent on voluntary contributions. Each exists as an independent charity, although organisations like ACH and ACT have brought cohesion to the children's hospice movement, as well as working collaboratively with wider organisations such as the National Council for Hospice and Specialist Palliative Care, and the Royal College of Paediatrics and Child Health. The growing strength of the movement has fostered political support and MP Lindsay Hoyle yet again offered a voice of support in the House of Commons:

'I have campaigned for many years, urging the Government to increase funding to hospices, particularly children's hospices such as Derian House based in my constituency, which is a leader in children's care. We must ensure that the Government release more funding. It is alarming that children's hospices are the poor relation in palliative care.'

'First, there is an acute shortage of paediatric palliative care medicine consultants. Secondly, children's hospices receive only in the region of 5% of funding from official sources, compared with 30% for adult hospices, so we can already see the vast difference in funding from the NHS. I want that anomaly to be addressed, in addition to the clear postcode lottery that exists with palliative care.' (Hoyle 2007)

Recognition of the funding shortfall is growing and 2004–2006 saw Big Lottery Funding (formerly New Opportunities Fund) support a variety of initiatives within the children's hospice movement, incorporating in-house services as well as community nursing projects. Other major funding sources have directly or indirectly supported the children's hospice movement, including Diana Community Nursing Teams, Macmillan nurses and Sargent Cancer Care; and the recent Department of Health publication, 'Better care: better lives' (2008, p. 3), insists that 'the Government is investing heavily in supporting all families with disabled children, including those who need palliative care services.'

Interestingly, the respite philosophy of children's services has also begun to materialise in adult hospices and the prior public conviction that hospice care was purely end stage is perhaps diminishing. Bed occupancy in children's hospices is largely respite care owing to the prolonged duration of many of the conditions, despite an ultimately terminal prognosis. Similarly, the concept of respite admission to an adult unit in order to access the expertise in pain relief and improved quality of life has developed.

Practice Point 15.1

Where is your nearest children's hospice? How much funding does it get from statutory sources? Does it have a dedicated palliative medicine physician?

Commentary:

As shown in this chapter your local children's hospice may be round the corner; however it may be many miles away. Would we expect adults to travel this distance for the care they require? You may also find that the support this hospice receives from the Health Authority is poor with the majority of funding coming from private donation. It makes stark reading to find out the total amount required to keep children's' hospice services going with such little support. The Children's Hospice Scotland declares on its website that it needs £5 million per year to keep all their services running with most of this coming from public and private donations (www.chas.org.uk/fundraising). In all areas of palliative care there is a shortage of experienced palliative medicine physicians, although NICE (2004) suggests that in adult hospices there should be one whole time equivalent consultant in palliative medicine per eight beds. Does it then seem sensible to suggest the same is required in children's hospice? So given that in 2004 there were 229 beds in children's hospice is the UK it means there should be around 29 paediatric palliative medicine consultants to support services adequately, not six as previously shown.

Medical conditions requiring palliative care

Medical conditions encountered within paediatric units differ widely from those seen in adult units. Clearly, there are some conditions well known to children's hospices that are never seen in adulthood simply because children do not survive the illness. Where adult hospices are still overwhelmingly utilised by cancer patients, children with cancer form only approximately 30% of children's hospice patients. The rationale for this is the criteria stipulated by children's hospices, the support service being accessible to any child with a life-limiting or life-threatening condition. These broad criteria can be defined under four categories:

Group 1: Life-threatening conditions for which curative treatment may be feasible but can fail. Where access to palliative care services may be necessary when treatment fails. Children in long-term remission or following successful curative treatment are not included (e.g. cancer, irreversible organ failures of heart, liver, kidney).

Group 2: Conditions where premature death is inevitable, where there may be long periods of intensive treatment aimed at prolonging life and allowing participation in normal activities (e.g. cystic fibrosis).

Group 3: Progressive conditions without curative treatment options, where treatment is exclusively palliative and may commonly extend over many years (e.g. Batten disease, mucopolysaccharidoses, muscular dystrophy).

Group 4: Irreversible but non-progressive conditions causing severe disability leading to susceptibility to health complications and likelihood of premature death (e.g. severe cerebral palsy, multiple disabilities such as following brain or spinal cord insult).

(ACT 2003)

To consider some aspects of those groups in more detail:

Group 1: There has perhaps been reluctance in families of children with cancer to move from the hopefully curative environs of hospital care, believing that the term 'hospice' denotes failure of treatment and imminent death. The criteria above suggests that this need not be the case, but with the optimistically high rates of cure, or long-term remission, for childhood cancers, it is understandable that families may not wish to avail themselves of hospice services until they are convinced that no further curative treatment is possible. Sadly, this results in hospice referral sometimes coming at a very late stage in a child's life and families not having sufficient time to fully appreciate the supportive environment that a children's hospice can offer.

Group 2: Cystic fibrosis (CF) is a good example of the dilemmas facing families who may appreciate respite or other supportive interventions in the course of their child's illness, but simultaneously want to acknowledge that the majority of those with cystic fibrosis are now surviving well into adulthood with the average life expectancy being early thirties. Research and understanding is developing exponentially so children born now with this condition may face even more optimistic prognoses. Nevertheless, there are those situations where a child with CF requires palliative care and even end of life care including emotional support for both child and family.

Group 3: This group carries some similarities to Group 2 and may overlap in some respects. Boys with Duchenne muscular dystrophy, for example, constitute a substantial portion of children's hospice users and while the condition is degenerative and incurable, survival into adulthood is also increasing. This affirms the relationship between disability issues and hospice users as these young wheelchair users are entitled to access mainstream education and pursue recreational opportunities alongside their peers. The realisation that this might include, in later adolescence, access to sexual relationships has caused some discussion and debate within society (Asthana 2007, p. 21). Some of the conditions are also familial, resulting in more than one child in a family being affected, bringing additional psychosocial issues.

Group 4: This is, perhaps the greyest area of admission criteria. Many children with cerebral palsy, for example, have very active and fulfilled existences with no sense of life-limitation – and certainly no prospect of utilising palliative care services. However, some children with a severe form of the condition are profoundly compromised through feeding difficulties, respiratory difficulties or frequent seizures. Each situation must be judged individually with thoughtful discussion between family and practitioners. Other circumstances that may compromise a child's life expectation and quality of life include traumas such as near-drowning or spinal injury.

Practice Point 15.2

Go onto the National Statistics Office website at www.statistics.gov.uk
   Make a note of the five most common causes of death for adults and children. Are they similar or different?

Commentary:

What you will have found is that the majority of adults die of degenerative diseases such as heart failure, chronic obstructive pulmonary disease, stroke and cancer. Children on the other hand die in a variety of different ways. Indeed, as many children die accidentally as of cancer, while the third most common cause of death in children is classed as 'other' which includes murder and suicide. The next four listed causes of childhood death in England (in descending order) are neurological conditions, congenital deformities, circularity disease and respiratory disease. It is many of these children that require palliative care

Education and the dying child

It is not always feasible or desirable for a child receiving palliative care to continue with their schooling. Very often, though, maintaining the social and educational stimulus of school attendance is vital to a child's emotional and mental health. ACT (2001, p. 19) suggests:

> 'the child and family should continue educational input for as long as possible while an illness is progressing. Local authorities are responsible for arranging to provide suitable education at school or elsewhere for children of school age who because of illness might not otherwise receive appropriate education.'
>
> (ACT 2001, p. 19)

A French research project followed the educational career of 30 school children with incurable cancer and found 60% of the children showed a clear wish to go to school well into advanced disease (Bouffet 1997). Education, then, is another element to consider within paediatric palliative care. Just as adults with a terminal prognosis may yet wish to maintain their employment for as long as possible, so also would many children choose to maintain their 'non-sick' persona on a social and intellectual level.

Psychosocial issues

It becomes apparent that the population of children's hospice users is varied and complex. Although, thankfully, numbers of children dying are far less than adults, it is clear that there is a wide range of differing circumstances that families may find themselves in. Some families may have known since birth that their child had a poor prognosis; others may have received a devastating diagnosis during toddlerhood (Batten's disease and muchopolysaccharidosis, for instance, are not immediately apparent in a baby); yet others may have had the shock of discovering that their hitherto healthy child has an incurable cancer. Neurodegenerative conditions, cancers, mitochondrial diseases, neuromuscular conditions whether in an only child, a twin, an older brother, siblings, whether it be a genetic link or a random illness, there is no league table measuring levels of grief in families. The hollow truth is that no parent anticipates their child dying before them – it is an unnatural deviation in the cycle of life. For this reason, children's hospices have, from the outset, acknowledged the need for emotional support for families, continuing through bereavement. Parents, siblings and grandparents have found support both individually and through group meetings (Potts 2005). Supportive interventions have extended to schools and friends of a child who has died. Organisations like the Child Bereavement Charity, the Childhood Bereavement Network and Winston's Wish have raised the profile of work with bereaved children and adults. Collaboration between Great Ormond Street Hospital and the Alder Centre (at Royal Liverpool Children's Hospital) sustains the Child Death Helpline – a telephone support system where calls are always answered by a volunteer bereaved parent. Counselling skills have much to offer in palliative care and are a valuable addition to the proficiency of practitioners at all levels (Davy and Ellis 2000). Research with parents around the quality of end of life care has revealed how much parents value 'staff members' genuine expression of emotion and concern' (Meyer et al. 2006, p. 654).

Working with children – the dying or the bereaved – can be particularly challenging for practitioners and it is essential that those supporting children have an understanding of child development as well as bereavement issues (Turner 2006). A 3-year-old's understanding of death, for example, is vastly different to a 7-year-old's. Most 3- and 4-year-olds are still at a very egocentric stage of their development, termed 'magical thinking' by Piaget (1929), which inclines them to believe that they are a causative factor in the major events that happen around them.

The ethos of paediatric palliative care that demands a holistic consideration of a child's needs must also consider spirituality within the realm of psychosocial care. One of the dilemmas facing practitioners is the contradiction that may exist between a parent's waning belief system and a child's more trusting faith. 'Making assumptions about a child's spiritual beliefs and welfare based upon the stance of anguished parents is a dubious advocacy for the dying child. The challenge for practitioners is to remain supportive of the whole family while attending to the spiritual needs of the dying child' (Potts 2007).

In giving a child voice regarding their psychosocial issues, it is also pertinent to consider the rights of children in decision-making. Most paediatricians will involve the child as far as possible in decisions and discussions around the child's illness. This can be another area of tension between practitioners and parents when parents, with very sincere motivation, wish to shield their child from 'bad' news. This requires sensitive and skilful discussion and there is no overriding dictum that covers all eventualities. Suffice to say, most children are either directly or intuitively aware of their prognosis and to be excluded from all conversation or discussion concerning their illness can be a very isolating experience – and more frightening than an honest, open relationship at a time when sincerity is most valued.

The way ahead

Liben et al. (2008) speak of the challenges and emerging ideas facing paediatric palliative care. They suggest the goals are to:

- clearly define the population served; better understand the needs of children with life-threatening conditions and their families
- develop an approach that will be appropriate across different communities
- provide care that responds adequately to suffering; advance strategies that support caregivers and health care providers; and promote needed change by cultivating educational programmes

It is reassuring to note that these suggestions are already being considered in the UK but there are further advances to be made. Formal training in children's palliative care, though increasing, is not yet widely available – this is one key area for future development and the application of standards (ACT 2007b).

Additionally, analysis of causes of death for those between the ages of 0 and 30 reveals that around 22% were causes likely to have required palliative care. It is also clear that medical advancements and supportive interventions are increasing the life expectancy in some conditions that would previously have only been the remit of a paediatric unit. Excellent transitional care for those young people who survive into adulthood is a key objective in the evolution of paediatric palliative care. It is pertinent to conclude with some words from the Department of Health's recent 'Better care: better lives' document (2008, p. 15) which summarises the ethos and the practice of paediatric palliative care:

'The time span of many children's illnesses may mean that palliative care extends over many years. Moreover, children may continue to develop physically, emotionally and cognitively through the course of their condition, and this affects their health and social needs, as well as their understanding of disease and death. Healthy children and young people mainly live in families and are encouraged to be part of a wider community such as school and religious and recreational groups. The effect of a child or young person having a life-limiting or life-threatening condition impacts not only on the child themselves, but also on the whole family and the wider communities in which they live. This impact should not be underestimated.'

(DoH 2008, p. 15)

References

ACH (Association of Children's Hospices), ACT (Association for Children with Life-Threatening or Terminal Conditions) NCHSPCS (2001) *Joint Briefing: Palliative Care for Children*. London: National Council for Hospice and Specialist Palliative Care Services.

ACT (Association for Children's Palliative Care) and the Royal College of Paediatrics and Child Health (RCPCH) (2003) Children's palliative care: descriptions and definitions. Available at www.act.org.uk.

ACT (2003) A guide to the development of children's palliative care services. Available at www.act.org.uk.

ACT (2007a) Children's palliative care and adult palliative care: similarities and differences. Available at www.act.org.uk.

ACT (2007b) Curriculum in paediatric palliative medicine. Available at www.act.org.uk.

Asthana A (2007) Meet Tyran and Leanne. *The Observer*, 7th October 2007.

Barrie JM (1993) *Peter Pan*. London: Wordsworth Editions Ltd.

Bouffet E (1997) Schooling as a part of palliative care in paediatric oncology. *Palliative Medicine*. 11(2):133–139.

Brown E and Warr B (2007) *Supporting the Child and the Family in Paediatric Palliative Care*. London: Jessica Kingsley.

Davy J and Ellis S (2000) *Counselling Skills in Palliative Care*. Buckingham: Open University Press.

Department of Health (2008) Better care: better lives. Available at www.dh.gov.uk/publications.

Doyle D (2005) Palliative medicine: the first eighteen years of a new subspecialty of general medicine. *Journal of the Royal College of Physicians of Edinburgh.* 35:199–205.

Every Child Matters: Change for Children (2004). Available at www.everychildmatters.gov.uk.

Every Disabled Child Matters (EDCM) (2008) Available at www.edcm.org.uk.

Goldman A (1998) ABC of palliative care: special problems of children. *British Medical Journal.* 316:49–52.

Hoyle L (2007) Hansard. Available at www.parliament.uk.

Liben S, Papadatou D and Wolfe J (2008) Paediatric palliative care: challenges and emerging ideas. *Lancet.* 371(9615): 852–864.

Meyer EC, Ritholz M, Burns J and Truog R (2006) Improving the quality of end of life care in the pediatric intensive care unit: parents' priorities and recommendations. *Pediatrics.* 117:649–657.

NICE (2004) Palliative and supportive care for adults with cancer. *The Economic Review.* London: DoH.

Piaget J (1929) *The Child's Conception of the World.* London: Routledge.

Potts S (2005) *Everylife: Death, Bereavement and Life Through the Eyes of Children, Parents and Practitioners.* Wiltshire: APS Publishers.

Potts S (2007) Spirituality in paediatric palliative care: communicating ethically with dying children. *Ethical Space: The International Journal of Communication Ethics.* 3(4):10–14.

Turner M (2006) *Talking with Children and Young People about Death and Dying* (2nd edition). London: Jessica Kingsley.

Worswick J (2000) *A House called Helen* (2nd edition). Oxford: Oxford University Press.

Websites

www.chas.org.uk

www.childbereavement.org.uk

The Child Bereavement Charity (CBC) provides specialised support, information and training to all those affected when a baby or child dies, or when a child is bereaved.

www.childdeathhelpline.org.uk

The Child Death Helpline is a helpline for anyone affected by the death of a child of any age, from prebirth to adult, under any circumstances, however recently or long ago.

www.childhoodbereavementnetwork.org.uk

The Childhood Bereavement Network (CBN) is a national, multi-professional federation of organisations and individuals working with bereaved children and young people. It involves and is actively supported by all the major bereavement care providers in the UK.

www.winstonswish.org.uk

Winston's Wish helps children rebuild their lives after the death of a parent or sibling, enabling them to face the future with hope. We offer practical support and guidance to families, professionals and anyone concerned about a grieving child. We want children to avoid the problems that can occur in later life if they are unable to express their grief.

Chapter 16

Challenges of providing paediatric palliative care in the hospital setting

Jane Belmore

Introduction

This chapter discusses the unique issues which arise when paediatric palliative care is delivered in a hospital setting. It begins with a discussion of some of the general issues encountered, but concentrates on care planning for dying children. Areas covered include physical, psychological, spiritual and cultural needs. The chapter concludes with an examination of the special challenges faced by the team providing palliative care to children and young people in hospital.

Learning outcomes

Once you have read this chapter and completed the associated practice points, you will be able to:

- Discuss the principal issues around delivering paediatric palliative care in a hospital setting
- Discuss the principal components of a care plan for a dying child
- Identify the unique challenges facing the paediatric nurse providing palliative care in hospital

General issues around providing paediatric palliative care in a hospital setting

Successful paediatric palliative care demands that all providers work together to provide seamless services matched to the needs of medically vulnerable young people and their families (Brown 2007). Frequently, the move to palliative care is gradual, so that rather than a discernible shift of emphasis, there is an evolving change. However, many factors can act as obstacles to the adoption of a palliative care model (Hicks and Lavender 2001; Hilden et al. 2001). However, Stevens (2005) suggests that a smooth transition to palliative care can be achieved if good communication and support are experienced by the family from an early stage in the child's illness.

Whatever the journey into palliation entails, this is clearly a distressing time for the family and can prove difficult for the care team as they negotiate the way forward. To move from a 'curative' to 'palliative' phase can be very difficult for some professionals, especially in the hospital setting. The care plan now requires to reflect this change in circumstances and be tailored to the needs of the child and family. It requires taking into account their physical, emotional, spiritual and cultural needs. Professionals must acknowledge that the parents are the experts in their own child – they know their child's likes and dislikes, their daily care requirements and also their medical care.

Excellent communication and listening skills are essential in order to enter into meaningful discussion with families. Poor communication can inflict profound, long-term and personal damage on the child and family. The provision of information by a skilled professional must take into account the emotional and cognitive state of the parents. Previous studies have shown that although 95% of parents attended a discussion with their doctor about the child's prognosis, only 50% realised that the child had no chance of cure (Wolfe et al. 2000).

In order to achieve meaningful discussions, the children need to receive accurate, age-appropriate information in a clear language and at a pace that they can control (Hicks and Lavender 2001). Younger children, for example, will require simple explanations and exploration through play. Older children may need the opportunity to spend time alone with medical or nursing staff to allow deeper questioning and discussion. An environment where a child is able to express worries and concerns is consequently invaluable (Vickers and Carlisle 2000).

One of the major challenges in paediatric palliative care is the issue of communication between all the professionals who may be involved in a child's care and the family and child. Coordination, understanding of roles, developing of relationships and assessing which services are appropriate and bringing them all together can be confusing and time-consuming. Members of the team need to understand their own and other member's roles and respect those with different knowledge and experience. The identification of an appropriate person to act as key worker and as a co-coordinator is one suggestion to achieve effective teamwork to meet the palliative care needs of the child and of the family. This has been strongly recommended within palliative care documents (Yerbury 1997). Historically, especially within the hospital setting this has been the child's consultant; however, he or she may not be the most appropriate person when palliative care when required.

Care planning for the dying child in hospital

Planning for the physical needs of the dying child

When a transition is made from curative to palliative care in the hospital setting, there are practical issues that need to be addressed. Some of these may prove to be quite challenging for both staff and the family and will need to be addressed sensitively. Things may need to be changed gradually to allow time for readjustment. Allowances should be made when allocating staff to care for the child. Of all health professionals, nurses are in the most immediate position to provide care and comfort, and counsel patients and families (Mitka 2000).

Practice Point 16.1

Make a list of changes in the physical care of the child which are likely to be required as the emphasis of care shifts from curative to palliative. These will mainly be measures intended to promote physical comfort and respond to deterioration in the child's physical condition.

Commentary :

Specific issues that need to be considered are as follows:

- A 'Do not Resuscitate' (DNR) form may have to be completed by the consultant in charge. All hospitals will have a local policy for this which ensures that parents are fully informed and involved in the decision-making process
- Current medication will require to be reviewed with non-essentials being discontinued. The focus has changed to the child's present condition and some medications may now be inappropriate
- Other inappropriate interventions (e.g. recording of vital signs and oxygen saturation monitoring) should be discontinued
- The bed used by the child should be appropriate for his or her condition and if not, a new bed should be ordered
- Issues of feeding will require to be reviewed. Both families and staff will have to face the challenge of responding to changing nutritional requirements as the disease progresses (Thompson 2006). Decisions about whether feeding interventions should be begun, and if so, for how long, and with what aims, as well as decisions about whether to withdraw, will be required to be made
- Adequate oral care is of vital importance to ensure the mouth is kept clean and moist
- Urinary output will be monitored and in cases of urinary retention a catheter may need to be inserted for the child's comfort

- Although the patient is expected to die, the timing can be difficult to predict, so bowel care needs to continue with suppositories or enemas being used if required

(Royal Hospital for Sick Children 2008)

The family may be willing to participate in some or all of these comfort measures for their child and it is important that they are allowed to do so. If siblings are present, they may also be included, depending on their age and ability.

Symptom control

Expected symptoms should be discussed with the family and child as appropriate and dealt with as they arise, with intervention being as rapid as possible in order that these symptoms do not become distressing. This can prove to be very challenging in a busy hospital setting and can lead to conflict between staff and parents. Therefore, pain control should be discussed openly with the family, as this is often the symptom that parents dread most (McGrath and Brown 2005). Routes of administration need to be reviewed and often analgesia will be given either intravenously or subcutaneously. The use of the World Health Organization (1990) analgesic ladder as described in detail in Chapter 8 (heart failure) is used managing pain in children, along with specific adjuvants that focus on neuropathic systems (McGrath and Brown 2005). The hospital pain control team can be invaluable in these situations to provide advice and support. Other symptoms including nausea and vomiting, increased respiratory secretions, seizures and terminal agitation can be very distressing for the family to witness. The goal here is to continuously assess symptoms and manage in accordance of the wishes of the child and family (Goldman and Burne 1994).

Admission to hospital inevitably may involve interaction with a greater number of health care professionals than in the community, while subtle differences in treatment approach or explanation can result in confusion and lack of trust (Contro et al. 2002). Ideally, a symptom control plan will be put in place with drugs and doses prescribed in advance of symptoms arising. Many hospitals are now developing their own end of life care pathways for symptom control, and the *Oxford Textbook of Palliative Care for Children* is an invaluable resource in this respect.

Care of the family

The nurse looking after the child must be sensitive to support the needs of parents and families, particularly around the transition from a curative to palliative approach. Later, the nurse may also be responsible for ensuring that the family are prepared for the child or young person's imminent death and advise them of what signs to look out for (i.e. changes in colour, breathing and conscious level).

The needs of the family require to be accommodated with offers of food and drink, offers to sit with the child if they want a break and offering time to talk. Some discussion needs to take place with the family about what they want their child to be told, especially if the child is older and aware of what is happening. The needs of the siblings also need to be addressed and explanations given appropriate to age and understanding.

If English is not the family's first language, it is extremely important to ascertain the family understands what is happening, and, if necessary, an interpreter should be booked when any discussions are taking place.

As already stated, discussions should have taken place with the family so that no resuscitation measures are attempted when the child dies. This needs to be clearly conveyed to all staff who are involved in the child's care. The nurse attending the child needs to remain calm and confident at the time of death, as the family will be looking to them for support and there is no way of predicting how families will react. The needs of parents are often overlooked, misinterpreted, minimised or underestimated by many health care professionals. This is often as a result poor knowledge and understanding regarding parents' grief reactions and the impact that health care professionals' interventions have on bereaved parents (Davies 2001). The family should be given as much time and privacy as they require to carry out the rituals that they view as important. When possible a member of staff should explain the procedure following death to parents, including the fact that their child can be returned home if they wish (Curnick and Harris 2000).

Responding to spiritual and cultural needs

Spirituality and spiritual care are the proper concern of all who work with dying children and their families. It must be recognised that spirituality and religion are very important to a number of people. However, they are two different aspects of care to consider:

1. Spirituality is what gives a person's life meaning, how he views the world he finds himself in and this may or may not include a 'God' or religious conviction
2. Religious care relates more to the practical expression of spirituality through a framework of beliefs, often pursued through rituals and receiving of sacraments

(Francis 2006).

Practice Point 16.2

What spiritual care services are available for children with life-limiting diseases and their families in hospital? How can these services be tailored to meet the needs of people from a range of belief systems and none? What is the role of the paediatric nurse in providing spiritual care?

Commentary:

Each child and each family are unique; they come into hospital with different backgrounds and different life experiences. For many families this will be their first experience of death and how it is handled will have a lasting impression on each member of that family. They may well then express 'existential distress' where they question why such an event has happened to them. The child may also ask questions about spiritual issues such as 'how will I die' which can be extremely upsetting for families and professional caregivers. However, good spiritual care allows the professional carer to journey along with each dying child and their family by providing comfort, support and the opportunity to try and make sense of their situation (Davies et al. 2002).

Supporting a child as they approach death can be made even more difficult if the assumption is made that the child is too young to understand what is happening to them. However, substantial literature is now available to show how and when children develop their concepts of death. For instance, in a study of 105 children aged between 5 and 9 years, Lansdown and Benjamin (1985) discovered that 60% of 5-year-olds, 70% of 6-year-olds, 66% of 7-year-olds and nearly 100% of 8–9 year olds had a complete or almost complete understanding of death. Newer literature continues to support this finding and suggests that with the ill child professionals are able to assess their psychological adaptation through art, music and books, so the team knows exactly what they understand about their illness (Stevens 2005).

The issue of culturally competent care, important in all aspects of health service provision, is particularly important in palliative care where alliances between professional caregivers and families are crucial to the delivery of the care (Randhawa et al. 2003). As our society becomes increasingly diverse, it is difficult for nurses to be aware of the needs of every cultural tradition. However, in the area of palliative care it is vital that nurses act sensitively and appropriately, and not cause additional distress, even by thoughtlessness or ignorance rather than malice. Information about beliefs and practices can easily be accessed through reference books or the Internet, and most hospitals will have this information available through their chaplaincy department. Gentle questioning of relatives will also assist the team in ensuring they provide culturally appropriate care.

Challenges facing the paediatric nurse and the multidisciplinary team providing palliative care in hospital

A large number of communication challenges are faced by those providing paediatric palliative care in a hospital setting.

- These include the breaking of bad news, discussions of limits of care or treatment, resolving conflicts among family members, exploring options for end of life care, interactions with parents at the time of death, pronouncing the death and managing the death certificate, dealing with avoidance of patient and family, finding out about cultural practices and supporting parents from different ethnic and cultural backgrounds (DeVita et al. 2003).

Communication skills, like any others, must be learned and continually updated. It should not be assumed that these skills can be simply 'picked up' in the course of working with children and families. Much has been written on the impact of poor communication with dying patients of all ages and clear guidance has been formulated to ensure professionals converse with patients and families in a holistic way, taking into account their values, beliefs and abilities (Buckman 2000; Judd 2000).

It is also important to consider the effect on the ward team of caring for a dying child in the hospital setting. Good paediatric palliative care should involve realistic goal setting, the recognition of one's limitations and the need for emotional support (Stevens 2005). However, it is acknowledged that a nurse's anxiety about their competence can manifest itself in distancing themselves from the patient and their family. Indeed, Curnick and Harris (2000) suggest that support may help staff recognise these patterns of behaviour and develop strategies to deal with them. Some team members may also have unrealistic expectations of what they are able to achieve and some may become over-involved in the care of the dying child. Therefore, the ward team may benefit from more formal support from either peer supervision or clinical supervision from outside the team. A multi-professional review of the patient's care as soon after death as possible is helpful both as a learning experience and to bring that case to a close. Finally, a good work/life balance is required to maintain the enjoyment in what is a rewarding but often emotionally charged occupation (Stevens 2005).

Conclusion

To ensure optimal palliative care is provided to all dying children and their families being cared for in the hospital setting, everyone involved needs to be working with identical aims and have a mutual acceptance of the inevitability of death. Clear aims and objectives relating to symptom management, family care, spiritual care and care in the terminal phase of life will help to ensure that the palliative phase of an child's illness is managed well by the nursing team and other professionals involved in the child's care.

References

Brown E (2007) *Supporting the Child and the Family in Paediatric Palliative Care*. London: Jessica Kingsley Publishing.

Buckman R (2000) Communication in palliative care: a practical guide. In: Dickenson D, Johnson M and Katz JS (Eds), *Death, Dying and Bereavement* (2nd edition). London: Sage, pp. 146–173.

Contro N, Larson J, Scofield S and Sourkes B (2002) Family perspectives on the quality of paediatric palliative care. *Archives of Paediatric and Adolescent Medicine.* 156(1): 14–19.

Curnick S and Harris A (2000) The dying child. In: Langton H (Ed), *The Child with Cancer: Family Centred Care in Practice*. Edinburgh: Bailliere Tindall, pp. 355–385.

Davies AM (2001) Death of adolescents: parental grief and coping strategies. *British Journal of Nursing*. 10(20):1332–1342.

Davies B, Brenner P, Orloff S, Sumner L and Worden W (2002) Addressing spirituality in pediatric hospice and palliative care. *Journal of Palliative Care*. 18(1):59–67.

DeVita MA, Arnold RM and Barnard D (2003) Teaching palliative care to critical care medicine trainees. *Critical Care Medicine*. 31(41):1257–1262.

Francis BR (2006) The spiritual life. In: Goldman A, Hain R and Liben S (Eds) *The Oxford Textbook of Palliative Care for Children*. Oxford: Oxford University Press, pp. 74–84.

Goldman A and Burne R (1994) Symptom management. In: Goldman A (Ed), *Care of the Dying Child*. Oxford: Oxford Medical Press, pp. 52–75.

Hicks MD and Lavender R (2001) Psychosocial practice trends in paediatric oncology. *Journal of Paediatric Oncology Nursing*. 18(4):143–153.

Hilden J, Emanuel EJ, Fairclough DL, Link MP, Foley KM, Clarridge BC, Schnipper LE and Mayer RJ (2001) Attitudes and practices among pediatric oncologist regarding end-of-life care: results of the 1998 American Society of Clinical Oncology Survey. *Journal of Clinical Oncology*. 19(1):205–212.

Judd D (2000) Communicating with dying children. In: Dickenson D, Johnson M and Katz JS. *Death, Dying and Bereavement* (2nd edition). London: Sage, pp. 176–182.

Lansdown R and Benjamin G (1985) The development of the concept of death in children aged 5–9 yrs. *Child: Care, Health and Development*. 11(1):13–20.

McGrath PA and Brown SC (2005) Paediatric palliative medicine; pain control. In: Doyle D, Hanks G, Cherny N and Calman K (Eds). *Oxford Textbook of Palliative Medicine* (3rd edition). Oxford: Oxford University Press, pp. 775–778.

Mitka M (2000) Suggestions for help when the end is near. *Journal of the American Medical Association*. 284(19):2441–2442.

Randhawa G, Owens A, Fitches R and Khan Z (2003) Communication in the development of culturally competent palliative care services in the UK: a case study. *International Journal of Palliative Nursing*. 9(1):24–30.

Royal Hospital for Sick Children (2008) *'Care of the Dying Child' Policy*. Glasgow: Royal Hospital for Sick Children.

Stevens MM (2005) Care of the dying child and adolescent: family adjustment and support. In: Doyle D, Hanks G, Cherny N and Calman K (Eds), *Oxford Textbook of Palliative Medicine* (3rd edition). Oxford: Oxford University Press, pp. 806–821.

Thompson A, MacDonald A and Holden C (2006) Feeding and nutrition. In: Goldman A, Hain R and Liben S (Eds), *The Oxford Textbook of Palliative Care for Children*. Oxford: Oxford University Press, 374–386.

Vickers JL and Carlisle C (2000) Choices and control: parental experiences in paediatric terminal home care. *Journal of Paediatric Oncology Nursing*. 17(1):12–21.

Wolfe J, Klar N, Grier HE, Duncan J, Salem-Schatz S, Emanuel EJ and Weeks JC (2000) Understanding of prognosis among parents of children who died of cancer. *Journal of the American Medical Association*. 284(19):2469–2475.

World Health Organization (1990) Cancer pain relief and palliative care. Report of an expert WHO committee. *Technical Support Series 804*. Geneva: WHO.

Yerbury M (1997) Issues in multidisciplinary teamwork for children with disabilities. *Child: Care, Health and Development*. 23(1):77–86.

Chapter 17

Children's palliative care in the hospice and the community

Elizabeth-Anne (Libby) Gold

Introduction

This chapter describes children's hospice care and how other professionals provide specialist and generic paediatric palliative care in the community. It begins by providing a background to the issues before looking first at children's hospices and the service they provide.

Learning outcomes

Once you have read this chapter and completed the associated reflective practice points, you will be able to:

- Discuss the services that children's hospices offer to dying children and their families
- Give examples of the needs dying children and their families in the community
- Describe the different models of palliative care that are available to dying children across the UK

Background

Palliative care for children has evolved over the last 20–30 years as those caring for life-limited children recognise the particular needs of the whole family. For children where there is no cure there has been a recognition of the need to shift the emphasis from the high-tech, invasive investigation and treatment to a style of care that embraces the emotional, psychological and spiritual aspects of a child's life as well as the physical condition (Hain 2002).

'Palliative care for children and young people with life-limiting conditions is an active and total approach to care, embracing physical, emotional, social and spiritual elements. It focuses on enhancement of quality of life for the child and support for the family and includes the management of distressing symptoms, provision of respite and care through death and bereavement.'

(ACT and RCPCH 2003, p. 9)

Children's hospices have a unique style of care that offers practical help and emotional support to the whole family from the day they are referred until the death of their child and beyond. The service has to be flexible to respond to the particular needs of the child, mother, father, brothers and sisters as well as the extended family. It has a home-like atmosphere, accommodation for all the family and a multidisciplinary team. But there are others who provide equally effective care in the community setting.

Children's hospices

Practice Point 17.1

Think about the role of children's hospices in the provision of care for children with life-limiting diseases and their families. What services can children's hospices provide which would otherwise not be available? What areas of expertise can children's hospice teams contribute to overall care provision?

Commentary:

Children's hospices are purpose built and provide most or all of the following to families with children with a life-limiting disease which will cause death in childhood:

- Specialist respite care and emergency care
- Terminal care in the hospice or family home
- Family and bereavement support for the whole family
- Home support
- Friendship, information, advice and practical support for families
- Play and recreation and the opportunity to make the most of life
- Symptom control to provide comfort and aid quality of life

The first children's hospice was opened in 1982 in Oxford by Sister Frances Dominica, an Anglican nun and children's nurse. As she cared for Helen, who as the result of a brain tumour was left with complex nursing needs, she recognised the overwhelming need of her family for respite care and practical support. Sister Frances provided this for the family and they found it beneficial. Recognising that other families in the same position might need this kind of help and recognising that a building was required for this purpose, Helen House was built. This was the first of many children's hospices. The philosophy which guides them is essentially the same as that which inspired Helen House – to embrace flexibility, sensitivity and dignity (Worswick 2000).

In Scotland Rachel House in Kinross opened to children and families in 1996 and Robin House in Balloch followed in 2005. The hospice services are run by the charity, Children's Hospice Association Scotland (CHAS). There are now over 40 children's hospice services in the UK. Although the UK is widely recognised as pioneering the children's hospice movement, there are such services in other parts of the world, for example America, Canada, Australia and Germany (Price et al. 2005).

Although Helen House has been a model for most of the children's hospices, each has developed its own particular character and strengths with some now having close links with an adult hospice or local children's hospitals and others have developed outreach and home care teams or day care facilities. Recently, hospices focusing specifically on the needs of adolescents and young adults have opened (Lenton et al. 2006).

There is no charge to the families who use a children's hospice in the UK. The funding comes largely from charitable donations although the state does provide a percentage of the running costs. The amount and how it is collected from government varies across Scotland, England, Wales and Northern Ireland. In Scotland the Scottish Government when it was known as the Scottish Executive made a strong case for health and social care commissioners to provide 25% of the funding requirements of the children's hospices through service level agreements (George 2005). This has been secured from the Health Boards and is in the process of being negotiated with local authorities.

Children likely to need palliative care

The definition of the term 'life-limiting' is commonly acknowledged as describing those illnesses for which there is no reasonable hope of a cure and from which children and young people will suffer an early death (ACT 2003).

ACT and RCPCH (2003) have categorised the conditions of children or young people that require palliative care. These were described in the previous chapter. However, it is important to note that not all children will need active care all the time – some may have periods of reasonable health whereas others with the same condition may be more vulnerable and the family will require more support (Elston 2003).

Children with congenital abnormalities and babies born early who survive with complex needs may require hospice care (Overton 2001). Rachel and Robin House have cared for neonates with significant cardiac abnormalities not compatible with life which were diagnosed in utero. The families were given support during pregnancy and then after the birth. Through sensitive symptom control in comfortable surroundings they were able to spend what little time they had with their babies.

Relatively few children and young people with cancer are supported by a children's hospice. In 1982 soon after Helen House opened they conducted research finding that only 7% of the young people admitted had cancer-related illnesses (Overton 2001). It is often children suffering from brain tumours that benefit best from hospice care because they tend to have significant disabilities as a result of the disease and/or treatment. When treatment has failed or is not possible the palliative phase is usually longer than for children with other cancers, necessitating the need for support.

Respite care

The degenerative nature of the illnesses the children and young people suffer from result in them being involved with palliative care services for a long time and the fact that many are genetic can result in a family having more than one child with terminal illness (Price et al. 2005). Families therefore require respite services that give them a break from the daily physical strain that caring for a highly dependent individual can bring (Rowse 2006). There is a scarcity of efficient, ongoing respite services that can cope with nursing tasks such as tube feeding, management of seizures and care for children with complex care needs (George 2005; Rowse 2006). Because children's hospices provide accommodation for the whole family where there is 24-hour nursing support and access to specialist medical care, the child or young person can have appropriate care and not have to be separated from the family.

Multidisciplinary working

The complex needs that children and young people with life-limiting conditions have require a multidisciplinary approach. Effective multidisciplinary working requires good communication and sharing of information with the family and all those involved (Elston 2003). Children's hospices have a number of staff of different disciplines, for example physiotherapists, social workers, play specialists, chaplains and occupational therapists.

Occupational therapists will build on the existing skills of the child or young person or find a different technique to maintain a skill such as playing computer games or self-feeding (Tester 2006). Physiotherapists as well as providing relief from chest symptoms also have a valuable role in pain relief through correct positioning and passive movements.

The team members within the hospice each have their own skills; however professional roles overlap and complement each other such as the family support provided by the social worker, chaplain, play specialist and bereavement support worker. They care for, provide advice and can act as an advocate and/or a key worker for families.

Volunteers work closely with the hospice teams and all the departments within CHAS. They offer valuable help in the kitchen and offices and many other areas within the hospice. CHAS currently has 865 volunteers throughout Scotland (from Shetland to Dumfries and Galloway), who in 2007 donated over 73 000 hours of their time. CHAS was the first organisation in Scotland to receive the Investing in Volunteers Award which is an accredited award for quality. The use of highly skilled volunteers is reflected in other children's hospices across the UK.

Symptom control

Children with life-limiting disease usually have symptoms in varying degree of severity throughout their life. Their treatment needs regular adjustment particularly in the terminal phase of the illness.

Most parents say that symptom control and ensuring their child's comfort is vital (Brown 2007a). Paediatric palliative care teams find that administrating opioids and/or benzodiazepines for symptom relief improves the quality of life of affected children and as a result they can live longer than expected and in greater comfort (Friedrichsdorf et al. 2007).

It is always useful to have a plan of action. Although pain, breathlessness or nausea might be associated with an attribute of an illness it is reassuring to know they can be controlled and it allows the parent to continue to parent and support the child through hard times (Frager and Collins 2006).

Pain assessment is really important and although many children with communication problems cannot express their pain verbally their non-verbal signs and behaviours can demonstrate how they feel (Brown 2007a). Pain assessment in children with special needs remains an uncertain and complex process. However, there is now more knowledge on the types of behaviour suggestive of pain in this group, and measurement tools are being developed (Hunt et al. 2004). Distress can be caused by a variety of different factors including psychological, social and spiritual aspects; it is therefore best to observe the child carefully and take note of what the parents say (Brown 2007a).

Sibling support

Siblings require specialist care. Brothers and sisters of life-limited children may grow up in an abnormal environment (Brown 2007b). They often have to make sacrifices because of their brother or sister's illness which can cause resentment. They may feel guilty that they are well and their brother or sister is not. Siblings do not always receive the same support as their parents or their ill brother or sister (Zirinsky 1994). They often need someone of their own age and/or in the same position as them to talk to. Visits to a children's hospice can provide such opportunities. Siblings support groups can provide an environment to encourage siblings to express their fears and emotions in a safe place (Overton 2001).

Care of young people

Statistical evidence available from children's hospices shows that between 26 and 54% of their clients are in their teenage years (Thornes 2001). With improved care and medical technology to support their needs children are surviving longer into teenage years and young adulthood. This gives rise to particular needs. Young people begin to gain some independence from their families as they grow older but for those with terminal illness with progressive symptoms resulting in complex nursing needs they become more dependent. Children's hospices have long since provided care for teenagers recognising that they have different needs from children, for example by staging specialist teenage weekends when parents do not usually stay and providing youth workers and social workers with the specialist skills for communicating and understanding this age group.

Some of these young people outgrow the services of a children's hospice. Adult hospices that mostly care for those with cancer and the elderly are not suitable (Rowse 2006). Children's hospice services are, therefore, evaluating the kind of care they provide for young adults and looking at the alternatives. Helen House in 2004 opened Douglas House a 'respice' for the care of young people aged 16–40 years (Rowse 2006) and Acorns in Walsall have incorporated an adolescent unit into their service (Overton 2001).

Bereavement support

Losing a child has been considered as the most painful of all bereavements; parents have said that the experience is like having part of them removed (Brown 2008). Ruth Davies (2005) conducted a small-scale study of 10 mothers who had lost a child in either hospital, home or in a children's hospice. Their stories reflect a need for time, space and privacy with their dying child and their child's body after death. A children's hospice has the facility of a special bedroom that can be specially cooled in order for a child or young person to remain in the hospice until the funeral. The mothers of those children who were in the special bedroom described how they and their families furnished the room with toys, photographs and their child's duvet. One mother also took her child out into the private garden. The opportunity for a slow and gentle separation from their child's body provided them with bittersweet memories that were a contrast to the distressing memories of the mothers who had little chance to be with their child's body because it was quickly removed to the hospital mortuary. This study recommends that hospitals should have good standards of accommodation for families within the hospital when it is known a child is dying and a special bedroom to allow unhurried time with their child's body after death.

Memories are a vital link for bereaved parents and talking about their child who has died makes the death real. They need people who recognise that the bond they have with their child is an ongoing relationship (Brown 2008). Children's hospices facilitate this through a variety of support mechanisms. Families can come together in groups to share their experiences under the guidance of hospice social workers and staff who are experienced in sibling support. Group and individual support can help foster coping mechanisms. The CHAS bereavement service use a change and loss peer support programme called Seasons for Growth (www.seasonsforgrowth.co.uk) from Australia. It is licensed to the Notre Dame Centre (www.notredamecentre.org.uk) in Glasgow which is a registered charity that provides assessment and treatment of emotionally disturbed children, young people and their families, and training and consultancy to parents and professionals (Kennedy et al. 2008). Seasons for Growth trains companions who regularly work with children to facilitate small groups of people experiencing change and loss to work through their own grief and support each other (Kennedy et al. 2008).

Most children's hospices have a remembering day or memorial day when bereaved families are invited back to the hospice for the purpose of remembering their dead child, meeting up with other families and talking to staff that cared for their child.

Children's palliative care in the community

Although hospices offer a valuable service, for the majority of time children with prolonged terminal illness are cared for at home by their families. They therefore need guidance and support from community based professionals who are willing to work with them in a collaborative way (Steele 2002).

> **Practice Point 17.2**
>
> Think about the pressures faced by the family of a child living at home with a life-limiting illness. Make a list of the support needs that a family might have. What are some of the ways in which services could be organised to ensure those needs are met?

Commentary:

It is likely, until the terminal stages of the illness, that families will spend only a small percentage of time in the hospice. It is also recognised that the home is the most preferred and comfortable place for children to die (Sentilhes-Monkam et al. 2003). Providing support for the family of a child with a life-threatening condition is a highly challenging aspect of health service delivery (Andrews and Hood 2003). In their approach to caring for children with complex needs practitioners have tended to work separately which has resulted in fragmented service provision (Warr 2007). However, it has been recognised that a more holistic and coherent approach is required in service provision (DoH 2008; Scottish Government 2008) and agencies have committed to working more collaboratively with families and with each other (Warr 2007).

Many of the children's hospices provide community support. Helen House was built principally to provide respite care whereas Acorns in the West Midlands incorporated community support and Martin House in Yorkshire was the first children's hospice to develop an outreach service which became the blueprint for other organisations (Overton 2001).

CHAS offers home support to families across Scotland. The services are based at the two hospices and a small service based in the north of Scotland that was originally funded by the New Opportunity Fund or Big Lottery Fund as it is now known. The home care from the two hospices is provided by multidisciplinary staff from within the care team. The service in the north of Scotland provides non-nursing practical and bereavement support to families in their own homes on an individual basis and also offers support to families on a group basis through social events they call 'ceilidhs'. The staff link closely with the children's community nursing team and other services in the Highlands.

The home care service was developed in 1999 to be responsive to family need but not to duplicate existing service provision or remove the responsibilities from the statutory service for local provision. The aim of home support is to:

- Work alongside the family in a way that best suits them
- Provide care for a set period of time in order to allow local services to organise appropriate care
- Act as an advocate for the family to secure appropriate care
- Provide crisis care in situations such as when the child/young person is particularly unwell, or if another member of the family is unwell or if there is a problem with the child's usual home care
- Provide care in the final stages of a child's/young person's life
- Support the family if the child/young person is in hospital
- Facilitate fun activities e.g. taking a young person to the ballet or to see a favourite band
- Facilitate children to get home after long periods in hospital
- Support carers from the statutory service when they are first introduced to a family
- Provide professional advice to families

The service has its limitations as CHAS covers the whole of Scotland. It can be difficult to support families who live outwith the central belt particularly in end of life situations where there might be a lack of supportive medical and nursing care to work in partnership with the hospice team. The service in the Highlands was evaluated recently and was found by families and professionals outwith CHAS to be a unique and flexible service. However, the size of the team was thought to be too small resulting in a lack of service capacity. CHAS has therefore made the decision to develop the home care service to meet the need more effectively. Sharing care with hospital, hospice and home is an ideal situation. Andrews and Hood (2003) describe a model of care where children and young people have been able to be discharged home from hospital using the hospice as a stepping stone. The 'hospice at home' team have then worked in partnership with local community staff once the child or young person is at home.

New opportunity fund (NOF)

NOF has funded a number of other palliative care services for children across the UK. In 2002 NOF offered £40 million for the development of paediatric palliative care services. The aims were to:

- Extend or create home-based palliative care teams for children with life-limiting or life-threatening conditions, building on the work of the Diana Community Nursing Teams
- Increase the overall provision of home-based palliative care and bereavement services in areas where access is limited
- Sustain or develop existing good quality provision in hospices

(NOF 2002)

Professionals and Carers Together (PACT) developed through NOF funding. The service was established in 2004 and aims to increase in quality and quantity the provision of respite to children with life-threatening and life-limiting illness and complex health and social care needs in Ayrshire and Arran. Child health care workers work with and are supported by the Community Paediatric Team and enhance the local authority services that provide existing services.

The Winchester Paediatric Palliative Care Team were also funded in this way and shaped their service around the child and family (Rowse 2006). They are also supported by the community children's nursing team which allows for integration of care and additional support for the team members. Other teams in the surrounding areas of Salisbury, Southampton, Portsmouth and Basingstoke have different models of provision, for example respite in the home, clinical nursing support, mental health professionals, play therapists, nursery nurses and social and financial expertise. A small local clinical network has therefore been established to ensure quality and share good practice.

Oxfordshire secured the funding to extend existing specialist children's palliative care to provide a 7 days a week, 24 hours a day service (Brombley 2006). Although Oxford had a wide range of services which could be involved in the care of a child with life-limiting illness none had the capacity to support a child at home out of hours. These services were integrated to create a service available for children (0–18) with community children's nurses, a lead nurse who provides a single point of contact, 24-hour medical support from the Helen House doctors as backup to the community children's nurses and other Oxfordshire health care professionals. There is also access to 24-hour medical palliative care assessment and treatment at Helen House and use of their 'Little Room' – the refrigerated special bedroom.

These services have audited favourably indicating that they are beneficial to families and other professionals in providing support, information and a prompt response to queries and problems. Children have been able to remain at home during acute illness instead of going into hospital and children have been brought home to die at their and their parent's request.

Paediatric oncology outreach

Children and young people with cancer who require terminal care and want to be at home are usually cared for by the hospital oncology outreach nurses (Brewis 2000). They will have supported the family from diagnosis and throughout active treatment providing hands on care, teaching and liaising with the community and hospital staff. These nurses enable the child to return to school and other activities during remission, reducing their involvement as active treatment is completed. At relapse, contact is re-established with the child and family and other relevant agencies.

During terminal care the nurse supports the family to do as much of the child's care as they wish and are able to do. They coordinate input from other services and support the family into bereavement. Establishing terminal care at home requires a community multidisciplinary and multi-agency meeting to identify who will do what and when in order to ensure continuity of care. There needs to be a continuous review of progress and professional motivations. This model of allowing the specialist medical and nursing expertise to be taken from the hospital to the child is usually described as the 'oncology' model because it happens in most paediatric oncology centres in the UK (Hain 2002).

Diana nurses (England)

The Diana, Princess of Wales, Memorial Committee agreed funding to develop a palliative care team with nursing, physiotherapy, respite care, bereavement support and any other services that might be pertinent in a local area. Professionals were invited to apply for the money. Many of these services now have statutory funding and have developed beyond their original form to provide a multiprofessional approach for families (Rowse 2006).

Community children's nurses

This service has evolved rapidly since the 1990s and most areas now have a team that will care for children in the community with a wide range of health care needs. Many of these teams provide care for children with acute and chronic conditions and for children who are ventilator-assisted or technology dependent (Myers 2005). These services aim to bring nursing care to sick children in their own homes, preventing and minimising children's stay in hospital (Walmsley 2006). Children's community nurses spend a significant amount of time, in partnership with other professionals, supporting children and families when a child is dying and after a child has died (Tuffrey et al. 2007).

Conclusion

Different disciplines have developed different models of care to achieve a style of care that recognises the holistic needs of children where there is no cure (Hain

2002). Children's hospices provide a rounded service for families, but they are there to augment statutory provision so it is best when there is collaborative working between all agencies including hospices, the community and hospitals.

References

Andrews F and Hood P (2003) Shared care: hospital, hospice, home. *Paediatric Nursing*. 15(6):20–22.

Association for Children with Life-threatening or Terminal Conditions and their Families (ACT) and Royal College of Paediatrics and Child Health (RCPCH) (2003) *A Guide to the Development of Children's Palliative Care Services* (2nd edition). Bristol: ACT.

Brewis E (2000) Oncology outreach history in the making. *Paediatric Nursing*. 16(9):24–27.

Brombley L (2006) Children's integrated palliative care services, Oxfordshire. *Linchpin* 9(1):2.

Brown E (2007a) Managing children's pain. In: Brown E (Ed), *Supporting the Child and the Family in Paediatric Palliative Care*. London: Jessica Kingsley Publishers, pp. 49–58.

Brown E (2007b) Working with siblings of life-limited children. In: Brown E (Ed), *Supporting the Child and the Family in Paediatric Palliative Care*. London: Jessica Kingsley Publishers, pp. 144–154.

Brown E (2008) Continuing parenting a child after their death. *Linchpin*. 11(1):12–13.

Davies R (2005) Mother's stories of loss: their need to be with their dying child and their child's body after death. *Journal of Health Care*. 9(4):288–300.

Department of Health (2008) *Better Care, Better Lives – Paediatric Palliative Care Strategy*. London: DoH.

Elston S (2003) *A Guide to Effective Care Planning Assessment of Children with Life-Limiting Conditions and their Families*. Bristol: Association for Children with Life-threatening or Terminal Conditions and their Families (ACT).

Frager G and Collins JJ (2006) Symptoms in life-threatening illness: overview and assessment. In: Goldman A, Hain R and Liben S (Eds), *Oxford Textbook of Palliative Care for Children*. Oxford: Oxford University Press, pp. 233–247.

Friedrichsdorf SJ, Remke S, Symalla B, Gibbon C and Chrastek J (2007) Developing a pain and palliative care programme at a US children's hospital. *International Journal of Palliative Nursing*. 13(11):534–542.

George M (2005) A home from home. *Children Now* 21st Sept. 22–23.

Hain R (2002) The view from a bridge. *European Journal of Palliative Care*. 9(2):75–77.

Hunt A, Goldman A, Seers K, Chrichton N, Mastroyannopoulou K, Moffat V, Oulton K and Brady M (2004) Clinical validation of the paediatric pain profile. *Developmental Medicine and Child Neurology*. 46(1):9–18.

Kennedy C, McIntyre R, Worth A and Hogg R (2008) Supporting children and families facing the death of a parent: part 1. *International Journal of Palliative Nursing*. 14(4):162–168.

Lenton S, Goldman A, Eaton N and Southall D (2006) Development and epidemiology. In: Goldman A, Hain R and Liben S (Eds), *Oxford Textbook of Palliative Care for Children*. Oxford: Oxford University Press, pp. 3–13.

Myers J (2005) Community children's services in the 21st century. *Paediatric Nursing*. 17(2):31–34.

New Opportunity Fund (2002) *Community Palliative Care – Children*. London: NOF.

Overton J (2001) The development of children's hospices in the UK. *European Journal of Palliative Care.* 8(1):30–33.

Price J, McNeilly P and McFarlane M (2005) Paediatric Palliative Care in the UK: past, present and future. *International Journal of Palliative Nursing.* 11(3):124–126.

Rowse V (2006) Home-based palliative care for children: the case for funding. *Paediatric Nursing.* 18(7):20–24.

Scottish Government (2008) *National Delivery Plan for Children and Young People's Specialist Services in Scotland. Draft for Consultation.* Edinburgh: Scottish Government.

Sentilhes-Monkham A, Limagne MP, Bercovitz A and Serryn D (2003) Caring for terminally ill children in the home setting. *European Journal of Palliative Care.* 10(5):209–211.

Steele RG (2002) Experiences of families in which a child has a prolonged terminal illness: modifying factors. *International Journal of Palliative Nursing.* 8(9):418–434.

Tester C (2006) Occupational therapy and paediatric oncology. In: Cooper J (Ed), *Occupational Therapy in Oncology and Palliative Care.* Chichester: Whurr Publishers Limited, pp. 107–124.

Thornes R (2001) *Palliative Care for Young People Aged 13–24 Years.* Bristol, London and Edinburgh: Published jointly by Association for Children with Life-threatening or terminal Conditions and their Families (ACT), National Council for Hospice and Specialist Palliative Care Services, and Scottish Partnership Agency for Palliative and Cancer Care (SPAPCC).

Tuffrey C, Finlay F and Lewis M (2007) The needs of children and their families at end of life: an analysis of community nursing practice. *International Journal of Palliative Nursing.* 13(1) 64–71.

Walmsley C (2006) Setting up a minor illness and injury service for children up to 5 years. *Paediatric Nursing.* 18(3):30–33.

Warr B (2007) Working collaboratively. In: Brown E (Ed), *Supporting the Child and Family in Paediatric Palliative Care.* London: Jessica Kingsley, pp. 26–37.

Worswick J (2000) *A House Called Helen: The Development of Hospice Care for Children* (2nd edition). Oxford: Oxford University Press.

Zirinsky L (1994) Brothers and sisters. In: Hill L (Ed), *Caring for Dying Children and Their Families.* London: Chapman and Hall, pp. 67–74.

PART THREE

EDUCATION AND RESEARCH

Chapter 18

Palliative nursing education and continuing professional development

Elaine Stevens

Introduction

This chapter discusses issues relating to palliative care education and the role of continuing professional education, including the roles of specialist and advanced practice. It begins by providing an overview of palliative care education before reviewing the current thinking in terms of the subjects that should be contained within a palliative care educational initiative and also the different educational levels programmes that should be delivered. The last section of the chapter focuses on professional development, looking at the different levels of nursing practice and the roles of different nurses working within specialist palliative care.

Learning outcomes

Once you have read this chapter and completed the associated practice points, you will be able to:

- Discuss the competencies required by nurses in order to provide both general and specialist palliative care
- Describe the palliative care courses that are available in your own local area
- Discuss your own learning needs and what you need to do to ensure you are competent to practice the level of palliative care delivered within your role

Background

In keeping with other palliative care services, education on care of the dying began within the hospice movement. Indeed, much of the early work of Cicely Saunders was educating other professionals about the ethos of hospice care (Clark 2002). As new hospices developed across the UK in the 1970s and

1980s it was recognised that hospice professionals required the knowledge and skills to ensure patients and families were cared for using the current under-pinning evidence. To this end many hospices developed their own in-house education to meet these needs. Many of the educators within the hospices at this time were nurse teachers who had moved from teaching within colleges of nursing. These educators not only recognised the benefits of palliative care education for the multi-professional hospice team but also acknowledged that it was nurses who had most contact with the dying patient. Therefore, the focus of much of the education provided by hospices was directed at the nursing team.

The importance of end of life care was also recognised to be a fundamental nursing skill by the Royal College of Nursing (RCN) that developed a Care of the Terminally Ill nursing group in 1984 (RCN 1994). In conjunction with nurse leaders and policy makers this group began promoting good practice in end of life care. One facet of this was to encourage new educational initiatives for nurses to allow them to meet each dying patient's needs. By the end of the 1980s a number of nursing courses were available within colleges of nursing that led to a palliative care qualification which could be registered with nursing's professional body. These qualifications allowed nurses to gain more specialised posts within the field of care of the dying and continued until the dissolution of the national boards. The advent of the Specialist Practitioner Qualification also allowed nurses wishing to practice at a higher level to do so by receiving education which was not only accredited by the professional body but also had academic credits attached to it (Wallace 1999).

By the mid 1990s the political landscape had changed and it was evident that palliative care should also be available to dying people in care settings other than hospices (Expert Advisory Group on Cancer 1995). Hospices there-fore began to provide more study days and short courses for nurses involved in care of the dying from other institutions and from primary care. However, with the move of nurse training into higher education, palliative care learn-ing for nurses continued to evolve and many hospices sought accreditation for their courses. As nurses needed to prove that the education they had un-dertaken met agreed standards, now today we see that many palliative care course are delivered by the expert hospice team while students receive aca-demic accreditation for their learning from their local university. Other edu-cational models now also exist and a number of universities have their own palliative care programmes. Many of these courses are delivered by hospice professionals, under the guidance of the university team, while other universi-ties offer joint appointments between themselves and the hospice or specialist palliative care team to ensure the clinical credibility of their courses. With the development of post registration standards of education nurses have to confirm that they have undertaken education pertinent to their practice (Wallace 1999). To meet these standards a number of palliative care educational model have evolved.

But what of the pre-registration nursing student?

So far we have shown that palliative care education for post-registration nurses has evolved to meet the needs of the dying patient; however, there is still some dubiety on how much palliative care education is provided in the undergraduate curriculum (Sherman et al. 2004). As these are our nurses of the future they need to be provided with education that allows the provision of high-quality, individualised, holistic end of life care and as such palliative care education should be integrated more fully into the undergraduate nursing programme (Paice et al. 2007). Indeed Paice et al. (2007) go on to say that well-trained nurses have the greatest potential to transform the delivery of care within organisations. Therefore, the palliative care education of our student nurses is of paramount importance and we need to ensure that they receive the education that will equip them with the knowledge and skills required to provide high-quality palliative care as and when it is required.

In conclusion as palliative nursing continues to evolve, so will the educational initiatives that are required to allow nurses to practice at different levels thus ensuring patients and families receive the palliative care they require, regardless of diagnosis or place of care. This chapter now proceeds to discuss the current thinking that underpins best practice in palliative care education at the time of writing.

Palliative nursing education

The provision of general palliative care is now seen as an integral clinical skill within national documents (Department of Health (DoH) 2000; National Institute of Clinical Excellence (NICE) 2004; Scottish Executive Health Department (SEHD) 2001) and as such all nurses working in clinical areas where patients die need to have the knowledge and skills to do so. This means that everyone in the nursing team, from the support worker to the most senior nurse, needs to be equipped with the knowledge and skills of the palliative care approach so that they can provide quality palliative care within their own clinical role. It is also known that nurses working in specialist palliative care require education which is suited to higher levels of practice and which meets standards for specialist palliative care provision (Clinical Standards Board for Scotland 2002; Welsh Assembly Government 2005). This means that those practicing in specialist areas or in a specialist role require more in-depth education to meet the needs of what might be a more complex patient population. This section of the chapter reviews the current ideas in terms of the content of palliative care courses and the professional and academic level that initiatives should be delivered at. This will help educators to develop initiatives which meet the needs of nurses working in different areas where palliative care is provided. It will also help the individual nurse to select courses in their own locality which provide education that meets current palliative care educational standards.

> **Practice Point 18.1**
>
> Before reading the next section make a list of the topics you think should be included in a palliative care course.

Commentary:

Keep your list to hand as you read the next section. As the topics you have listed come up tick them off. You may find you have others on your list that are not incorporated into the broad headings of the documents reviewed. If this is the case you could review the finer content of the documents further. Here are the contact details for the three main documents:

- ISNCC – email: secretariat@isncc.org
- EAPC Taskforce – http://www.eapcnet.org/download/forTaskforces/NurseEducationGuide.pdf
- West of Scotland Managed Clinical Network for Palliative Care – http://www.palliativecareglasgow.info/pdf/Education_Competencies_Final_Version_24_March_06.doc

The main point of this exercise is to allow to choose a course that contains subjects you require for your practice and that is in keeping with current best evidence. The following section should provide you with the information to do this.

The content of palliative nursing courses

In 2002 The International Society for Nurses in Cancer Care (ISNCC) in conjunction with the World Health Organization (WHO) updated their core curriculum for palliative nursing to meet the changing needs of global health care systems (ISNCC 2002). This document clearly shows the required content of a programme of study that characterises the fundamental knowledge that all nurses require to provide quality palliative nursing care. These eight fundamental subject areas are then divided into ten modules where the content is more fully described. Table 18.1 shows the ten core modules.

Following this The European Association for Palliative Care (EAPC) produced guidance on the development of palliative nurse education across Europe

Table 18.1

Module name	
Death, society and palliative care – a global perspective	Emergencies in palliative care
Experience of the patient and his or her family	Therapeutic communication
Nursing in palliative care	Care in the last hours of life
Managing clinical symptoms 1	Loss, grief and bereavement
Managing clinical symptoms 2	Ethics at the end of life

Adapted from ISNCC (2002).

Table 18.2

Nursing interactions occur with
The patient The family/carer The team Society Health care systems

Adapted from De Vlieger et al. (2004).

(De Vlieger et al. 2004). As well as discussing levels of practice they suggested that there were interactions that occurred in palliative nursing and suggested palliative care educational initiatives should include these in their curriculum. These are listed in Table 18.2.

From these five aspects of nursing interaction De Vlieger et al. (2004) show the detailed content of a fundamental palliative care educational initiative. The detailed subject areas are very similar to the areas developed by the ISNCC (2002), that is communication, symptom management, ethics, palliative care emergencies, death and society and loss, grief and bereavement.

In 2002 The Royal College of Nursing (RCN) Nurses Managing Hospices Forum developed a competency framework for nurses working in specialist palliative care, showing the knowledge, skills and behaviours needed to provide optimal care within this specialist setting. This framework shows, using a number of subject areas, what is expected of nurses practicing at different levels. These subject areas and description of levels of achievement could easily be used to develop an educational programme aimed at nurses working at higher levels of practice in specialist palliative care. These can be seen in Table 18.3.

Using both the ISNCC (2002) and the EAPC (De Vlieger et al. 2004) criteria reviewed above as well as the RCN (2002) competency descriptors, The West of Scotland Managed Clinical Network for Palliative Care (WoSPCMCN) (2006) developed a comprehensive set of competencies required by nurses (and other professionals) working with dying patients to ensure they had the knowledge, skills and behaviours to provide optimal palliative care within their role. The suggested core content for educational programme is divided into nine areas, and is shown in Table 18.4. This framework also suggests that as well as teaching

Table 18.3

RCN competency areas	
Communication Quality assurance Clinical practice	Management and leadership Research and development Grief, loss and bereavement

Adapted from the RCN (2002).

Table 18.4

WoSPCMCN core content	
Rehabilitation	End of life care
Pain and symptom management related to disease process	Ethical and legal issues
Spirituality	Communication skills
Quality of life	Multidisciplinary team working
Loss, grief and bereavement	

Adapted from WoSPCMCN (2006).

knowledge, palliative care courses should teach skills and behaviours within each subject area. This will allow a nurse to not only learn underpinning knowledge but also apply this to practice and be able to use behaviours consistent with good palliative care.

Finally, the most recent suggestions for the content of palliative care educational programmes have come from The International End of Life Nursing Education Consortium (Paice et al. 2007). The aim of this group is to introduce a curriculum for palliative nursing education in order to reduce global suffering. They suggest that palliative care training from undergraduates through to senior nurses should include nine core topics. These can be seen in Table 18.5.

In conclusion, from this review it would appear that there is a well-recognised, core content for palliative care courses. Indeed the content suggested in this section mirrors the facets of palliative care discussed in Chapter 2. Therefore, educators should incorporate these subjects into their curriculum, whether it is education for nursing assistants, student nurses or post-registration nurses. As well as this all nurses wishing to embark on palliative care education should ensure these topics feature in the course they choose. It would be advisable to check with the education provider to ensure a well-balanced course is being offered which meets the needs of the learner and their employer.

As well as the content of courses current thought indicates that nurses should learn at different levels depending on their role within palliative care (De Vlieger et al. 2004). The next section reviews the current thinking on the different levels

Table 18.5

Core topics	
Overview of palliative care	Communication
Pain management	Loss, grief and bereavement
Symptom management	Terminal phase
Cultural issues	Achieving quality
Ethical and legal issues	

Adapted from Paice et al. (2007).

of palliative care education to help both educators and students determine the correct levels for course provision.

Levels of knowledge and skill

It is generally agreed that qualified nurses work in cancer and palliative care practice at three distinct levels: core level, specialist level and advanced level (EAPC 2004; ISNCC 2002; NHS Education for Scotland 2006). However, the role of higher level skills is not standardised (DoH 2006) and as such there is ambiguity in the meaning of the titles of nurses practicing at specialist or advanced level and also the level of academic achievement that is required. This can be seen in the key documents that discuss palliative nursing education. The EAPC (2004) discuss three levels of practice: basic, advanced, with specialist at the top of the scale. However, the ISNCC (2002) suggests that specialist practice comes at a lower level than advanced practice and that nurses working in advanced practice should have a superior breadth and depth in the theories underpinning palliative care practice. Further discussion of the different levels of nursing practice in the UK is provided later in this chapter.

However, what we do know is that nurses work at different levels in palliative care and as such palliative care education should be delivered at different levels to meet the needs of a dynamic nursing workforce. Indeed, the *Modernising Nursing Careers* (DoH 2006) document states that one of the key priorities of nursing in the UK is to develop a competent and flexible workforce by providing education that is built around patient pathways and not like the current system where 'one size fits all'. To ensure that the palliative care workforce, including nurses, are educated to a level that is required for their role, the WoSPCMCN (2006) devised a five-level competency framework, which has partly been described above. This multi-layered framework begins by describing the attributes required by lay carers to allow them to care for a loved one effectively before describing four levels of attributes required by professional carers, beginning with support workers, that is the nursing assistant, and finishing with the most senior practitioner, that is the senior nurse or nurse specialist. The knowledge, skills and behaviours required by professional carers are then described in terms of job title, that is qualified nurse, and academic level, that is Scottish Qualifications Framework level 7/8, to allow both educators and learners to see the level of learning that is required. By using the framework everyone involved with palliative care education, whether in the academic sector or continuing professional development department and whether as an educator, manager or learner, all can determine whether a course is fit for purpose and meets the required needs. Table 18.6 shows the WoSPCMCN (2006) competency framework for teaching ethical and legal issues in palliative care. The whole document can be viewed at http://www.palliativecareglasgow.info/pdf/Education_Competencies_Final_ Version_24_March_06.doc.

Table 18.6 West of Scotland managed clinical network for palliative care education – ethical and legal issues.

Scottish credit and qualifications framework	Knowledge and understanding	Competency and skills	Behaviour
Level 1/4 Informal carer; Administration and ancillary staff. Volunteers	Awareness of the complexities of ethical and legal decision-making in palliative care	Recognises and communicates ethical and legal issues to the appropriate personnel Responds within their own abilities to the ethical and legal issues that arise	Observant Communicates observation
Level 5/6 Support worker: Health care assistant or Social carer E.g. N/SVQ level 2/3	Basic knowledge and understanding of the concepts and complexities, ethical and legal issues related to palliative care Gives an account of appropriate theoretical components related to ethical and legal matters	Applies knowledge and understanding to practice skills Observes, monitors and accurately reports areas of concern to senior staff Uses policies and protocols to guide practice Acts under supervision to promote best practice in ethical and legal dilemmas Utilises oral and written communication	Responsible Aware of own role within the multidisciplinary team Some supervisory responsibility Aware of own learning needs
Level 7/8 Qualified nurse or Health care professional Certificate/Diploma in post registration studies	Applies a broad knowledge of the concepts and complexities of ethical and legal issues to Palliative Care Detailed knowledge of some issues within ethical/legal dilemmas Knowledge and understanding of the research process	Utilises a range of simple, complex or advanced techniques in ethical/legal decision-making Investigates legal & ethical issues relating to palliative care utilising evidence-based literature Adapts and improves practice within a dynamic evidence-based framework Utilises a variety of communication methods effectively	Exercises autonomy and initiative Supervisory responsibility Shares knowledge and skills with others
Level 9/10 Senior qualified nurse or Health care professional Degree level studies in palliative care	Develops critical analysis of principles and theories related to ethical and legal issues in Palliative Care Broad integrated knowledge of the complexities of ethical and legal issues in Palliative care Specialist knowledge informed by research and development	Utilises advanced and specialist knowledge and techniques to practice Critically analyses and develops best practice through clinical governance strategies Contributes to the clinical governance strategy	Supervisory responsibility Managerial skills Innovator of evidence-based practice Skilled practitioner Addresses and facilitates the educational needs of self and others

Table 18.6 (*Continued*)

Scottish credit and qualifications framework	Knowledge and understanding	Competency and skills	Behaviour
Level 11 Specialist nurse or Health care professional Medical staff Postgraduate or Masters level	Develops critical analysis of specialised ethical and legal principles to inform practice Maintains extensive, detailed knowledge and understanding within the specialised area of ethical and legal decision-making Maintains critical analysis of current ethical and legal issues	Leadership skills in team management and practice development Practices within currently accepted best practice guidelines High standards of interpersonal skills Utilises IT skills within specialist role	Leads and motivates team members Managerial responsibility Skilled communicator Practices at a high level of skill Utilises expert knowledge to contribute to the delivery of palliative care education (WoSPCMCN 2006)

Reproduced from MCN Competence Framework with the kind permission of West of Scotland Managed Clinical Network for Palliative Care.

Suggested content dependent of level of entry and professional background: The principles of medical ethics; The processes of ethical decision-making; ethical and legal issues relating to artificial nutrition and hydration; resuscitation; end of life planning; euthanasia; opioid analgesics; informed consent; advance directives and truth telling (WoSPCMCN 2006).

It can be seen from Table 18.6 that nurses should have different levels knowledge, skills and behaviours depending on their level of practice.

Practice Point 18.2

Before reading the next section on continuing professional development review the West of Scotland MCN document in full and decide where your post sits within the framework. What knowledge, skills or behaviours do you need to ensure you are working effectively at this level? Look out for palliative care courses that are available in your area – would they help you to enhance your practice?

From this exercise you should now be aware of your own learning needs. As an accountable practitioner the nurse should possess the knowledge and skills to ensure they provide safe, effective, evidence-based care (Nursing and Midwifery Council (NMC) 2008). By using the above information you should now be able to choose palliative care courses that best meet your needs. The next section will discuss the importance of continuing professional development and how to prepare yourself for a career working at higher levels of practice within a palliative care environment.

Continuing professional development

It is your responsibility, as a registered nurse, to ensure you keep your knowledge and skills up to date throughout your nursing career (NMC 2008) and as such there should be a system in place within your organisation to allow you to do this. Gone are the days when nurses did not require to update their skills following registration. Lifelong learning is now seen as an integral part of practice (Wallace 1999). In response to the ideal that all staff should participate in lifelong learning and to ensure all staff are able to perform safely and effectively within their roles, the National Health Service Agenda for Change system developed a separate framework to ensure all staff have the knowledge and skills required to do their job effectively (DoH 2004a). This framework is called The National Health Service Knowledge and Skills Framework (NHS KSF) (DoH 2004a) and together with its associated development review process forms the basis of the career progression pathway within the NHS.

Most post should now have NHS KSF outlines that sit alongside the job description to allow nurses to see clearly what is expected of them in their role. Also by looking at other NHS KSF outlines which can be accessed through managers it can give nurses an idea of how to progress their career in palliative care. The framework is not intended to describe the exact knowledge and skills that nurses working with dying patients need to develop to do their job competently and as such more specific standards and competences developed for palliative care, such as those already reviewed in the Section 'The content of palliative nursing courses', would help to do this. The NHS KSF will now be reviewed to show how it can be used within palliative nursing to aid professional development and career progression.

The National Health Service Knowledge and Skills Framework

The NHS KSF (DoH 2004a) provides a single, constant, all-inclusive framework on which to base and review the development of all NHS staff members. The purpose of the NHS KSF is to facilitate the development of services so that they better meet the needs of users and the public through investing in the development of all members of staff. The NHS KSF is based on the principles of good people management – how people like to be treated at work and how organisations can enable people to work effectively. It aims to:

- support the effective learning and development of individuals and teams – with all members of staff being supported to learn throughout their careers and develop in a variety of ways, and being given the resources to do so
- support the development of individuals in the post in which they are employed so that they can be effective at work – with managers and staff being clear about what is required within a post and managers enabling staff to develop within their post

- promote equality for and diversity of all staff – with every member of staff using the same framework, having the same opportunities for learning and development open to them and having the same structured approach to learning, development and review.

(DoH 2004a)

The NHS KSF is made up of 30 dimensions, with six of these being core to every job. These core dimensions are:

1. Communication – this domain is highly pertinent to caring for dying people as the majority of complaints received by the NHS are about poor communication between staff and dying patients and their families (Mayor 2007)
2. Personal and people development – the job you have will dictate whether you are only responsible for your own learning needs or whether you are responsible for the learning needs of junior team members such as care assistants and nursing students
3. Health, safety and security – this domain centres on the notion that everybody within the NHS whether a staff member, patient or visitor has the right to be kept safe and well. Again your post outline will dictate how much responsibility you have for your own and the safety of others
4. Service improvement – as an evolving speciality palliative care provision needs to keep abreast of new evidence as do all other areas of care. This domain helps to ensure that nurses are equipped with current knowledge to underpin their practice
5. Quality – quality assurance is a big part of ensuring that palliative care is provided in an effective way. Indeed, NICE (2004) suggests to ensure effective palliative care provision that individual practitioners need to have the knowledge and skills to do this
6. Equality and diversity – one of the criticisms of palliative care service in the past is that they do not cater well for ethnic minorities (Robinson 2001). However, this domain makes it clear that all care services should be provided equitably and no group should be disadvantaged

(DoH 2004a)

The other 24 dimensions are only specific to particular roles. The overarching dimension entitled 'Health and Wellbeing', contains 10 specific domains which are mainly concerned with planning, evaluating and implementing different aspects of care. It is these specific domains that should be utilised to formulate NHS KSF outlines for nursing posts to ensure they are able to provide high-quality patient care. Throughout this book it has been shown that high-quality planning of individualised, holistic palliative care is required to ensure it is available to all dying people regardless of place of care or diagnosis. Therefore, NHS KSF outlines for posts should encompass the knowledge and skills required by nurses to provide this care effectively.

Each dimension, whether core or specific, has four levels and a title which describes what each level is about. The higher the level the greater the skill

Table 18.7

	Level 1	**Level 2**	**Level 3**	**Level 4**
Dimension 1. Communication	Communicate with a limited range of people on day-to-day matters	Communicate with a range of people on a range of matters	Develop and maintain communication with people about difficult matters and/or in difficult situations	Develop and maintain communication with people on complex matters, issues and ideas and/or in complex situations

Adapted from DoH (2004a). Reproduced under the terms of the Click-Use licence.

and knowledge required by the post holder. Table 18.7 shows the criteria for dimension 1 – communication.

Interestingly this four level design echoes the format of palliative nursing competency frameworks previously reviewed in this chapter. This means that frameworks can be used together to show nurses the knowledge and skill they require when providing different levels of palliative care.

Within the NHS KSF some examples of application are provided to show how these might be applied in different posts and are purely for illustrative purposes to allow those developing the outline to see what type of evidence would be required to show the attainment of knowledge. In palliative care settings it may be that the NHS KSF frameworks for nursing posts use examples of application to show the specialised knowledge and skills required for a post. For example, using one of the palliative care frameworks reviewed earlier the statements of competence could be used to give examples of the evidence that is required by nurses to prove they have the knowledge and skills to do their job effectively.

Evidence of learning

The development review (sometimes referred to a performance appraisal) is the way in which those with a NHS KSF outline will be measured against the knowledge and skills required for their post. The process will initially focus on helping the nurse develop to meet the demands of their NHS KSF outline. Once the nurse has shown they meet the demands of their current post the focus of learning may then shift to career development, whether this is upwards or sideways. The NHS KSF, and related post outlines, should be available to every nurse in an organisation so that they are able to think about their next career steps. Nurse's Personal Development Plans can focus on future career development, once they have shown that they can apply the knowledge and skills necessary for their current post. Appraisal is your opportunity to tell your manager what you would like to achieve in the next year. Prepare for the exercise well and before the interview decide on which course you feel you suit your needs best. These can then be negotiated with you manager. The next section discusses the importance of recording evidence of learning and how this can be achieved.

Keeping a portfolio

Since the development of the Post-registration Education and Practice standards (UKCC 1994) nurses have had to declare that they have attended 5 days of training relating to their current role within each 3-year registration period. In order to evidence this ongoing training the UKCC (1994) stated that nurses should keep a 'Personal Professional Profile'. The governing body could then request to see the portfolio as evidence of learning each time a nurse re-registered. However, there was never an 'official' UKCC profile (Wallace 1999) and many nurses over the years in conjunction with their employers have developed their own profiles as evidence of learning. This portfolio should not just contain factual information about the courses or study days attended but should also contain a reflection of how the learning has impacted on practice. It is evidence of how new knowledge and skills relate to clinical practice that demonstrates the nurse has understood how the new knowledge is pertinent to their role.

As as well as providing the nurse with evidence of learning a good portfolio can also be used at interview to show prospective employees that education has been undertaken and that the nurse has the knowledge and skills to take on a new role. This can be especially helpful if the nurse wants to move from providing general palliative care to working within a specialist palliative care team.

e-Portfolios

Within the NHS e-portfolios that give evidence of knowledge and skill attainment have been successfully piloted with junior doctors and are now being rolled out across the UK and to other health care professionals (www.nhseportfolios.org). This system will save professionals having to keep ever-growing paper portfolios and also because of their electronic format they will be able to be moved from employer to employer. This will allow the employee to provide evidence of their continuing professional development at appraisal and to provide evidence that they are working well within their NHS KSF outline. Other education providers are now also moving towards the use of easily accessible e-portfolios, including the university sector. This hopefully in the future will allow all learning to be updated within one electronic record that can be used for nurses' continuing professional development as well as their academic achievements.

Practice Point 18.3

Review your Personal, Professional Profile. Would it give accurate and current evidence of lifelong learning for either your performance appraisal or for a prospective employer?

Commentary:

Keeping a portfolio up to date is often a task that is forgotten about. As previously mentioned your professional body, appraiser or prospective employer is not just interested in the course you have been to but also in how this has influenced your practice. Make sure you have current reflective accounts within your portfolio in preparation for the next time you are required to provide evidence of this. If you have never used a reflective cycle, a simple one can be found in Marks-Maran and Rose (1996).

Higher levels of nursing practice

This section discusses the higher levels of nursing practice and the roles that currently exist within palliative care settings in the UK. The aim of this section is to allow nurses to determine what they would need to do in terms of professional development to gain employment in a more senior role.

Specialist practitioner qualification

Specialist practitioners are depicted as nurses that will apply higher levels of judgement, prudence and decision-making in their area of practice. They will be able to review and progress standards of care through the supervision and clinical audit and lead the development of practice through research, teaching and support of other nurses (UKCC 1994). Education to allow nurses to practice at this level has been available since the mid 1990s and the academic standards for such programmes must meet the following strict criteria and be:

- An academic year in length
- No less than first degree level study
- Modular where possible
- Flexible
- Accessible full or part time
- Approved by the professional body
- Arranged round a common core framework with specialist modules
- Linked to a higher education accreditation system

(Adapted from Wallace 1999)

In Scotland this qualification has been used as a benchmark for the standards for specialist palliative care (Clinical Standards Board for Scotland (CSBS) 2002) to ensure nurses working in specific specialist roles, such as palliative care community nurse specialists, are educated to an agreed level. This use of the qualification as a role benchmark is useful to ensure nurses working at this level have the knowledge and skills to do so. However, there is evidence to suggest that nurses working at this level may not have access to courses that allow them to have the credibility they require in order to practice at specialist level (Jones

2005). It is also noted that role ambiguity has resulted from different expectations of the role of the specialist nurse and that this has impacted on the motivation of some nurses (Jones 2005). During the last few years nursing's professional body has been reviewing the higher levels of nursing practice, and although at the time of writing no firm decision has been made, the consultation documents seem to favour the title advanced nurse practice rather than specialist practice (NMC 2005).

Advanced nursing practice

From its consultation mentioned above the NMC (2005) has provided a definition of advanced practice which is shown below.

> 'Advanced nurse practitioners are highly experienced, knowledgeable and educated members of the care team who are able to diagnose and treat your health care needs or refer you to an appropriate specialist if needed.'
>
> (NMC 2005)

In the outcome of their consultation on higher levels of practice the NMC (2005) also provides a list of skills required by the advanced practitioner. These are the ability to:

- carry out physical examinations
- use their expert knowledge and clinical judgement to decide whether to refer patients for investigations and make diagnoses
- decide on and carry out treatment, including the prescribing of medicines, or refer patients to an appropriate specialist
- use their extensive practice experience to plan and provide skilled and competent care to meet patients health and social care needs, involving other members of the health care team as appropriate
- ensure the provision of continuity of care including follow-up visits
- assess and evaluate, with patients, the effectiveness of the treatment and care provided and make changes as needed
- work independently, although often as part of a health care team that they will lead and
- as a leader of the team, make sure that each patient's treatment and care is based on best practice

(NMC 2005)

This definition may help to resolve the issues surrounding different ideas of what is expected of nurses working at higher levels. As well as their definitions the NMC (2005) has eluded to the notion that nurses working at this level should be educated to Masters level and they have aligned the skills and knowledge listed above to the NHS KSF previously reviewed in this chapter. This would be in keeping with other countries where it is expected that nurses working at higher levels of practice are educated to Master or indeed in the US nurses working at this level are required to be educated to doctoral level (Clinton 2008).

Practice Point 18.4

Review the annex to the NMC's (2005) document *Implementation of a Framework for the Standard for Post-registration Nursing* to see how they have mapped the role of the advanced nurse practitioner to the NHS KSF. You can find this at http://www.nmc-uk.org/aFrameDisplay.aspx?DocumentID=1324 – just click on the button marked save and the document will open. How does this set of KSF competencies match with your current NHS KSF outline?

Commentary:

This exercise will allow you to focus on where you are now and where you need to be in terms of the competencies that you would be required to give evidence of if you wish to progress to a more specialised nursing role within palliative care.

The final part of this section will review the roles of advanced nurse practitioners, educators and research nurses working in palliative care to help you to decide which career pathway suits your needs and aspirations.

The clinical nurse specialist

As previously noted the clinical nurse specialist (CNS) is a registered nurse who has obtained higher level knowledge, skills and experience, together with a professionally and/or academically accredited post-registration qualification in palliative care. Many of these nurses have traditionally worked as site-specific cancer nurses, for example breast care and colorectal CNS, where they follow the patient's journey from pre-diagnosis, through treatments to survivorship or palliative care. However, with the move to providing palliative care for all regardless of diagnosis there are other CNS posts being developed that care specifically for groups with non-malignant diseases, for example heart failure and Huntington's disease. The largest group of CNS that work in specialist palliative care are community palliative care nurse specialists (who may be termed Macmillan nurses if their post is funded by Macmillan Cancer Support). However, many of these CNS are now funded by an independent hospice or the NHS. As well as having expertise in palliative care many employers also ask for these practitioners to have either experience and/or a qualification in community nursing. Other palliative care CNSs who are employed within the NHS may work as part of a hospital palliative care team. These nurses are highly experienced hospital nurses who once again have achieved specialist qualifications in palliative care.

The community matron

The Community Matron's role was developed in response to the government's plans for the management of long-term conditions (DoH 2004b). From earlier chapters in this book it has become clear that the provision of palliative care for people diagnosed with long-term conditions such as multiple sclerosis and Parkinson's disease improve quality of life. It is therefore reasonable to suggest that Community Matrons will require a high level of palliative care knowledge and skills. In fact there is some emerging anecdotal evidence to suggest that community specialist palliative care nurses are taking on this new role, following education in areas such as nurse prescribing and advanced clinical assessment skills. As part of their role, the Community Matron will be expected to use case management techniques to:

- use data to actively seek out patients who will benefit
- combine high level assessment of physical, mental and social care needs
- review medication and prescribe medicines via independent and supplementary prescribing arrangements
- provide clinical care and health-promoting interventions
- coordinate inputs from all other agencies, ensuring all needs are met
- teach and educate patients and their carers about warning signs of complications or crisis
- provide information so that patients and families can make choices about current and future care needs
- are highly visible to patients and their families and carers, and are seen by them as being in charge of their care
- are seen by colleagues across all agencies as having the key role for patients with very high intensity needs

(DoH 2004b)

From this list of attributes it can be seen that this nurse requires a high level of knowledge and skills to manage patients' whose conditions are complex, the main aim of which is to try and prevent recurrent hospital admissions (DoH 2004b).

The nurse consultant

The Nurse Consultant post was developed in 2000 following the Department of Health (1999a) report on *Strengthening the Nursing, Midwifery and Health Visiting Contribution to Health and Healthcare* which recognised that nurses had a pivotal role in the NHS that needed to be strengthened. Following this report a Health Service Circular (DoH 1999b) provided guidance to employers on the role and employment of the Nurse Consultant and stated –

'Establishing nurse, midwife and health visitor consultant posts is intended to help provide better outcomes for patients by improving services and quality, to strengthen leadership and to provide a new career opportunity to help retain experienced and expert nurses, midwives and health visitors in practice.'

(DoH 1999b)

At this time it was acknowledged that posts could be introduced into any areas of practice where it was felt a nurse consultant would be beneficial in meeting the intended outcomes (DoH 1999b). To this end there are a number of Nurse Consultant posts within the palliative care arena. Some of these posts are within the NHS and others which have been developed by independent hospices. Some are combined with cancer care while others are purely palliative care. At the time of writing there is one nurse consultant in the UK with a specific remit to provide expertise in the provision of palliative care to people who have a life-limiting illness that is not cancer. However, it does not matter where the Palliative Care Consultant Nurse is employed; all these posts have the same core functions as described in the NHS circular (DoH 1999b). These are:

- an expert practice function (which should be the majority of the role)
- a professional leadership and consultancy function
- an education, training and development function
- a practice and service development, research and evaluation function

(Adapted from DoH 1999b)

As well as determining the core function of each post, the guidance also gives clear information about the level of academic achievement the Consultant Nurse should have attained and states that this should be at Masters level and above. However, Woodward et al. (2005) suggest that some appointed Nurse Consultants have not reached this academic level which has led to them struggling with their new role. These authors go on to suggest that in order to fulfil the role fully Consultant Nurses should be educated to at least Masters level (Woodward et al. 2005). As well as this academic attainment Cox (2000) also suggests that part of the Consultant Nurse role is to have diagnostic skills and be a nurse prescriber. This would be much in keeping with the Community Matron role.

To secure a post at this level it can be seen that the nurse needs to have expert clinical skills combined with educational abilities and leadership expertise and as such continuing professional development should be focused on attaining the skills listed in the DoH (1999b) guidance.

Working in palliative care education and research

As well as describing the core content for palliative nursing education, The EAPC (De Vlieger et al. 2004) goes one step further and suggests the content of courses that should be available to nurses wishing to become palliative care educators and those wishing to become researchers. The overarching content for both these educational programmes can be viewed in Table 18.8.

Nurses wishing to become educators or researchers in palliative care may already be working in a more specialised role. They should certainly have received palliative care education at a postgraduate level and even at Masters level before embarking on this career path. Many of the postgraduate level

Table 18.8

Content of a palliative care educators course	Content of a course for nurses wishing to work in palliative care research
Fundamental principles of adult education	Ethical and methodological principles for research in palliative care including:
Education specifically applied to palliative care	Critical reading and academic writing skills
Evaluation of education and training	Application and limitations in palliative care research
	Developing and using a research tool
	Methods of data collection
	Multidisciplinary research

Adapted from De Vlieger et al. (2004).

palliative care courses within the UK deal specifically with palliative care research methodology while others offer a more generic research module. Therefore, if a nurse is wishing to pursue a career in palliative care research, course content should be scrutinised to see which meets their needs best. Most nurses entering the palliative care education arena in the UK will have to gain a generic teaching qualification that allows them to be registered with their professional body. These courses however focus on generic teaching and learning methodology, although there is usually scope to carry out the course assessments in the development, delivery and evaluation of palliative care education. Again, it would be wise for a nurse to find out this information to ensure the course being applied for meets their learning needs.

Conclusion

From the discussion in this chapter it can be seen that within the modern health care arena it is important for nurses to keep their knowledge and skills up to date to allow them to provide the highest quality of palliative care when it is required. The NHS KSF is the most common framework that employers use to ensure they have a skilled workforce. However, nurses can utilise this framework, not only to ensure they are competent in their current role but in achieving career progression. Keeping evidence of lifelong learning is the key to career progression, whether using a traditional portfolio or a newer, electronic one. However, at the time of writing there is no coherent pathway for registering nurses with their professional body when practicing at an advanced level. Although many nurses working in palliative care are already employed in extended roles, they are waiting to see how they will be affected when a decision is made on how to regulate these posts in the future. Finally, it is up to each individual nurse to take responsibility for their career progression and to develop an ongoing plan to allow them to achieve their envisaged role.

References

Clark D (2002) *Cicely Saunders: Founder of the Hospice Movement. Selected letters 1959–1999.* Oxford: Oxford University Press.

Clinical Standards Board for Scotland (2002) *Clinical Standards for Specialist Palliative Care.* Edinburgh: NHSQIS.

Clinton J (2008) Latest developments in advanced nursing practice. *Journal for Specialists in Pediatric Nursing.* 13(2):123–125.

Cox C (2000) The nurse consultant: an advanced nurse practitioner? *Nursing Times.* 96(13):48.

De Vlieger M, Gorchs N, Larkin, PJ and Porchet F (2004) A guide to the development of palliative nurse education in Europe. Palliative nurse education: Report to the EAPC task force. Milan: EAPC.

Department of Health (1999a) *Making a Difference: Strengthening the Nursing, Midwifery and Health Visiting Contribution to Health and Healthcare.* London: DoH.

Department of Health (1999b) *Nursing, Midwifery and Health Visiting Consultants: Establishing Posts and Making Appointments. Health Service Circular 1999/217.* Leeds: NHS Executive.

Department of Health (2000) *The NHS Cancer Plan: A Plan for Investment; a Plan for Reform.* London: DoH.

Department of Health (2004a) *The NHS Knowledge and Skills Framework (NHS KSF) and the Development Review Process.* London: DoH.

Department of Health (2004b) *NHS Improvement Plan.* London: DoH.

Department of Health (2006) *Modernising Nursing Careers: Setting the Direction.* London: DoH.

Expert Advisory Group on Cancer (1995) A policy framework for commissioning cancer services: A report by the Expert Advisory Group on cancer to the Chief Medical Officers of England and Wales. The Calman-Hine Report. London: DoH.

International Society for Nurses in Cancer Care (2002) *A Core Curriculum for Palliative Nursing* (2nd edition). Macclesfield: ISNCC.

Jones M (2005) Role development and effective practice in specialist and advanced practice roles in acute hospital settings: systematic review and meta synthesis. *Journal of Advanced Nursing.* 49(2):191–209.

Marks-Maran M and Rose P (1996) *Reconstructing Nursing.* London: Balliere Tindall.

Mayor S (2007) Care of the dying patients and safety dominate report on NHS complaints. *British Medical Journal.* 334(7588):278.

National Institute for Clinical Excellence (2004) *Improving Supportive and Palliative Care for Adults with Cancer.* London: NICE.

NHS Education for Scotland (2006) *Working with Individuals with Cancer, Their Families and Carers.* Edinburgh: NES.

Nursing and Midwifery Council (2005) *Implementation of a Framework for the Standard for Post-registration Nursing.* London: NMC.

Nursing and Midwifery Council (2008) *The Code: Standards of Conduct, Performance and Ethics for Nurses and Midwives.* London: NMC.

Paice JA, Ferrell BR, Coyle N, Coyne P and Calloway M (2007) Global efforts to improve palliative care: the international end of life nursing education consortium training programme. *Journal of Advanced Nursing.* 61(2):173–180.

Robinson MRD (2001) *Palliative Care, Cancer and Minority Ethnic Communities: A Literature Review. Working Paper No5*. Leicester: Mary Seacole Research Centre, De Montfort University.

Royal College of Nursing (1994) *The Palliative Nursing Forum Introductory Leaflet*. London: RCN.

Royal College of Nursing (2002) *A Framework for Nurses Working in Specialist Palliative Care*. London: RCN.

Scottish Executive Health Department (SEHD) (2001) *Cancer in Scotland – Action for Change*. Edinburgh: SEHD.

Sherman DW, Matzo ML, Coyne P, Ferrell BR and Penn BK (2004) Teaching symptom management in end of life care: the didactic content and teaching strategies based on end of life nursing education curriculum. *Journal of Nurses in Staff Development*. 20(3):103–115.

UKCC (1994) *The Future of Professional Practice: The Council's Standards for Education and Practice Following Registration (PREP) – A Position Statement (Number 1)*.London: UKCC.

Wallace M (1999) *Lifelong Learning: PREP in Action*. Edinburgh: Churchill Livingstone.

Welsh Assembly Government (2005) *National Standards for Specialist Palliative Care Cancer Services*. Cardiff: Cancer Services Co-ordinating Group.

West of Scotland Managed Clinical Network for Palliative Care (2006) *Palliative Care Educational Core Competencies*. Glasgow: NHS.

Woodward VA, Webb C, and Prowse M (2005) Nurse consultants: their characteristics and achievements. *Journal of Clinical Nursing*. 14(7):845–854. Available at www.nhseportfolios.org. Accessed on 01 May 2008.

Chapter 19

Palliative care research

Stuart Milligan

Introduction

The aim of this chapter is to provide the reader with an introduction to the place of research in contemporary palliative care. As well as considering the current state of palliative care research, the chapter identifies barriers and challenges to effective research practice and ways in which these might be overcome.

Learning outcomes

Once you have read this chapter and completed the associated practice points, you will be able to:

- Explain why palliative care requires a sound research base
- Discuss the current state of palliative care research from both a UK and a European perspective
- Describe the principal barriers and challenges encountered in palliative care research
- Identify ways in which these barriers and challenges are being addressed

The need for palliative care research

In 1978, Cicely Saunders wrote 'It is only by asking questions and attempting to solve them, that advances can be made in the practical management of advanced malignant disease' (Saunders 1978, p. 37). True to this statement, Saunders had already established St Christopher's Hospice on the three pillars of clinical practice, education and research (Clark et al. 2005; Kaasa et al. 2006). Indeed, it is not difficult to imagine the intense atmosphere of inquiry which must have pervaded St Christopher's in the 1960s and 1970s, with studies on topics as diverse as the side effects of morphine and human responses to bereavement going on side by side (Saunders 2000).

It goes without saying that all clinical practice should be underpinned by evidence, but this is perhaps particularly the case in relatively new spheres of practice such as palliative care (Higginson 2003; Lee and Kristjanson 2003). New treatments are being proposed with unanswered questions about efficacy, dose response and side effects (Jubb 2002; Wilkinson 1998). At the same time, new services are being funded from limited resources, with a pressing demand for evidence that need exists, and that interventions are effective (Higginson 2003). Palliative care research must respond to both these and other agendas (Royal College of Physicians 2007).

The primary aim of health care research is to generate empirical evidence which can be used to inform practice. However, since the main purpose of palliative care is the relief of suffering, there is a particular imperative to investigate the needs and preferences of patients and their families (Addington-Hall 2007; European Association for Palliative Care (EAPC) and International Association for Palliative Care (IAPC) 2006; Mularski et al. 2007). What is ultimately needed is a body of evidence which will ensure that all patients and their families receive the care most appropriate to their needs and most likely to deliver their preferred outcomes (Murray 2008).

This broad scope presents challenges in itself. Palliative care is not a narrow field of practice that might lend itself well to intensely focused investigation with highly standardised research methods and processes (Addington-Hall 2007). Instead, it requires the input of a range of professionals across a range of theoretical disciplines employing a range of approaches and methodologies. The challenge of joining up that research activity into an integrated whole is enormous, touching on issues such as government policy, funding, identification of research priorities, ethical issues, relationships between researchers and subjects, and the attitudes of practitioners towards research (Christakis 2006; EAPC and IAPC 2006).

The current state of palliative care research in the UK and abroad

There is no doubt that there has been considerable progress made in palliative care research over recent years. The number of palliative care articles listed on *Medline*, although still small, increased by over 100% between 1987 and 2005 (Addington-Hall 2007). The number of palliative care journals available continues to grow, submissions of palliative care abstracts to research conferences have also risen and there is evidence of increased interest in palliative care projects from funding bodies (Davies 2001; Froggatt et al. 2003). However, it is also the case that the number of researchers engaged in palliative care research is relatively low, and concerns continue to be expressed over the quality of some of the research being produced (Addington-Hall 2007).

In 2004, the National Cancer Research Institute (NCRI) published a landmark report on supportive and palliative care research in the UK (NCRI 2004). The report revealed that spending on palliative care research accounted for around

4% of the total of cancer research spend in the UK. Around 330 researchers distributed between 43 teams were identified, with most activity in London, followed by Manchester and other major UK cities. Although small in number, UK researchers performed relatively strongly in terms of publications, coming second only to the US in terms of global research output. Interestingly however, other countries produced more research papers per head than the UK.

The NCRI (2004) study confirmed that palliative care research in the UK is a multidisciplinary endeavour with a wide range of professional groups contributing to the research workforce. The provision of PhD training is good and there is evidence of good links between research groups and clinical areas. However, many of the research groups identified were critically small and relatively isolated from others. The report also identified other organisational, financial, methodological and clinical challenges.

Subsequent to the NCRI study, a Scotland-wide scoping exercise was carried out in 2005 (Johnston et al. 2006). The smaller scale of this study enabled it to capture some interesting information about the many small, mostly unfunded studies which make an unknown contribution to palliative care research. The principal aim of the exercise was to identify all planned, current and recently completed palliative care research in Scotland. However, it was also intended that the exercise would give a measure of the strength of the Scottish research base and identify future priorities for palliative care research. The exercise covered a relatively long (15-year) period and both published and unpublished research was included. It is surprising therefore that the total number of studies found was only 44. This is a disappointingly small number, even though an unknown number of studies may have been missed.

The report demonstrates that the Scottish research base is not only small but also relatively narrow in scope. Half of all studies addressed only two research areas: models of palliative care/provision and pain and/or symptom control. Methodological quality was also variable, with only two of the studies using the 'gold standard' of the randomised controlled trial (RCT). Sample size was variable and sometimes appeared not to be decided in a rigorous way (Bakitas et al. 2006). Also, most samples were relatively small. One particularly interesting finding was the extent to which gaps exist in the Scottish research base. For instance, although patient involvement and non-malignant palliative care are amongst the most important themes in contemporary palliative care policy, only 10% of studies specifically addressed either of these issues.

Practice Point 19.1

Find out what palliative care research is (or has been) taking place in your local health authority. You may have to contact your local institutions of higher education, the health authority's research and development department and national funding bodies.

Commentary:

Although the findings of the Scottish scoping exercise are a little disappointing, there is anecdotal evidence that the situation in Scotland and elsewhere in the UK is improving. Increasing numbers of palliative care nurses, doctors and other professionals are undertaking research as part of higher degrees and, on a larger scale, efforts are being made regionally and nationally to stimulate collaboration and build research capacity (Bailey et al. 2006; Davies 2001; Payne et al. 2007).

The picture of palliative care research across Europe is also one of gradual improvement from a relatively low starting point. Kaasa et al. (2006) conducted a review of European research activity and organisation and concluded that palliative care research should be regarded as still in its infancy. Nevertheless, gradual improvements were noted. For instance, the number of oral and poster presentations at the European Association of Palliative Care research congresses rose steadily from 200 in 2000 to 480 in 2006. Research capacity is uneven across Europe with only the UK having more than one research grouping of significant size, and many countries have only small, isolated research teams. Degree of organisation is limited (only the UK was found to have a national research strategy for palliative care) and funding levels are low.

European palliative care research like that in the UK is variable in quality with relatively few RCTs. Also, researchers tend to focus on certain topics, and consistent with the findings of the Scottish study, the two main areas for research were service development and symptom control.

The body of palliative care evidence gathered to date

It has been argued that some of the reasons why the research base of palliative care might be relatively underdeveloped are linked to the way in which the speciality developed (Kaasa and Radbruch 2008). In its early years, palliative care was primarily concerned with the setting up of hospice and other care programmes. Although research was integral to that process, the relative lack of links with academic institutions may have influenced research direction and priorities. Organisation of research along academic lines appears only to have gathered momentum in the 1990s, with the establishment of the UK Palliative Care Research Society and the European Association for Palliative Care Research Network (Kaasa and Radbruch 2008).

In spite of this relatively short history of organised research, the body of evidence to support palliative care is steadily growing. The last 10–15 years have seen a sustained increase in the number of palliative care journals available to English-speaking readers, and a recent survey identified 15 journals exclusively or mainly publishing papers on palliative care (Stevens et al. 2008). There are also many other publications which cover palliative care research including general medical, oncological, general nursing and oncology nursing journals (Kaasa et al. 2006). The advent of online, searchable research databases has greatly aided the process of finding useful published evidence. In the UK, online resources have been usefully gathered together by the National Library for Health's Supportive and Palliative Care Specialist Library (accessible at http://www.library.nhs.uk/palliative/).

Another useful point of access for current palliative care research is the palliative care conference. Both Europe in general and the UK in particular are well served in this respect. For instance both the European Association for Palliative Care and the Palliative Care Research Society (the later in conjunction with the Association of Palliative Medicine and the Royal College of Nursing) organise biennial research conferences. There also seems to be no shortage of smaller events. All will include talks on current or recently completed research and most will also have displays of research posters (Palliative Care Congress 2008).

Some topics receive more attention in the palliative care literature than others. A review of palliative care research reviews found a predominance of papers on pain and symptom management (DePalma 2006). However, across the literature as a whole, studies of services and other aspects of care provision dominate the knowledge base (Johnston et al. 2006; NCRI 2004). Some topics seem to fluctuate in popularity. For instance, articles on spirituality and spiritual care seem to have become more common recently, and there has been a plethora of descriptive studies of health professionals' roles.

In terms of methodology, the evidence base for palliative care is largely composed of reviews, surveys and retrospective, descriptive or observational studies (Kaasa et al. 2006). On the whole, RCTs and prospective, interventional studies are still relatively uncommon, even in the most respected journals. For instance, a search of *Palliative Medicine* and the *Journal of Symptom Management* between 1998 and 2006 found only 16 RCTs out of over 500 papers (Kaasa et al. 2006). However, there is a large and growing body of qualitative, interpretative research evidence.

The use of qualitative research methods to describe and understand the human experience is well established in fields such as anthropology and sociology. Indeed, the ethnographic studies of Glaser and Strauss were an important milestone in the early development of modern ideas about the needs of the dying (Koenig et al. 2003). However, it has only been relatively recently that the potential of qualitative approaches to add unique insights into illness experiences has been widely recognised (Froggatt et al. 2003). A review of qualitative research in palliative care between 1990 and 1999 found an overall increase over the period from 9 published articles in 1990 to 24 in 1999 (Froggatt et al. 2003). Nurses were the main professional group publishing qualitative research. In terms of subject matter, the largest number of studies were concerned with issues of care delivery. Interestingly, given the findings of more general reviews, physical symptoms were relatively little studied.

Given their potential to contribute significantly to understanding practice, it is unfortunate that qualitative studies, even when well conducted, carry relatively little academic authority (Horne and Watson 2003; Jubb 2002). This may be partly because insufficient methodological rigour has been applied in some studies. It may also be related to the fact that many palliative care journals have low scientific standing. For instance, both the *International Journal of Palliative Nursing* and the *European Journal of Palliative Care* regularly publish qualitative studies, but neither has an Institute for Scientific Information impact factor (Stevens et al. 2008).

In spite of recent progress, there still remains a pressing need for more and better quality palliative care research (Addington-Hall 2007). In particular, attention must be paid to the methodological, organisational, attitudinal and financial barriers facing contemporary palliative care researchers.

Barriers and challenges in palliative care research

As already discussed, there is general agreement in the literature that a great deal of palliative care practice is inadequately researched (Hanks et al. 2005). However, numerous challenges face those who would attempt to rectify this situation.

Practice Point 19.2

Make a list of the barriers and challenges that might discourage nurses from taking part in palliative care research. You might choose to consider these under three main headings: factors specific to nurses as researchers, factors related to the organisation of research and factors pertaining to the use of patients as research subjects.

Commentary:

Check your list as you read through the following sections and reflect on which barriers and challenges you might have missed. Most nurses will anticipate the ethical and practical challenges likely to accompany studies involving dying people, but those not used to research work may not anticipate some of the other obstacles.

Cultural and practical barriers to palliative care research

It has been claimed that 'research has not yet become embedded in the culture of palliative care' (Hanks et al. 2005, p. 128). Indeed, a potential cultural conflict has been recognised between the imperative in palliative care to relieve suffering and the principle of evidence-based practice (Kaasa et al. 2006). Nurses, especially with their traditional role of patient advocate, may struggle to reconcile the need for research data with the potential to cause distress (Sorensen and Iedema 2007).

Leaving aside the ethical issues for a moment, conducting research with very ill people is fraught with practical difficulties. Many patients will be frail, tired, anxious or in pain, and may lack the concentration or energy reserves required to cooperate with data collection (Hopkinson et al. 2005). State of health can change over short periods of time, making an ideal subject suddenly unsuitable (Fowell et al. 2008). Recruitment may be difficult because of gatekeeping by health care professionals or discouragement from family members (Henderson et al. 2005). Then there is the very real risk that the patient might die before the study is complete.

Additional practical challenges come into play because of the unique nature of palliative care populations. Almost by definition, palliative care is delivered to groups of people who vary considerably in, for instance, diagnosis, stage of disease, psychosocial needs and symptom profile. This heterogeneity, combined with the fact that many palliative care units are small and isolated from others, presents a considerable challenge to the researcher attempting to define a population or recruit a representative cohort (Hanks et al. 2005; Mazzocato et al. 2001; Sentilhes-Monkam and Serryn 2004).

Ethical issues in palliative care research

There has traditionally been much opposition to the involvement of dying patients in palliative and end of life care research (Jubb 2002). As a result, many empirical and quality improvement studies have been based on data obtained from family members, patients' friends and even professionals (Takesaka et al. 2004). This is clearly unsatisfactory as none of these people can accurately replicate the patient's unique perspective (Hopkinson et al. 2005). Nevertheless there are several major ethical concerns which researchers must consider before they contemplate involving such potentially vulnerable individuals. First and foremost is the question of whether the likely benefits of the study justify the potential disruption and distress which might be caused to the patient (Takesaka et al. 2004). Dean and McClement (2002) have identified a number of potential detrimental effects of research participation including energy depletion, role conflict, emotional burden and obligation to report. However, other authors have argued that the risks to patients are exaggerated (Berry 2004). Indeed, surveys of dying patients and their families have suggested that at least some may have positive attitudes towards taking part in research (Henderson et al. 2005; Pautex 2005; Perkins et al. 2007).

Another concern is that decision-making capacity (including the decision to refuse to participate) might be compromised by the distress of dying (Casarett 2003; Casarett et al. 2003). In other words, dying patients may feel compelled to consent or may not be able to make fully informed choices about participation. A number of authors have suggested strengthening guidelines covering recruitment and consent to give added protection to potential research subjects (Koenig et al. 2003).

Perhaps the major question facing decision-makers in this field is whether palliative care does indeed raise unique ethical issues (Casarett et al. 2003). Or put another way, are palliative care patients especially vulnerable for purposes of research? Increasingly, commentators appear to be concluding that palliative care patients should not be considered as a special case (Berry 2004). Instead, the stringent ethical guidelines already in place to protect those involved in health research are being re-evaluated to ensure that they offer adequate protection to the palliative patient as well (Koenig et al. 2003; Lee and Kristjanson 2003; Peattie 2003).

Methodological challenges to palliative care research

Some of the methodological obstacles to palliative care research are related to the practical and ethical issues discussed above. For instance, the reason why small-scale descriptive designs are often chosen may be because they only require the recruitment of relatively few subjects, and the period of data collection is conveniently short. Interventional or longitudinal studies require larger patient numbers and perhaps impossibly long time scales for gathering data (Hanks et al. 2005). Achieving adequate recruitment into palliative care studies is another major methodological challenge as many studies could potentially be weakened by small sample size. However, some research groups have addressed this problem by developing a participatory approach where the patient engages in the research process and negotiates the level and nature of his or her participation (Hopkinson et al. 2005).

A final methodological issue is choice of data collection methods. Much criticism has been levelled at palliative care for placing too much emphasis on descriptive studies, surveys and reviews. Lack of infrastructure and perhaps some ideological concerns have meant that RCTs have yet to make the impact they have in other specialities, most notably oncology. Increasingly, however, this position is appearing indefensible.

One of the issues appears to be that although they are excellent at measuring discrete and specific outcomes such as symptom prevalence and symptom severity, RCTs are less effective at capturing aspects of suffering and quality of life (Crombie 2003). Some researchers have argued that it is possible to have both methodological rigour and accurate capture of the individual's experience, by designing RCT outcomes which are complex and subtle but also measurable (Mularski et al. 2007). Others have proposed alternative methodologies. For instance Fowell et al. (2008) designed a switchback cluster randomised design which may prove to be as rigorous as the RCT but with fewer issues around consent, gatekeeping and attrition. Still others have argued that regarding the RCT as the only 'gold standard' in palliative care research is damaging to the endeavour as a whole (Aranda 2008).

Because quantitative data can sometimes lack the depth or subtlety required to capture patients' and families' lived experience, palliative care researchers have tended to use qualitative methodologies which better capture the illness experience but attract criticism for lack of rigour (Seymour and Clark 1998). One solution is clearly to adopt approaches which increase the rigour of qualitative methods (O'Conner and Payne 2006; Pope et al. 2000). Another is to employ mixed methodologies, for example using quantitative data to complement and confirm qualitative findings (Corner et al. 2003).

Other organisational issues

Perhaps the single greatest barrier to effective palliative care research is the lack of organisation. Lack of infrastructure means that many researchers are working in isolation from potential collaborators. Lack of collaboration between palliative care and academic departments means there are problems attracting high-quality researchers into the speciality (Hanks et al. 2005). Opportunities for multi-centre work are limited, although improving, following recent attempts at capacity building (Bailey et al. 2006). There are also concerns that the level of funding which palliative care research currently receives is still too low (Kaasa et al. 2006).

Future directions for palliative care research

A number of key steps are required if palliative care research is to continue to progress towards delivering the evidence base which the speciality needs (Ahmedzai et al. 2004; Kaasa et al. 2006). In the first instance, agreement on priority areas for future research would be welcome. Different research authorities tend to produce their own lists, but recurring themes include user involvement, patient experience and non-malignant diseases (Addington-Hall 2007; Johnston et al. 2006). Some accommodation of national research priorities may be necessary if palliative care research is to consolidate its position on the NHS research and development agenda. Paying attention to stated NHS priorities such as social exclusion and patient involvement would seem to be a logical first step in this process (Davies 2001).

Sharing common priorities is one way of joining up research activity and building research capacity. Another is the formation of collaboratives between research groupings. The work of the National Cancer Research Institute in particular is to be applauded. However further national and international cooperation is also called for. None of this can be achieved without funding, so more investment in palliative care research is also required (Kaasa and Radbruch 2008).

Large-scale initiatives to build capacity must be complemented by local initiatives to stimulate interest in research. Nurses (especially those practising at clinical nurse specialist level) and other health care professionals should be encouraged to participate in research as part of their clinical role (Daniels and Exley 2001). Nurses who have developed skills in audit may find that many of those skills are transferable to research practice (Gould 2008). Skills in database searching and reading research should also be encouraged, and more attention paid to incorporating the findings of research into clinical practice (Hughes and Addington-Hall 2005).

Choice of research methodology continues to be a sticking point as attempts are made to advance and coordinate palliative care research. A glance through any of the major palliative care research journals will reveal that researchers employ a bewildering array of different study designs. This diversity is partly due to the variety of professional backgrounds and philosophical leanings represented within the palliative care research community. It is also indicative of the vast range of phenomena covered by the palliative care research 'umbrella'. Perhaps the best that can be hoped for is that methodology should be consistent with the underlying research paradigm. Nevertheless, new methodologies which better capture the subjective experiences of people at the end of life are also being developed (Christakis 2006).

Finally, if palliative care research is to flourish and make a more effective contribution to practice, it must engage more fully with its research subjects (Hopkinson et al. 2005; Hubbard et al. 2008). There is a need for researchers to work more collaboratively with patients and families, involve them more fully in the research process, and take a more proactive role in supporting their participation. Numerous benefits are likely to follow these efforts including improvements in recruitment, identification of more appropriate outcomes and greater empowerment of the individuals concerned.

References

Addington-Hall JM (2007) Introduction, Chapter 1. In: Addington-Hall JM, Bruera E, Higginson IJ and Payne S (Eds), *Research Methods in Palliative Care*. Oxford: Oxford University Press, pp. 1–9.

Ahmedzai SH, Costa A, Blengini C, Bosch A, Sanz-Ortiz J, Ventafridda V and Verhagen SC (2004) On behalf of the international working group convened by the European School of Oncology. *European Journal of Cancer*. 40(15):2192–2200.

Aranda S (2008) Current issues in palliative care research. Keynote Address at Palliative Care Congress, Glasgow, 29th April 2008.

Bailey C, Wilson R, Addington-Hall J, Payne S, Clark D, Lloyd-Williams M, Molassiotis A and Seymour J (2006) The cancer experience research collaborative (CECo): building research capacity in supportive and palliative care. *Progress in Palliative Care*. 14(6):265–270.

Bakitas MA, Lyons KD, Dixon J and Ahles TA (2006) Palliative care programme effectiveness research: developing rigor in sampling design, conduct, and reporting. *Journal of Pain and Symptom Management*. 31(3):270–284.

Berry SR (2004) For purposes of research, palliative care patients should not be considered a vulnerable population. *Clinical Oncology*. 16(3):223–224.

Casarett DJ (2003) Assessing decision-making capacity in the setting of palliative care research. *Journal of Pain and Symptom Management*. 25(4):S6–S13.

Cassarett DJ, Knebel A and Helmers K (2003) Ethical challenges of palliative care research. *Journal of Pain and Symptom Management*. 25(4):S3–S5.

Christakis NA (2006) Advances in palliative care research methodology. *Palliative Medicine*. 20(8):725–726.

Clark D, Small N, Wright M, Winslow M and Hughes N (2005) *A Bit of Heaven for the Few?* Lancaster: Observatory Publications.

Corner J, Halliday D, Haviland J, Douglas HR, Bath P, Clark D, Normand C, Beech N, Hughes P, Marples R, Seymour J, Skilbeck J and Webb T (2003) Exploring nursing outcomes for patients with advanced cancer following interventions by Macmillan specialist palliative care nurses. *Journal of Advanced Nursing.* 41(6):561–574.

Crombie I (2003) Evidence in medicine: the randomised control trial – past, present and future. In: Scottish Partnership for Palliative Care (2003) *Beyond the Randomised Controlled Trial: Evidence and Effectiveness in Palliative Care.* Edinburgh: SPPC, p. 6.

Daniels LE and Exley C (2001) Preparation, information and liaison: conducting successful research in palliative care. *International Journal of Palliative Nursing.* 7(4):192–197.

Davies SC (2001) Palliative care research for the National Health Service. *Journal of the Royal Society of Medicine.* 94(9):483.

Dean RA and McClement SE (2002) Palliative care research: methodological and ethical challenges. *International Journal of Palliative Nursing.* 8(8):376–380.

DePalma JA (2006) Palliative care published research reviews, 2000 to 2005. *Home Healthcare Management Practice.* 18(10):482–485.

European Association for Palliative Care and International Association for Palliative Care (2006) Declaration of Venice: adoption of a declaration to develop a global palliative care research initiative. *Progress in Palliative Care.* 14(5):215–217.

Fowell A, Johnstone R, Finlay I, Russel D and Russel I (2008) Novel approaches to trials in palliative care. In: *Abstracts of the 5th Research Forum of the European Association for Palliative Care (EAPC)*, Trondheim, Norway, 28–31 May 2008, p. 429. Also *Palliative Medicine.* 22:399–558. Accessible at http://www.eapcnet.org/download/forCongresses/Trondheim/Trondheim2008AbstractBookPallMed.pdf. Accessed on 22 November 2008.

Froggatt KA, Field D, Bailey C and Krishnasamy M (2003) Qualitative research in palliative care 1990–1999: a descriptive review. *International Journal of Palliative Nursing.* 9(3):98–104.

Gould D (2008) Audit and research: similarities and differences. *Nursing Standard.* 22(37):51–56.

Hanks G, Kaasa S and Robbins M (2005) Research in palliative care: getting started, Chapter 5.2. In: Doyle D, Hanks G, Cherny N and Callman K (Eds), *Oxford Textbook of Palliative Medicine* (3rd edition). Oxford: Oxford University Press, pp. 128–137.

Henderson M, Addington-Hall JM and Hotopf M (2005) The willingness of palliative care patients to participate in research. *Journal of Pain and Symptom Management.* 29(2):116–117.

Higginson IJ (2003) Effectiveness in palliative care: gathering the evidence. In: Scottish Partnership for Palliative Care (2003) *Beyond the Randomised Controlled Trial: Evidence and Effectiveness in Palliative Care.* Edinburgh: SPPC, pp. 7–9.

Hopkinson JB, Wright DNM and Corner JL (2005) Seeking new methodology for palliative care research: challenging assumptions about studying people who are approaching the end of life. *Palliative Medicine.* 19(7):532–537.

Horne C and Watson H (2003) Qualitative research: how can we maximise its potential to improve our understanding of issues in palliative care? In: Scottish Partnership for Palliative Care (2003) *Beyond the Randomised Controlled Trial: Evidence and Effectiveness in Palliative Care.* Edinburgh: SPPC, pp. 21–22.

Hubbard G, Kidd L and Donaghy E (2008) Involving people affected by cancer in research: a review of the literature. *European Journal of Cancer Care.* 17(3):233–244.

Hughes RA and Addington-Hall JM (2005) Feeding back survey research findings within palliative care: findings from qualitative research. *International Journal of Nursing Studies.* 42(4):449–456.

Johnston B, Nimmo S, Baughan P, Kearney N, Roe L and Fraser M (2006) *A Scoping Review of Palliative Care in Scotland: Final Report.* Stirling: Cancer Care Research Centre.

Jubb AM (2002) Palliative care research: trading ethics for an evidence base. *Journal of Medical Ethics.* 28(6):342–346.

Kaasa S, Hjermstad MJ and Loge JH (2006) Methodological and structural challenges in palliative care research: how have we fared in the last decades? *Palliative Medicine.* 20(8):727–734.

Kaasa S and Radbruch L (2008) Palliative care research – priorities and the way forward. *European Journal of Cancer.* 44(8):1175–1179.

Koenig BA, Back AL and Crawley LM (2003) Qualitative methods in end of life research: recommendations to enhance the protection of human subjects. *Journal of Pain and Symptom Management.* 25(4):S43–S52.

Lee S and Kristjanson L (2003) Human research ethics committees: issues in palliative care research. *International Journal of Palliative Nursing.* 9(1):13–18.

Mazzocato C, Sweeney C and Bruera E (2001) Clinical research in palliative care: patient populations, symptoms, interventions and endpoints. *Palliative Medicine.* 15(2):163–168.

Mularski RA, Rosenfeld K, Coons SJ, Dueck A, Cella D, Feuer DJ, Lipscomb J, Karpeh MS, Mosich T, Sloan JA and Krouse RA (2007) Measuring outcomes in randomised prospective trials in palliative care. *Journal of Pain and Symptom Management.* 34(Suppl 1):S7–S19.

Murray MA (2008) A question of evidence: decision-making in palliative care nursing. *International Journal of Palliative Nursing.* 14(1):45–47.

National Cancer Research Institute (2004) *Supportive and Palliative Care Research in the UK: Report of the NCRI Strategic Planning Group on Supportive and Palliative Care.* London: NCRI.

O'Connor M and Payne S (2006) Discourse analysis: examining the potential for research in palliative care. *Palliative Medicine.* 20(8):829–834.

Palliative Care Congress (2008) *The 7th Palliative Care Congress: Abstracts of Oral and Poster Presentations.* Bournemouth: PCC.

Pautex S (2005) Is research really problematic in palliative care? A pilot study. *Journal of Pain and Symptom Management.* 30(2):109–111.

Payne S, Addington-Hall J, Richardson A and Sharpe M (2007) Supportive and palliative care research collaboratives in the United Kingdom: an unnatural experiment? *Palliative Medicine.* 21(8):663–665.

Peattie P (2003) Issues for research ethics committees. In: Scottish Partnership for Palliative Care (2003) *Beyond the Randomised Controlled Trial: Evidence and Effectiveness in Palliative Care.* Edinburgh: SPPC, p. 12.

Perkins P, Barclay S and Booth S (2007) What are patients' priorities for palliative care research? Focus group study. *Palliative Medicine.* 21(8):219–225.

Pope C, Ziebland S and Mays N (2000) Qualitative research in health care: analysing qualitative data. *British Medical Journal.* 320(7227):114–116.

Royal College of Physicians (2007) *Palliative Care Services: Meeting the Needs of Patients.* London: RCP.

Saunders C (Ed) (1978) *The Management of Terminal Disease.* London: Edward Arnold.

Saunders C (2000) The evolution of palliative care. *Patient Education and Counselling.* 41(1):7–13.

Sentilhes-Monkam A and Serryn D (2004) Conducting research in the palliative care population. *European Journal of Palliative Care.* 11(1):23–26.

Seymour J and Clark D (1998) Phenomenological approaches to palliative care research. *Palliative Medicine.* 12(2):127–131.

Sorensen R and Iedema R (2007) Advocacy at the end of life. Research design: an ethnographic study of an ICU. *International Journal of Nursing Studies.* 44(8):1343–1353.

Stevens RJ, Brady D, Hodson M and Ahmedzai SH (2008) Comparative analysis of the top 50 journals in palliative and supportive care using data from preferences amongst professionals weighted for impact factor scores. Poster presented at 7th Palliative Care Congress, Glasgow, 29th April–1st May 2008.

Takesaka J, Crowley R and Casarett D (2004) What is the risk of distress in palliative survey research? *Journal of Pain and Symptom Management.* 28(6):593–598.

Wilkinson S (1998) The importance of evidence-based care. *International Journal of Palliative Nursing.* 4(4):160.

Index